Baillière's

CLINICAL HAEMATOLOGY

INTERNATIONAL PRACTICE AND RESEARCH

Volume 5/Number 2
April 1992

Epidemiology of Haematological Disease: Part II

A. F. FLEMING
Guest Editor

Baillière Tindall
London Philadelphia Sydney Tokyo Toronto

This book is printed on acid-free paper.

Baillière Tindall 24–28 Oval Road,
W.B. Saunders London NW1 7DX

The Curtis Center, Independence Square West,
Philadelphia, PA 19106–3399, USA

55 Horner Avenue
Toronto, Ontario M8Z 4X6, Canada

Harcourt Brace Jovanovich Group (Australia) Pty Ltd,
30–52 Smidmore Street, Marrickville, NSW 2204, Australia

Harcourt Brace Jovanovich Japan, Inc.
Ichibancho Central Building, 22–1
Ichibancho, Chiyoda-ku, Tokyo 102, Japan

ISSN 0950-3536

ISBN 0-7020-1627-6 (single copy)

Baillière's Clinical Haematology is published four times each year by Baillière Tindall. Annual subscription prices are:

TERRITORY	ANNUAL SUBSCRIPTION	SINGLE ISSUE
UK and Europe	£65.00 post free	£27.50 post free
All other countries	Consult your local Harcourt Brace Jovanovich office for dollar price	

The editor of this publication is Stephen Handley, Baillière Tindall,
24–28 Oval Road, London NW1 7DX.

Baillière's Clinical Haematology was published from 1972 to 1986 as *Clinics in Haematology*.

Typeset by Phoenix Photosetting, Chatham.
Printed and bound in Great Britain by Mackays of Chatham PLC, Chatham, Kent.

Contributors to this issue

E. M. ESSIEN MD, FMCPath, FWACP, MRCPath, FAS, Professor of Haematology, University of Ibadan; Director, National Institute for Medical Research, Edmond Crescent, P.M.B. 2013, Yaba, Lagos, Nigeria.

ALAN F. FLEMING MA, MD, FRCPath, FMCPath(Nigeria), FWACP(West Africa), Professor, Department of Haematology, School of Pathology of the South African Institute for Medical Research and University of the Witwatersrand; Honorary Consultant Haematologist, Baragwanath Hospital, P.O. Bertsham, Soweto 2013, South Africa.

EDWARD COLIN GORDON-SMITH MA, MSc, FRCPath, FRCP, Professor of Haematology, St George's Hospital Medical School, Cranmer Terrace, Tooting, London SW17 0RE, UK.

PETER B. HESSELING, Professor and Head of Department of Paediatrics and Child Health, PO Box 19063, Tygerberg 7505, Republic of South Africa.

JONATHAN R. HIBBS MD, National Research Service Award Fellow, Clinical Haematology Branch, National Heart, Lung and Blood Institute, Bldg 10, Room 7C-103, 9000 Rockville Pike, Bethesda, MD 20892, USA.

GERHARD HUNSMANN Professor, MD, Head of Department of Virology and Immunology, German Primate Centre, Kellnerweg 4, 3400 Göttingen, Germany.

SURAPOL ISSARAGRISIL MD, Department of Medicine, Division of Haematology, Mahidol University Faculty of Medicine, Siriraj Hospital, Bangkok 10700, Thailand.

RONALD L. NAGEL MD, Professor of Medicine, Head of Division of Hematology, Albert Einstein College of Medicine and Montefiore Medical Center, 1300 Morris Park Avenue, Bronx, NY 10461, USA.

A. C. NATHWANI MD, MB, ChB, MRCP, Haemostasis Research Group, Clinical Research Centre, Watford Road, Harrow, Middlesex HA1 3UJ, UK.

GEOFFREY PASVOL DPhil, FRCP, Department of Infectious Diseases and Tropical Medicine, St Mary's Hospital Medical School, Lister Unit, Northwick Park Hospital, Middlesex HA1 3UJ, UK.

RODNEY E. PHILLIPS MD, Molecular Immunology Group, Institute of Molecular Medicine, John Radcliffe Hospital, Oxford OX3 9DU, UK.

O. SODEINDE MB, BS(Ibadan), FMC Paed(Nig), FWACP, Senior Lecturer and Consultant Paediatrician, University College Hospital, College of Medicine, University of Ibadan, P.M.B. 5116, Ibadan, Nigeria.

WENDY STEVENS Registrar, MB, BCh, Department of Haematology, South African Institute for Medical Research, Baragwanath Hospital, P.O. Bertsham, Soweto 2013, South Africa.

E. G. D. TUDDENHAM MD, FRCP, FRCPath, Director of Haemostasis Research Group, Clinical Research Centre, Watford Road, Harrow, Middlesex HA1 3UJ, UK.

THOMAS WEBER MD, Neurologist, Neurologische Klinik und Poliklinik der Universität Göttingen, Robert-Koch-Str. 40, 3400 Göttingen, Germany.

NEAL S. YOUNG MD, Chief, Cell Biology Section; Head, Clinical Services, Clinical Hematology Branch, National Heart, Lung and Blood Institute, Bldg 10, Room 7C-103, 9000 Rockville Pike, Bethesda, MD 20892, USA.

Table of contents

PREVIOUS ISSUES

January 1990
Haematology in HIV Disease
C. COSTELLO

April 1990
Blood Transfusion: The Impact of New Technologies
M. CONTRERAS

July 1990
Antithrombotic Therapy
J. HIRSH

October 1990
Advancing Haematological Techniques
I. CAVILL

January 1991
Chemotherapy of Malignant Blood Diseases
R. A. ZITTOUN

April 1991
Paediatric Haematology
I. M. HANN & B. E. S. GIBSON

July 1991
Minimal Residual Disease in Leukaemia
S. J. PROCTOR

December 1991
Molecular Immunohaematology
A. E. G. KR. VON DEM BORNE

January 1992
Epidemiology of Haematological Disease: Part I
A. F. FLEMING

FORTHCOMING ISSUES

July 1992
Growth Factors in Haemopoiesis
B. I. LORD & T. M. DEXTER

October 1992
The Molecular Genetics of Haematological Malignancy
B. D. YOUNG

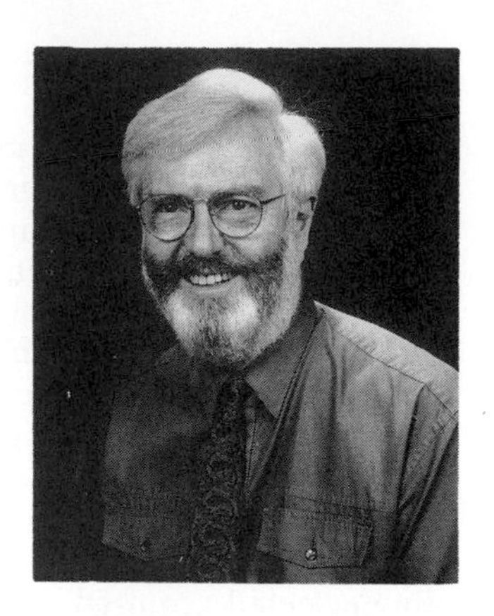

Foreword

This is the second of two volumes devoted to the global epidemiology of haematological disorders. The need to meet strict deadlines has meant that the logical ordering of the chapters has been largely disrupted.

Many haematologists are not well informed about the epidemiology of microorganisms which have profound direct or indirect influences on the distribution of disorders of the blood. In the first two chapters, the epidemiologies of selected viruses are discussed per se: their causative associations with myelosuppression, leukaemias and lymphomas are touched on, and these are discussed further in the chapters on these diseases. Drs Hibbs and Young have selected viruses which typify certain characteristics of myelosuppressive viral disease. Dengue is probably the most important of the haemorrhagic fevers today, and its incidence is growing. Parvovirus B19 and the Epstein–Barr virus are amongst those ubiquitous infections which cause bewilderingly wide spectra of diseases, from the trivial to the life-threatening, depending on the pre-existing immunological and haematological status of the host. Human retroviruses were unknown until just over a decade ago, but now they impinge on every aspect of the study and practice of medicine. The human T-cell lymphotropic virus type 1 (HTLV-1) has a far wider endemic distribution than was first thought and is showing epidemic spread through intravenous drug use and blood transfusion. The study of the epidemiology of HTLV-2 is only just beginning with the application of serology based on synthetic antigens and the polymerase chain reaction. The pandemic of the human immunodeficiency viruses (HIV-1 and to a lesser extent HIV-2) is spreading inexorably, so that AIDS in Asia, reported rarely up until now, is likely to overshadow even Africa in the coming decades. Dr Weber and colleagues conclude with a concise review of the haematological consequences of HIV infection.

It is probable that AIDS will assume first place, but today malaria remains the greatest infectious biological burden carried by man. Drs Phillips and Pasvol review only one aspect, malarial anaemia, its pathophysiology and its importance as a cause of morbidity and mortality. The sickle-cell gene arose at least once in Asia and four times in Africa: Drs Nagel and Fleming hypothesize that the expansion of these mutations in populations can be linked to the prehistoric introduction of agriculture, which favours the transmission of malaria. The spread by gene flow can also be linked historically to the trans-Saharan and Atlantic slave-trades over the centuries. Dr Sodeinde's chapter completes the discussion of malaria-dependent balanced polymorphisms, by describing the biological advantages and disadvantages of glucose-6-phosphate dehydrogenase (G6PD) deficiencies: he speculates that G6PD-deficient subjects could be especially vulnerable to the action of oxidative pollutants in the environment.

Three chapters are devoted to haemostasis. Drs Nathwani and Tuddenham contribute a comprehensive and definitive review of epidemiology of coagulation disorders, both congenital and the more common but scientifically neglected acquired conditions, such as hypoprothrombinaemias, disseminated intravascular coagulation and snake-envenomation. Platelet function and platelet disorders in tropical Africa present fascinating and important features: Dr Essien reviews platelets, especially in relation to malaria in west Africa; Dr Hesseling establishes onyalai as an epidemiological, clinical and pathological entity in southern Africa, after many years during which its identity separate from idiopathic thrombocytopenic purpura was denied.

Drs Gordon-Smith and Issaragrisil contradict many inaccurate statements concerning the epidemiology of aplastic anaemia in the western world and Asia, and their section on viral aetiology closes the circle by linking with the first chapter.

Eric Arthur Beet died on 28 April 1989. He had been a Medical Officer in the British Colonial Service, Northern Rhodesia (now Zambia) in the late 1940s. While posted to the remote Balovale District (now Luvale), then about 770 km (480 miles) by earth road from the nearest railway station, he observed that children less than 5 years of age with positive sickling tests enjoyed a partial protection against malarial parasitaemia (*East African Medical Journal* (1946) **23:** 75–86). He was transferred to the marginally less remote Fort Jameson (now Chipata) in the Eastern Province, where he reported that positive sickling was associated with less frequent palpable splenomegaly (*East African Medical Journal* (1947) **24:** 212–222). Both differences approached statistical significance, but Beet's observations were largely ignored for more than a decade, until they were confirmed by A. C. Allison. He completed family studies of up to five generations amongst Lalas of Serenje and Mkushi Districts, under what must have been extremely difficult conditions, and showed (independently from J. V. Neel who published in the same year) that sickle-cell trait behaved as a Mendelian dominant and that sickle-cell anaemia occurred only in homozygotes (*Annals of Eugenics* (1949) **14:** 279–284). He published only a handful of articles, of which three are classics, and his death went unmarked by any obituary in a leading medical journal. This volume is dedicated to his memory.

ALAN F. FLEMING

1

Viruses and the blood

JONATHAN R. HIBBS
NEAL S. YOUNG

Several virus families are associated with bone marrow suppression. The purpose of this chapter is to acquaint the reader with epidemiological characteristics of selected viruses and their pathophysiological implications for bone marrow suppression. These syndromes are chosen because they typify certain characteristics of myelosuppressive viral illness; an exhaustive discussion of each myelotoxic virus is beyond the scope of this review. Myeloproliferative disorders, platelet disorders and retroviruses are discussed elsewhere in these two volumes.

DENGUE VIRUS

Dengue is one of the diverse group of haemorrhagic fever viruses (World Health Organization, 1985; LeDuc, 1989). The exotic names of haemorrhagic fever agents often signify our limited understanding of the causative organisms (Young, 1990). Diseases caused by these agents are usually characterized by insect vectors, defective haemostasis not necessarily due to disseminated intravascular coagulation (Kuberski et al, 1977; Lange et al, 1985; Fisher-Hoch et al, 1987) and a non-human host (World Health Organization, 1985; LeDuc, 1989). In some cases (Work et al, 1959) much of our knowledge of the epidemiology of an agent derives from descriptions of a single epidemic. Generalizations regarding these viruses must be circumspect because of the limited information available and the phylogenetic diversity of the agents. Next to yellow fever, dengue is the best studied of the haemorrhagic fever viruses. Dengue may be the most important of the haemorrhagic fevers from the viewpoint of public health officials and clinicians in the 1990s. No effective vaccine is available, and dengue incidence is large and growing (Halstead, 1981; World Health Organization, 1986).

Virology

Dengue is a member of the flavivirus family. The flaviviridiae include agents of many inflammatory arthropod-borne encephalidities such as Japanese

Baillière's Clinical Haematology—
Vol. 5, No. 2, April 1992
ISBN 0–7020–1627–6

encephalitis (Umenai et al, 1985) and St Louis encephalitis (Monath and Tsai, 1987). The family also includes three other haemorrhagic fever agents: Kyasanur Forest (Work et al, 1959), Omsk fever, and yellow fever (Monath, 1987) viruses. Typical of flaviviruses (Rice et al, 1985), the dengue genome is approximately 10 kilobases of positively stranded RNA. A single open reading frame is transcribed into a polyprotein which is subsequently cleaved into three structural and seven non-structural proteins; the entire genome has been sequenced (Deubel et al, 1988; Hahn et al, 1988). Dengue has four recognized serotypes (Halstead et al, 1970a).

Transmission

Half of all recognized flaviviruses are transmitted by mosquitoes, although some species are transmitted by ticks, and many have no known vector (Monath, 1990). Dengue is transmitted by *Aedes* mosquitoes, particularly *A. aegypti* and *A. albopictus* (Gubler, 1988); epidemics can be sustained by small vector populations (Gilbertson, 1945). In the western hemisphere, the significance of animal hosts has not been documented; monkeys can sustain the dengue life cycle in south-east Asia (Rudnick et al, 1967). Patients develop clinical illness within 1 week of being bitten by an infected mosquito (Siler et al, 1926; Simmons et al, 1931; Sabin, 1952). Patients are viraemic (and can presumably transmit the disease to mosquitoes) for 3–5 days during febrile illness (Gubler et al, 1981). Mosquitoes remain infected for life, and transovarian transmission occurs (Gubler, 1987). Infection with one serotype confers lifetime immunity against reinfection with that serotype only (Sabin, 1952; Halstead, 1981).

Clinical syndromes

Eighty per cent of seropositive persons could not recall any dengue fever symptoms after a dengue-2 epidemic (Guzman et al, 1990), implying that the great majority of dengue virus infections are asymptomatic. A high rate of asymptomatic infection also occurs with other arboviruses (Benenson et al, 1975; Monath et al, 1980; Grimstad et al, 1987). Dengue causes two recognizable clinical syndromes. In classical dengue, the patient develops high fever, chills, and excruciating headaches, myalgias and arthralgias ('breakbone fever'); these symptoms resolve spontaneously, usually within 5 days of onset, and are followed by a diffuse maculopapular rash; mortality is rare or nil (Siler et al, 1926; Neff et al, 1967; World Health Organization, 1986; Centers for Disease Control, 1990). In dengue haemorrhagic fever (which can occur with or without shock) the patient develops symptoms of classical dengue and then defervesces. Two or three days following defervescence, a bleeding diathesis occurs, sometimes accompanied by intravascular volume depletion and shock (Hammon et al, 1957; Nimmannitya et al, 1969; World Health Organization, 1986; Diaz et al, 1988). Hydration and supportive care can reduce mortality in haemorrhagic fever, but the case fatality rate has been as high as 10% in some epidemics (Halstead, 1981, 1988).

Haematology and diagnosis

Classical dengue patients typically have mild to moderate thrombocytopenia and neutropenia (Halstead, 1972; Mas, 1979), and a hypoplastic marrow (Bierman and Nelson, 1965). During dengue haemorrhagic fever, the platelet count falls below 100×10^9/litre, and the haematocrit typically rises 20% or more of its initial value due to haemoconcentration (Cohen and Halstead, 1966; Halstead, 1972; Edelman et al, 1975; World Health Organization, 1986). Acute viraemia can be diagnosed by culture of the virus from body fluids in insects (Kuberski and Rosen, 1977) or insect cell cultures (Kuno et al, 1985), and serotypes can be identified by plaque reduction neutralization (Sangkawibha et al, 1984; Morens et al, 1985). Haemagglutination-inhibition and enzyme-linked immunosorbent assays are available for detection of dengue antibodies (Chungue et al, 1989).

Epidemiology

World incidence

In 1988, it was estimated that 100 million cases of dengue infection occur annually, and that dengue haemorrhagic fever had caused 1.5 million hospitalizations and 33 000 deaths over the previous 20 years (Halstead, 1988).

Variations in time

A syndrome resembling classical dengue has been described in the Americas and the Pacific basin since the eighteenth century (Carey, 1971). Anecdotal evidence suggests a worldwide secular trend toward increased incidence (World Health Organization, 1986; Halstead, 1988). Certainly this is the case in Thailand (Kitayaporn et al, 1989) and in the western hemisphere (see below). Dengue epidemics coincide with periods of peak mosquito activity, usually during the summer in subtropical countries or the rainy season in the tropics. This may be due not only to vector density but also to more rapid growth of the virus in the vector with high ambient temperatures (Watts et al, 1987; Koopman et al, 1991).

Variations in place

Dengue is hyperendemic in south-east Asia, where epidemics of dengue haemorrhagic fever have increased in frequency and severity over the past decade. The annual incidence of dengue haemorrhagic fever in Thailand (age-adjusted to 1983) was 345 per 100 000 in 1987 (Kitayaporn et al, 1989). Up to 1% of the population of some Thai villages develops dengue haemorrhagic fever during the course of a single epidemic (Eamchan et al, 1989). Within the past 5 years, dengue haemorrhagic fever outbreaks have also been described in Asian countries remote from Thailand, including India (Srivastava et al, 1990), Indonesia (Samsi et al, 1990), and Taiwan (Liu et al, 1991). After more than 30 years of absence, epidemics of classical dengue returned to the People's Republic of China in 1978, and cases of haemorrhagic fever have followed (Fan et al, 1989). In the western hemisphere, although sporadic dengue epidemics occurred in the Caribbean basin in the three decades following World War II (Neff et al, 1967; Ehrenkranz et al, 1971), no dengue haemorrhagic fever outbreaks were documented. In 1977, the first outbreak of classical dengue in over 30 years was reported in Cuba, infecting approximately 45% of the population (Cantelar et al, 1981). Four years later, the first dengue haemorrhagic fever outbreak ever reported in the western hemisphere occurred in Cuba (Kouri et al, 1986). Since that time, classical dengue epidemics have been documented in Brazil (Dietz et al, 1990), Ecuador (Centers for Disease Control, 1989b), and Peru (Centers for Disease Control, 1991a), and a second dengue haemorrhagic fever outbreak has occurred in Venezuela (Pan American Health Organization, 1990). *A. albopictus* mosquitoes have entered the continental United States, possibly by means of eggs imported on tyres from Asia (Centers for Disease Control, 1989c), and efforts to eradicate *A. aegypti* from the western hemisphere have not been successful (Slosek, 1986). During 1990 most dengue cases in the United States continued to be imported (Centers for Disease Control, 1991b), but it is likely that indigenous epidemics will soon occur there (Halstead, 1981). Foci of dengue also exist in Africa (Botros et al, 1989; Johnson et al, 1990).

Host characteristics

Dengue haemorrhagic fever occurs principally among persons who have been infected previously with another serotype (Halstead et al, 1970b; Halstead, 1981; Diaz et al, 1988; Guzman et al, 1990). Thai children are most likely to die of dengue haemorrhagic fever at 6–8 months of age (when non-protective levels of maternal antibodies are present) or after 2 years of age (when they have had at least one rainy season in which to develop a primary infection) (Halstead et al, 1969). Although gender-specific rates of exposure appear to be similar, the rate of shock due to dengue haemorrhagic fever appears twofold higher in females than in males in Thailand (Halstead et al, 1970b). The age-stratified attack rate was also higher among females during the classical dengue epidemic in Puerto Rico in 1964–1965 (Neff et al, 1967); the cause of this gender differential is unknown. During the 1981 dengue haemorrhagic fever epidemic in Cuba, Whites were no more likely than Blacks to be infected, but were 3.5 times as likely to be hospitalized with findings of dengue haemorrhagic fever (Bravo et al, 1987), and infected Whites were twice as likely to recall being symptomatic as were infected Blacks (Guzman et al, 1990). Variation in incidence by HLA type, or other immunological characteristics, has not been adequately investigated.

Pathophysiology

Despite a hypoplastic marrow (Bierman and Nelson, 1965), the major haematological consequences of dengue are due not to myelosuppression but to capillary leakage and bleeding diathesis (Halstead, 1981; World Health Organization, 1986; Halstead, 1988). These findings are disproportionate to the degree of thrombocytopenia, and are not due to defects in the kinin system (Edelman et al, 1975). Based on the greater risk of haemorrhagic fever in previously exposed patients, Halstead and others hypothesize that non-protective antibodies opsonize the virion, allowing it to penetrate easily into macrophages and resulting in rapid and massive dissemination (Halstead et al, 1970b; Halstead and O'Rourke, 1977a, 1977b; Halstead, 1981, 1988). A single laboratory has provided evidence that non-protective antibodies do increase uptake of virions by macrophages (Halstead and O'Rourke, 1977a, 1977b), but strain-specific differences in virulence have not been excluded as the cause of dengue haemorrhagic fever (Rosen, 1977, 1989). Although the highest incidence of dengue haemorrhagic fever in Cuba during the 1981 epidemic occurred among persons infected previously (Bravo et al, 1987; Guzman et al, 1990), a dengue haemorrhagic fever epidemic occurred on the island of Niue more than 25 years after the last previous dengue exposure (Barnes and Rosen, 1974). This suggests that host characteristics besides prior exposure might allow haemorrhagic fever to develop. The host immune system appears to play a role in these events, possibly involving histamine and other soluble factors (Tuchinda et al, 1977; Bhamarapravati, 1989; Khanna et al, 1990) as final mediators. Dengue virus activates both helper and suppressor human T lymphocytes in vitro, promoting the release of γ-interferon and other lymphokines (Kurane et al, 1989). The appearance of haemorrhagic fever several days after the patient has defervesced, and more than a week after initial infection, is consistent with a host immune response rather than direct viral toxicity as the cause of haemorrhagic phenomena. Since dengue virus can be cultured in human marrow cells with minimal cytotoxicity (Nakao et al, 1989), it is likely that the host immune system plays a critical role both in the mild myelosuppression of classical dengue and the pathophysiology of haemorrhagic fever.

HEPATITIS-ASSOCIATED APLASIA

Since its initial description (Ehrlich, 1888), the aetiology of aplastic anaemia has been unclear. Clinical observations have suggested a causal link with a variety of viral infections (Young, 1990), especially hepatitis (Zulik and Bako, 1971; Böttiger and Westerholm, 1972; Ajlouni and Doeblin, 1974; Hagler et al, 1975). Hepatitis-associated aplasia was first described in 1955 (Lorenz and Quaisar, 1955). A viral cause of hepatitis-associated aplasia has not been proved, but is considered a strong possibility (Hagler et al, 1975; Young, 1990), and an animal model exists for a virus which causes both hepatitis and bone marrow failure (Piazza et al, 1965).

Virology

Although a few cases following hepatitis A and B infection have been reported (Casciato et al, 1978; McSweeney et al, 1988; Smith et al, 1978), hepatitis-associated aplasia is most often associated with non-A, non-B hepatitis (Perillo et al, 1981; Bannister et al, 1983; Campbell and Freedman, 1983; Cargnel et al, 1983; Zeldis et al, 1983; Stock et al, 1987; Pikis et al, 1988; Tzakis et al, 1988; Liang et al, 1990). This raised the possibility that the recently discovered flavivirus-like hepatitis C virus (Choo et al, 1989) could be the cause. Hepatitis-associated aplasia is associated neither with hepatitis C seropositivity (Pol et al, 1990) nor with viraemia (our laboratory, unpublished data). If hepatitis-associated aplasia has a viral aetiology, therefore, it is most likely a non-A, non-B, non-C hepatitis virus. Possible agents that have not yet been investigated in association with hepatitis-associated aplasia include the calcivirus-like agent of hepatitis E (Bradley, 1990) and the paramyxovirus-like agent of giant-cell hepatitis (Phillips et al, 1991).

Transmission

Like fulminant hepatitis (Bernau et al, 1986), hepatitis-associated aplasia is rarely if ever associated with prior transfusion or other parenteral exposure (Perillo et al, 1981; Zeldis et al, 1983; Stock et al, 1987; Pikis et al, 1988; Tzakis et al, 1988).

Clinical syndrome

Most cases conform to a stereotypical pattern. Aplasia follows onset of jaundice by less than 2 months; the hepatitis is not always severe, but the subsequent aplastic anaemia is often fatal (Hagler et al, 1975; Perillo et al, 1981; Foon et al, 1984; Stock et al, 1987; Pikis et al, 1988; Tzakis et al, 1988). Recent advances in therapy may make survival comparable to that of other aplastic anaemia patients (Liang et al, 1990).

Haematology and diagnosis

Patients present with laboratory findings typical of aplastic anaemia, usually at a time when hepatitis is resolving and transaminase levels are returning to normal (Perillo et al, 1981; Bannister et al, 1983; Campbell and Freedman, 1983; Cargnel et al, 1983; Zeldis et al, 1983; Stock et al, 1987; Pikis et al, 1988; Tzakis et al, 1988; Liang et al, 1990).

Epidemiology

World incidence and variations in time

Annual incidence of hepatitis-associated aplasia is less than one case per 10 million persons (see below). Because of its rarity, 'clusters' of hepatitis-associated aplasia consist of only two or three patients, and it is difficult to distinguish such small clusters from chance occurrences. There is no reported seasonal or secular variation in hepatitis-associated aplasia incidence.

Variations in place

Incidence of aplastic anaemia generally, and hepatitis-associated aplasia in particular, is thought to be higher in east Asia than in north America and western Europe (Young et al, 1986). The annual incidence of aplastic anaemia is estimated to be 1.4–3.1 per million in Israel and western Europe (International Agranulocytosis and Aplastic Anemia Study Group, 1987; Mary et al, 1990), of which approximately 5% are hepatitis-associated (Mary et al, 1990). In Thailand, the annual incidence of aplastic anaemia is approximately 3.7 per million (Issaragrisil et al, 1991). The incidence of hepatitis-associated aplasia among the Thai patients has not yet been reported; however, a study of children in Taiwan found that 23% of aplastic anaemia cases were hepatitis-associated (Liang et al, 1990).

Host characteristics

Hepatitis-associated aplasia usually occurs in patients with non-A, non-B hepatitis which is not transfusion acquired (Perillo et al, 1981; Zeldis et al, 1983; Stock et al, 1987; Pikis et al, 1988). In a large series of liver transplant patients, aplastic anaemia followed transplantation in nine (28%) of 32 patients transplanted for fulminant non-A, non-B hepatitis, but none of 1436 patients transplanted after liver failure from other causes (Tzakis et al, 1988). Case patients are predominantly young males (Hagler et al, 1975; Perillo et al, 1981; Bannister et al, 1983; Campbell and Freedman, 1983; Cargnel et al, 1983; Zeldis et al, 1983; Stock et al, 1987; Pikis et al, 1988; Tzakis et al, 1988; Liang et al, 1990). It is interesting to note that aplastic anaemia patients in Thailand also have a higher male : female ratio, and are younger, than aplastic anaemia patients in the United States or Europe (Issaragrisil et al, 1991). No racial predilection of hepatitis-associated aplasia has been described.

Pathophysiology

Geographic variation in hepatitis-associated aplasia is consistent with infectious or environmental causes, or genetic susceptibility. Genetic susceptibility appears less likely because no increased incidence in Asian emigrants to other continents has been described. The available epidemiological evidence does not distinguish between environmental and infectious causes. A viral agent is an attractive hypothesis because the dense human and animal populations of south-east Asia, combined with the warm, humid climate, support a plethora of viral agents known to suppress marrow, including non-A, non-B hepatitis and many of the haemorrhagic fever viruses (World Health Organization, 1985; LeDuc, 1989). The increase in activated cytotoxic T lymphocytes in aplastic anaemia is consistent with an immunological mechanism (Zoumbos et al, 1985a). Hepatitis-associated aplasia also has some features of immunologically-mediated disease, including a 2 month interval between inflammatory illness and myelotoxicity (Hagler et al, 1975; Perillo et al, 1981; Bannister et al, 1983; Campbell and

Freedman, 1983; Cargnel et al, 1983; Zeldis et al, 1983; Stock et al, 1987; Pikis et al, 1988; Tzakis et al, 1988; Liang et al, 1990), impaired cell-mediated immunity (Foon et al, 1984), diminished T4:T8 lymphocyte ratio (Wang et al, 1986), and the response of some patients to immunosuppression (Foon et al, 1984; Tzakis et al, 1988; Liang et al, 1990). These findings imply that a cytotoxic immune response to an unknown (possibly viral) stimulus may cause hepatitis-associated aplasia.

PARVOVIRUS B19

Discovered in normal donor serum in 1975 (Cossart et al, 1975), B19 is the only parvovirus proven to cause human disease. The closely related feline panleucopenia virus (Siegl et al, 1985) causes suppression of leukocyte progenitors in the marrow and lymph nodes of cats (Lawrence and Syverton, 1938; Hammon and Enders, 1939a, 1939b; Lawrence et al, 1940), and provides an animal model for cytotoxic viral diseases of bone marrow (Kurtzman et al, 1981).

Virology

Like other parvoviridiae, B19 has a single-stranded genome 5000 bases long, which has been cloned (Cotmore and Tattersall, 1986; Deiss et al, 1990) and sequenced (Shade et al, 1986; Deiss et al, 1990). One non-structural and two coat protein genes have been identified (Cotmore and Tattersall, 1986; Ozawa et al, 1987, 1988a; Deiss et al, 1990). B19 packages positive and negative strands of DNA with equal frequency into capsids (Summers et al, 1983).

Transmission

B19 can be identified in nasal secretions (Plummer et al, 1985; Chorba et al, 1986) within 10 days of respiratory exposure (Anderson et al, 1985a; Potter et al, 1987). After exposure to an infected person, approximately 50% of susceptible household contacts become infected (Plummer et al, 1985; Chorba et al, 1986), probably by droplet transmission, personal contact or fomites. Factors contributing to the virulence of B19 include the fact that it is heat stable (Cossart et al, 1975; Bartolomei et al, 1988), and reaches very high titres in body fluids, up to 10^{14} virions per ml of serum (Young, 1988; Kurtzman et al, 1989a). It is not surprising, therefore, that B19 has been transmitted through transfusion (Bartolomei et al, 1988). Transplacental infection to the fetus occurs (Anand et al, 1987; Woernle et al, 1987; Franciosi and Tattersall, 1988; Maeda et al, 1988; Schwarz et al, 1988; Samra et al, 1989) and the rate has been estimated to be 33% in pregnancies among women who acquire B19 during pregnancy (PHLS Working Party on Fifth Disease, 1990). There is an incubation period of 1–3 weeks between exposure and clinical illness (Anderson et al, 1985b; LJ Anderson, 1987; Potter et al, 1987). The patient is viraemic (and presumably contagious) during the week prior to the onset of symptoms, but becomes aviraemic within a week thereafter (Anderson et al, 1985b; Saarinen et al, 1986; Potter et al, 1987). Patients with immunoglobulin (Ig)G antibody against parvovirus B19 are resistant to reinfection (Anderson et al, 1985b).

Clinical syndromes

The most commonly recognized syndrome of B19 infection is a childhood exanthem known as erythema infectiosum or fifth disease (Anderson et al, 1984). Approximately 20% of infected adults are asymptomatic (Plummer et al, 1985; Chorba et al, 1986). Symmetrical, large joint polyarthralgias are common, particularly among women, and may be the only clinical manifestation of infection; the characteristic 'slapped cheek' rash found in children is rare among infected adults (White et al, 1985; Woolf et al, 1989; Naides et al, 1990; Mayo and Vance, 1991). B19 infections are usually benign and self-limited. There are, however, at least three exceptions.

First, in patients with diminished erythrocyte survival, B19 infection causes erythroblastopenic crises, characterized by a precipitous and sometimes life-threatening drop in haematocrit, accompanied in some cases by congestive heart failure. Since 1948, when the misnomer 'aplastic crisis' was coined to describe this syndrome (Owren, 1948), erythroblastopenic crisis has been thought to be associated with an infectious illness of some kind, and has been known to occur in clusters (Hilkowitz, 1960). Clusters of erythroblastopenic crises in sickle-cell anaemia patients are now known to be associated in time and place with erythema infectiosum outbreaks (Chorba et al, 1986), but the geographical and temporal clustering of erythroblastopenic crises was unexplained for many years before an association with B19 was proven (Pattison et al, 1981; Serjeant et al, 1981; Chorba et al, 1986; Saarinen et al, 1986). B19 also causes erythroblastopenic crises in patients with other conditions in which erythroid survival is diminished (LeFrere et al, 1986a), including autoimmune haemolysis (Bertrand et al, 1985; Chitnavis et al, 1990), hereditary spherocytosis (Davidson et al, 1984), pyruvate kinase deficiency (Duncan et al, 1983) and thalassaemia (LeFrere et al, 1986b). It has been postulated that B19 may contribute to some of the life-threatening anaemias which are seen in young children with malaria in Africa (Jones et al, 1990). Immunosuppressed patients are a second group to suffer serious consequences from B19 infection. In particular, B19 infection is poorly cleared by patients infected with human immunodeficiency virus, in whom B19 can cause a chronic anaemia requiring multiple transfusions (Bowman et al, 1990; de Mayolo and Temple, 1990; Frickhofen et al, 1990; Mitchell et al, 1990). B19 causes similar problems in some patients with global immunodeficiency due to other causes (Van Horn et al, 1986; Kurtzman et al, 1987, 1988a; Smith et al, 1988; Carstensen et al, 1989; Weiland et al, 1989), as well as a small group of patients with a specific tolerance for B19 (Kurtzman et al, 1989a, 1989b). Finally, B19 infection during pregnancy can result in fetal loss due to hydrops fetalis (Anand et al, 1987; Woernle et al, 1987; Franciosi and Tattersall, 1988; Maeda et al, 1988; Schwarz et al, 1988; Samra et al, 1989).

Haematology and diagnosis

In the normal host, B19 infection rarely causes significant laboratory abnormalities (Young, 1988). Moderate thrombocytopenia or neutropenia occur occasionally (LeFrere et al, 1986a; Saarinen et al, 1986), and a case of vascular purpura coincident with B19 infection has also been described (Schwarz et al, 1989a). Patients with anaemia due to B19 infection have a diminished reticulocyte count, and marrow biopsy reveals greatly diminished or absent erythrocyte precursors and the presence of giant pronormoblasts (Van Horn et al, 1986; Kurtzman et al, 1987, 1989a, 1989b). Serum antibodies against B19 can distinguish between acute (IgM) and prior (IgG) infection (Cohen et al, 1983; Anderson et al, 1986), but at present this is primarily a research tool because of limited antigen supplies. B19 DNA can be detected in the serum (Anderson et al, 1985a; Clewley, 1985; Azzi et al, 1990), high-density peripheral blood leukocytes (Kurtzman et al, 1988a), and other tissues of infected patients by molecular hybridization. The polymerase chain reaction offers a detection mechanism that is approximately 30-fold more sensitive than hybridization alone (Salimans et al, 1989). Commercially licensed kits are not presently available for any of these detection techniques.

Epidemiology

World incidence

A study of 235 susceptible women of reproductive age in the United States, with a cumulative follow-up period of 280 woman-years, found that four women seroconverted, for an incidence of 1.4% per year (Koch and Adler, 1989). Prevalence of infection is strongly age dependent (see below); among persons over 70 years of age, more than 85% have been infected at some time during their lives (Cohen and Buckley, 1988).

Variations in time

Although B19 infection occurs throughout the year, it is commonly believed that most epidemics occur in late winter or early spring, with a 5–7 year periodicity (American Public Health Association, 1990). No secular trend in erythroblastopenic crises, non-immune hydrops fetalis or erythema infectiosum has been described.

Variations in place

Epidemics of erythema infectiosum are often centred in schools (Woolf et al, 1989; American Public Health Association, 1990). Distribution of the virus is worldwide. Reports from countries outside north America are relatively rare, but have included countries of Europe (Courouce et al, 1984), continental Africa and neighbouring islands (Schwarz et al, 1989b; Jones et al, 1990), south America (de Freitas et al, 1990; Nascimento et al, 1990) and Japan (Umene and Nunoue, 1990).

Host characteristics

The cumulative risk of B19 exposure increases with age throughout life. In Koch and Adler's serosurvey of two-parent families, prevalence was 28% among children and 50% among parents; prevalence by age group rose with each succeeding decade, from less than 20% among those 0–9 years old to more than 60% among those 50 years of age or over (Koch and Adler, 1989). Findings in a British serosurvey were similar (Cohen and Buckley, 1988). Koch and Adler found that women were more likely than men to be seropositive (Koch and Adler, 1989). This probably reflects a greater degree of contact between women and young children, who are at greatest risk for epidemics. Degree of contact with young children is strongly associated with B19 infection in school and day care personnel, among whom B19 infection is an occupational hazard (Gillespie et al, 1990). Risks of adverse sequelae from B19 infection among persons with underlying haematological disorders, immunocompromised patients and the fetus have not been well quantified. Occasionally sickle-cell anaemia patients have been acutely infected with B19 without developing erythroblastopenic crisis (Serjeant et al, 1981; Anderson et al, 1982). The risk of pregnancy loss attributable to B19 after intrapartum infection remains uncertain (Brown, 1989). A meta-analysis of pre-1988 studies of women infected during pregnancy implied the risk of early pregnancy loss to be as high as 50% (Samra et al, 1989), while a large German study in 1988 estimated the risk to be half that (Schwarz et al, 1988). Prospective studies organized by the British and United States Public Health Services found that among women infected with B19 during pregnancy the risk of fetal loss due to B19 was less than 10% (Centers for Disease Control, 1989a; PHLS Working Party on Fifth Disease, 1990). Factors influencing susceptibility to B19-induced marrow failure after infection in the presence of underlying haematological disorders or pregnancy remain unknown. At least one severely anaemic, chronically B19-infected patient had no other clinically apparent haematological or immunological disorders (Hamon et al, 1988), implying a specific tolerance for B19. The absence of HLA-DR1 is associated with persistence of B19-mediated arthropathy (Woolf et al, 1989), but no HLA associations with B19-mediated myelotoxicity have been documented.

Pathophysiology

B19 is directly toxic to erythroid progenitors in bone marrow culture (Mortimer et al, 1983; Young et al, 1984a, 1984b), and the non-structural protein gene is toxic when transfected into HeLa cells (Ozawa et al, 1988b). The same toxicity probably occurs to some degree in the marrow of all infected patients. In normal patients, the virus is cleared within 2 weeks (Anderson et al, 1985b; Potter et al, 1987) and erythrocytes outlive the viraemic period by 8- or 9-fold, resulting in minimal diminution of the number of circulating erythrocytes. Clinically significant anaemia occurs only when the erythrocyte life span is shortened or the viraemic period prolonged. Persistent infection occurs when the patient fails to mount an effective antibody response to the virus (Frickhofen and Young, 1989), for reasons including immunodeficiency diseases, immunosuppressive chemotherapy and specific tolerance to B19 (Van Horn et al, 1986; Kurtzman et al, 1987, 1988b, 1989a, 1989b; Smith et al, 1988; Carstensen et al, 1989; Weiland et al, 1989; Frickhofen et al, 1990). Patients who are anaemic due to persistent infection can be rendered transfusion independent by treatment with immune globulin (Frickhofen and Young, 1989; Frickhofen et al, 1990). Host-to-host variability in clearing the virus may explain some of the variations in morbidity after infection during pregnancy or in the presence of haemolytic anaemia. It is worth emphasizing that the potent myelotoxicity of B19 comes to clinical attention only sporadically because of host characteristics. It took many years before the common syndrome of erythema infectiosum was linked to the sporadic occurrence of erythroblastopenic crisis, and similar patience may be needed in order to identify other infectious causes of apparently idiopathic haematological disorders.

EPSTEIN–BARR VIRUS

Virology

Epstein–Barr virus (Epstein et al, 1964) is a member of the herpesvirus family. Its genome comprises 172 kilobases of double-stranded DNA (Wagner et al, 1970), which has been cloned (Dambaugh et al, 1980) and sequenced (Baer et al, 1984). Three major capsid proteins, two major envelope proteins, and a variety of minor proteins surround the core of the virion (Dolyniuk et al, 1976a, 1976b). Like other herpesviruses, Epstein–Barr virus can cause lytic or latent infections. Latent Epstein–Barr virus infection occurs in B lymphocytes, which are transformed and immortalized (Pope et al, 1968; Sudgen and Mark, 1977). In the latently infected cell, viral DNA persists in circular episomes and can also integrate with the host genome (Henderson et al, 1983). Integration does not appear to be site specific. Epstein–Barr virus also replicates in upper respiratory epithelia (Lemon et al, 1977; Sixbey et al, 1984), but latent infection and integration have only been proven in lymphocytes.

Transmission

Mononucleosis incidence peaks among United States military cadets within 2 months after they return from vacation, leading Hoagland (1955) to infer that the disease was spread by kissing. A case-control study supported this hypothesis (Evans, 1960). Epstein–Barr virus is present in the saliva of almost all mononucleosis patients for a minimum of 3 months after onset (Miller et al, 1973) and persists for years thereafter in the saliva of up to 20% of infected persons (Golden et al, 1973). Infected saliva probably transmits Epstein–Barr virus by multiple routes, including fomites (Ginsburg et al, 1976). Infection follows exposure in approximately 10% of household contacts (Fleisher et al, 1981; Sumaya and Ench, 1986), and clinical illness develops 6–9 weeks after exposure (Sumaya and Ench, 1986). The same Epstein–Barr virus strain which infects the oropharynx also establishes itself in blood lymphocytes (Yao et al, 1991), and transfusion-acquired infection has been documented (Gerber et al, 1969). Epstein–Barr virus has been recovered from the uterine cervix, although sexual transmission has not been proven to occur (Sixbey et al, 1986). Once infection has occurred, the host appears to be protected against re-infection, and two strains of the virus are not recovered from the same patient (Yao et al, 1991).

Clinical syndromes

Mononucleosis (Sprunt and Evans, 1920; Hoagland, 1960) is the most common clinical illness associated with acute Epstein–Barr virus infection. Pancytopenia is a rare complication (Read and Hellwig, 1945; Mir and Delamore, 1973; Jain and Sherlock, 1975; Martin, 1977; Van Doornik et al, 1978; Shadduck et al, 1979; Lazarus and Baehner, 1981; Ahronheim et al, 1983; Sullivan, 1984; Schooley et al, 1986; Sawaka et al, 1987; Baranski et al, 1988), occurring 7 days to 7 weeks after the onset of mononucleosis. Rarer still are pure red cell aplasia (Socinski et al, 1984; Baranski et al, 1988), neutropenia (Penman, 1968), and thrombocytopenic purpura (Ellman et al, 1973). Epstein–Barr virus infection is associated with Burkitt's lymphoma in Africa (Epstein et al, 1964; de Thé et al, 1978) and with nasopharyngeal carcinoma in east Asia (Zhu et al, 1986). In human immunodeficiency virus-infected patients, Epstein–Barr virus causes the distinctive syndrome of oral hairy leukoplakia (Resnick et al, 1990). A chronic fatigue syndrome may be associated with the host response to Epstein–Barr virus infection (Jones et al, 1985; Straus et al, 1985), although some controlled studies have failed to support this hypothesis (Hellinger et al, 1988; Gold et al, 1990; Matthews et al, 1991).

Haematology and diagnosis

Lymphocytosis with 10% or more atypical lymphocytes is characteristic of mononucleosis. Mild to moderate thrombocytopenia is also common (Carter, 1965), possibly because of platelet antibodies (Ellman et al, 1973). Haemolytic anaemia due to anti-i antibodies occurs in less than 5% of patients and is rarely of clinical significance (Jenkins et al, 1965; Wilkinson et al, 1973). Most patients with pancytopenia following Epstein–Barr virus infection have typical hypoplastic marrow; however, one case with granulomatous marrow disease has been reported (Martin, 1977). Epstein–Barr virus has been demonstrated in the marrow cells of seven aplastic anaemia patients by immunofluorescence (Ahronheim et al, 1983; Baranski et al, 1988), and in six of these patients Epstein–Barr virus DNA was also identified in marrow cells (Baranski et al, 1988). Serological diagnosis of acute Epstein–Barr virus infection relies on detection of IgM antiviral capsid antibody and the absence of antibody to Epstein–Barr virus-associated nuclear antigen; IgG antiviral capsid antibody persists indefinitely thereafter (Henle et al, 1974). Heterophil antibodies (IgM antibodies directed against certain xenogeneic antigens) generally correlate with mononucleosis symptoms in persons acutely infected with Epstein–Barr virus. Immune adherence haemagglutination appears to be the most sensitive and specific of the several heterophil antibody tests available (Lennette et al, 1978), but heterophil antibody titre elevations are less marked among symptomatic children under 5 years of age (Fleisher et al, 1979). Lymphocyte-transforming virus can be recovered from the saliva of infected patients, but virus recovery does not identify acute infections (Gerber et al, 1972; Chang et al, 1973).

Epidemiology

World incidence

Prevalence of Epstein–Barr virus infection is probably $> 90\%$ among adults, however, annual incidence varies by age, socioeconomic status and population density (see Host characteristics, below). Annual incidence of Epstein–Barr virus-associated pancytopenia is unknown, but the total number of reported cases is even less than those of hepatitis-associated aplasia, suggesting that annual incidence is $< 10^{-7}$.

Variations in time

Consistent seasonal or secular trends in lifetime prevalence of Epstein–Barr virus infection have not been identified. The incidence of symptomatic infection increases with the age at which infection occurs, which in turn depends on socioeconomic status (see Host characteristics, below). Therefore mononucleosis incidence tends to rise during socioeconomic improvements (Strom, 1960; Henke et al, 1973).

Variations in place

Prevalence of Epstein–Barr virus infection appears to be nearly universal in all regions for which reports are available (Pereira et al, 1969; Porter et al, 1969; Black et al, 1970; Kafuko et al, 1972; Golubjatnikov et al, 1973; Lang et al, 1977; Twai et al, 1989; Dan and Chang, 1990; Yadav et al, 1990). Geographical variations in the neoplastic sequelae of Epstein–Barr virus infection are striking. Epstein–Barr virus infection in Africa is associated with Burkitt's lymphoma (de Thé et al, 1978). The association of Epstein–Barr virus with Burkitt's lymphoma depends on the specific insertion site of the viral genome within a protooncogene (Shiramizu et al, 1991). An explanation for the geographical association of this insertion site remains uncertain, but there is some evidence that coinfection of Epstein–Barr virus with *Plasmodia* promotes carcinogenesis (Rickinson and Gregory, 1988). Anecdotal reports suggest that mosquito control reduces the incidence of Epstein–Barr virus-associated Burkitt's lymphoma (Miller, 1990). Migration studies adequate to separate the effects of heredity and environment are not available in the Medline literature, but the low incidence of Burkitt's lymphoma among

African-Americans is also consistent with the hypothesis that the association between this disease and Epstein–Barr virus may owe less to heredity than to environment. In Asia, Epstein–Barr virus is strongly associated with nasopharyngeal carcinoma (Zhu et al, 1986). There is no known geographical variation in the haematological consequences of acute infection. The reported cases of Epstein–Barr virus bone marrow failure syndromes have all been from the United States or western Europe, but the total number of such cases is very small and this may reflect ascertainment bias.

Host characteristics

Presumably because of overcrowding and poor personal hygiene, Epstein–Barr virus infection is thought to occur at lower ages in lower socioeconomic groups (Evans, 1982). The incidence of clinical illness among acutely infected persons increases with age. Mononucleosis is extremely rare among acutely infected infants but may occur in up to 66% of acutely infected adolescents (Sawyer et al, 1971; Biggar et al, 1978). In industrialized countries, mononucleosis incidence peaks in early adolescence (Davidson, 1970; Heath et al, 1972; Henke et al, 1973), although cases in adults do occur (Kirov et al, 1989; Schmader et al, 1989). Most patients with aplastic anaemia following acute Epstein–Barr virus infection (Read and Hellwig, 1945; Mir and Delamore, 1973; Jain and Sherlock, 1975; Martin, 1977; Van Doornik et al, 1978; Shadduck et al, 1979; Lazarus and Baehner, 1981; Ahronheim et al, 1983; Sullivan, 1984; Schooley et al, 1986; Sawaka et al, 1987; Baranski et al, 1988) are typical of mononucleosis patients generally. Patients with the rare X-linked immunoproliferative syndrome are particularly likely to develop aplastic anaemia following Epstein–Barr virus infection (Purtilo et al, 1982; Sullivan et al, 1983). In these patients, Epstein–Barr virus infection is unusually severe: half of the patients die during acute infection, and a majority of the survivors develop hypogammaglobulinaemia or lymphoma (Purtilo and Grierson, 1991). A second, autosomal immunodeficiency syndrome associated with severe Epstein–Barr virus infections is characterized by defective natural killer cell function, but these patients have not been noted to develop chronic myelosuppression following acute illness (Fleisher et al, 1982).

Pathophysiology

Unlike parvovirus B19, Epstein–Barr virus is not toxic to bone marrow cells in culture (Kurtzman and Young, 1989). Instead, it is likely that the pathology induced by Epstein–Barr virus is immune mediated. There is some evidence for this in nasopharyngeal carcinoma, in which malignant epithelial cells express a possibly pathogenic lymphocyte activation factor (Billaud et al, 1989). Patients with Epstein–Barr virus-mediated aplasia typically have dysfunction of the immune system (Fleisher et al, 1982; Purtilo et al, 1982; Sullivan et al, 1983; Purtilo and Grierson, 1991). Epstein–Barr virus stimulates the activation and proliferation of cytotoxic T lymphocytes (Tosato et al, 1979; Tosato and Blaese, 1985; Zoumbos et al,

1985b), a phenomenon also observed in aplastic anaemia (Zoumbos et al, 1985a; Herrman et al, 1986). Epstein–Barr virus-specific cytotoxic T lymphocytes are toxic to marrow cells in culture (Baranski et al, 1988), and lymphocytes capable of suppressing haematopoiesis have been isolated from the marrow of a patient with Epstein–Barr virus-mediated aplasia (Shadduck et al, 1979). Several cases of Epstein–Barr virus-mediated aplasia have been successfully treated with antithymocyte globulin (Shadduck et al, 1979; Lazarus and Baehner, 1981; Baranski et al, 1988). Given the ubiquity of Epstein–Barr virus infection and the rarity of Epstein–Barr virus-mediated bone marrow failure, there is reason to believe that a host or environmental cofactor is necessary for Epstein–Barr virus to trigger an immune response directed against the host bone marrow.

SUMMARY

Haematological syndromes attributed to viruses demonstrate geographical variations in incidence and great dependence on host factors. Severe haematological disease is the exception rather than the rule in dengue virus infection, and probably depends at least in part on the host immune response to the virus. The increased incidence of hepatitis-associated aplasia in east Asia may reflect distribution of an infectious agent, an environmental toxin, or genetic predisposition, but probably represents some combination of these factors. Agents with apparently universal distribution, such as parvovirus B19 and Epstein–Barr virus, are associated with bone marrow failure only in a very narrow range of hosts. These examples teach us that viral causes cannot automatically be excluded from the differential diagnosis of syndromes whose occurrence is rare or apparently sporadic. Further investigation of these syndromes should include more detailed characterization of host factors, particularly immunological characteristics, and possible infectious and toxic cofactors which are associated with morbidity.

REFERENCES

Ahronheim GA, Joncas JH, Ghibu R, Rivard G & Raab-Traub N (1983) Primary infection by Epstein–Barr virus presenting as aplastic anemia (letter). *New England Journal of Medicine* **309:** 313–314.

Ajlouni K & Doeblin TD (1974) The syndrome of hepatitis and aplastic anaemia. *British Journal of Haematology* **27:** 345–355.

American Public Health Association (1990) Erythema infectiosum. In Benensen AS (ed.) *Control of Communicable Diseases in Man* 15th edn, pp 159–161. Washington DC: APHA.

Anand A, Gray ES, Brown T, Clewley JP & Cohen BJ (1987) Human parvovirus infection in pregnancy and hydrops fetalis. *New England Journal of Medicine* **316:** 183–186.

Anderson LJ (1987) Role of parvovirus B19 in human disease. *Pediatric Infectious Disease Journal* **6:** 711–718.

Anderson LJ, Tsou C, Parker RA et al (1986) Detection of antibodies and antigens of human parvovirus B19 by enzyme-linked immunosorbent assay. *Journal of Clinical Microbiology* **24:** 522–526.

Anderson MJ, Davis LR, Hodgson J et al (1982) Occurrence of infection with a parvovirus-like

agent in children with sickle cell anaemia during a two-year period. *Journal of Clinical Pathology* **35:** 744–749.
Anderson MJ, Lewis E, Kidd IM, Hall SM & Cohen BJ (1984) An outbreak of erythema infectiosum associated with human parvovirus infection. *Journal of Hygiene* **93:** 85–93.
Anderson MJ, Jones SE & Minson AC (1985a) Diagnosis of human parvovirus infection by dot-blot hybridization using cloned viral DNA. *Journal of Medical Virology* **15:** 163–172.
Anderson MJ, Higgins PG, Davis LR et al (1985b) Experimental parvoviral infection in humans. *Journal of Infectious Diseases* **152:** 257–265.
Azzi A, Zakrzewska K, Gentilomi G, Musiani M & Zerbini M (1990) Detection of B19 parvovirus infections by a dot-blot hybridization assay using a digoxigenin-labelled probe. *Journal of Virological Methods* **27:** 127–134.
Baer R, Bankier AT, Biggin MD et al (1984) DNA sequence and expression of the B95-8 Epstein–Barr virus genome. *Nature* **310:** 207–211.
Bannister P, Mioszewski K, Barnard D & Losowsky MS (1983) Fatal marrow aplasia associated with non-A, non-B hepatitis. *British Medical Journal* **286:** 1314–1315.
Baranski B, Armstrong G, Truman JT, Quinnan GV, Straus SE & Young NS (1988) Epstein–Barr virus in the bone marrow of patients with aplastic anemia. *Annals of Internal Medicine* **109:** 695–704.
Barnes WJS & Rosen L (1974) Fatal hemorrhagic disease and shock associated with primary dengue infection on a Pacific island. *American Journal of Tropical Medicine and Hygiene* **23:** 495–506.
Bartolomei O, Assi A, Morfini M, Fanci R & Rossi P (1988) Human parvovirus infection in haemophiliacs first infused with treated clotting factor concentrates. *Journal of Medical Virology* **25:** 165–170.
Benenson MW, Top FJ Jr & Gresso W (1975) The virulence to man of Japanese encephalitis virus in Thailand. *American Journal of Tropical Medicine and Hygiene* **24:** 974–980.
Bernau J, Rueff B & Benhamou JP (1986) Fulminant and subfulminant liver failure: definitions and causes. *Seminars in Liver Disease* **6:** 97–106.
Bertrand Y, Lefrere JJ, Leverger G et al (1985) Autoimmune haemolytic anaemia revealed by human parvovirus linked erythroblastopenia. *Lancet* **i:** 382–383.
Bhamarapravati N (1989) Hemostatic defects in dengue hemorrhagic fever. *Reviews of Infectious Diseases* **11 (supplement):** S826–829.
Bierman HR & Nelson ER (1965) Haematodepressive diseases of Thailand. *Annals of Internal Medicine* **62:** 867–884.
Biggar RJ, Henle G, Bocker J et al (1978) Primary Epstein–Barr virus infections in African infants. II. Clinical and serological observations during seroconversion. *International Journal of Cancer* **22:** 244–250.
Billaud M, Busson P, Huang D et al (1989) Epstein–Barr virus (EBV)-containing nasopharyngeal carcinoma cells express the B-cell activation antigen blast2/CD23 and low levels of the EBV receptor CR2. *Journal of Virology* **63:** 4121–4128.
Black FL, Woodall JP, Evans AS et al (1970) Prevalence of antibody against viruses in the Tiriyo, an isolated Amazon tribe. *American Journal of Epidemiology* **91:** 430–438.
Botros BA, Watts DM, Soliman AK et al (1989) Serological evidence of dengue fever among refugees, Hargeysa, Somalia. *Journal of Medical Virology* **29:** 79–81.
Böttiger LE & Westerholm B (1972) Aplastic anemia. III. Aplastic anemia and infectious hepatitis. *Acta Medica Scandinavica* **192:** 323–326.
Bowman CA, Cohen BJ, Norfolk DR & Lacey CJ (1990) Red cell aplasia associated with human parvovirus and HIV infection. *AIDS* **4:** 1038–1039.
Bradley DW (1990) Enterically transmitted non-A, non-B hepatitis. *British Medical Bulletin* **46:** 442–461.
Bravo J, Guzman MG & Kouri G (1987) Why dengue hemorrhagic fever in Cuba? 1. Individual risk factors for dengue hemorrhagic fever/dengue shock syndrome (DHF/DSS). *Transactions of the Royal Society of Tropical Medicine and Hygiene* **81:** 816–820.
Brown KE (1989) What threat is human parvovirus B19 to the fetus? A review. *British Journal of Obstetrics and Gynaecology* **96:** 764–767.
Campbell AN & Freedman MF (1983) Fatal marrow aplasia associated with non-A non-B hepatitis. *British Medical Journal* **286:** 1820–1821 (letter).
Cantelar N, Fernandez A, Albert L & Perez E (1981) Circulacion de dengue en Cuba 1978–9. *Revista Cubana de Medicina Tropical* **33:** 72–78.

Carey DE (1971) Chikungunya and dengue: a case of mistaken identity? *Journal of the History of Medicine* **26:** 243–262.

Cargnel A, Vigano P, Davoli C, Morelli R, Perna MC & Mariscotti C (1983) Sporadic acute non-A, non-B hepatitis complicated by aplastic anémia. *American Journal of Gastroenterology* **78:** 245–247.

Carstensen H, Ornvold K & Cohen BJ (1989) Human parvovirus B19 infection associated with prolonged erythroblastopenia in a leukemic child. *Pediatric Infectious Diseases Journal* **8:**56.

Carter RL (1965) Platelet levels in infectious mononucleosis. *Blood* **25:** 817–821.

Casciato DA, Klein CA, Kaplonitz N & Scott JL (1978) Aplastic anemia associated with type B viral hepatitis. *Archives of Internal Medicine* **138:** 1557–1558.

Centers for Disease Control (1989a) Risks associated with human parvovirus B19 infection. *Morbidity and Mortality Weekly Report* **38:** 81–97.

Centers for Disease Control (1989b) Dengue epidemic—Ecuador, 1988. *Morbidity and Mortality Weekly Report* **38:** 419–421.

Centers for Disease Control (1989c) Update: Aedes albopictus infestation—United States, Mexico. *Morbidity and Mortality Weekly Report* **38:** 440, 445–446.

Centers for Disease Control (1990) Case definitions for public health surveillance. *Morbidity and Mortality Weekly Report* **39(RR13):** 10–11.

Centers for Disease Control (1991a) Dengue epidemic—Peru, 1990. *Morbidity and Mortality Weekly Report* **40:** 145–147.

Centers for Disease Control (1991b) Imported dengue—United States, 1990. *Morbidity and Mortality Weekly Report* **40:** 519–520.

Chang RS, Lewis JP & Abildgaard CF (1973) Prevalence of oropharyngeal excreters of leukocyte transforming agents among a human population. *New England Journal of Medicine* **289:** 1325–1329.

Chitnavis VN, Patou G, Makar YF & Kendra JR (1990) B19 parvovirus induced red cell aplasia complicating acute cold antibody mediated haemolytic anaemia. *British Journal of Haematology* **76:** 433–434.

Choo Q, Kuo G, Weiner AJ, Overby LR, Bradley DW & Houghton M (1989) Isolation of a cDNA clone derived from a blood-borne non-A, non-B viral hepatitis genome. *Science* **244:** 359–362.

Chorba T, Coccia P, Holman RC et al (1986) The role of parvovirus B19 in aplastic crisis and erythema infectiosum (fifth disease). *Journal of Infectious Diseases* **154:** 383–393.

Chungue E, Marché, G, Plichart R, Boutin JP & Roux J (1989) Comparison of immunoglobulin G enzyme-linked immunosorbent assay (IgG-ELISA) and haemagglutination inhibition (HI) test for the detection of dengue antibodies. Prevalence of dengue IgG-ELISA antibodies in Tahiti. *Transactions of the Royal Society for Tropical Medicine and Hygiene* **83:** 708–711.

Clewley JP (1985) Detection of human parvovirus using a molecularly cloned probe. *Journal of Medical Virology* **15:** 173–181.

Cohen BJ & Buckley MM (1988) The prevalence of antibody to human parvovirus B19 in England and Wales. *Journal of Medical Microbiology* **25:** 151–153.

Cohen BJ, Mortimer PP & Pereira MS (1983) Diagnostic assays with monoclonal antibodies for the human serum parvovirus-like virus (SPLV). *Journal of Hygiene* **91:** 113–130.

Cohen SN & Halstead SB (1966) Shock associated with dengue infection. I. Clinical and physiologic manifestations of dengue hemorrhagic fever in Thailand, 1964. *Tropical Pediatrics* **68:** 448–456.

Cossart YE, Field AM, Cant B & Widdows D (1975) Parvovirus-like particles in human sera. *Lancet* **i:** 72–73.

Cotmore SF & Tattersall P (1986) Characterization and molecular cloning of a human parvovirus genome. *Science* **226:** 1161–1165.

Courouce AM, Ferchal F, Morinet F et al (1984) Human parvovirus infections in France. *Lancet* **i:** 160.

Dambaugh T, Beisel C, Hummel M et al (1980) EBV DNA. VII. Molecular cloning and detailed mapping of EBV (B95-8) DNA. *Proceedings of the National Academy of Sciences of the USA* **70:** 2999–3003.

Dan R & Chang RS (1990) A prospective study of primary Epstein–Barr virus infections among university students in Hong Kong. *American Journal of Tropical Medicine and Hygiene* **42:** 380–385.

Davidson RJ (1970) A survey of infectious mononucleosis in the north-east regional hospital board area of Scotland. *Journal of Hygiene* **68:** 393–400.
Davidson RJ, Brown T & Wiseman D (1984) Human parvovirus infection and aplastic crisis in hereditary spherocytosis. *Journal of Infection* **9:** 928–930.
de Freitas RB, Wong D, Boswell F et al (1990) Prevalence of human parvovirus (B19) and rubella virus infections in urban and remote rural areas in northern Brazil. *Journal of Medicine and Virology* **32:** 203–208.
Deiss V, Tratschin J, Weitz M & Siegl G (1990) Cloning of the human parvovirus B19 genome and structural analysis of its palindromic termini. *Virology* **175:** 247–254.
de Mayolo JA & Temple JD (1990) Pure red cell aplasia due to parvovirus B19 infection in a man with HIV infection. *Southern Medical Journal* **83:** 1480–1481.
de Thé G, Geser A, Day NE et al (1978) Epidemiological evidence for causal relationship between Epstein–Barr virus and Burkitt's lymphoma from Ugandan prospective study. *Nature* **274:** 756–761.
Deubel D, Kinney KM & Trent DW (1988) Nucleotide sequence and deduced amino acid sequence of the nonstructural proteins of dengue type 2 virus, Jamaica genotype comparative analysis of the full length genome. *Virology* **165:** 234–244.
Diaz A, Kouri G, Guzman MG et al (1988) Description of the clinical picture of dengue hemorrhagic fever/dengue shock syndrome in adults. *PAHO Bulletin* **22:** 133–144.
Dietz VJ, Gubler DJ, Rigae-Perez JG et al (1990) Epidemic dengue 1 in Brazil, 1986: evaluation of a clinically based dengue surveillance system. *American Journal of Epidemiology* **131:** 693–701.
Dolyniuk M, Pritchett R & Kieff ED (1976a) Proteins of Epstein–Barr virus. I. Analysis of the polypeptides of purified enveloped Epstein–Barr virus. *Journal of Virology* **17:** 935–939.
Dolyniuk M, Wolff E & Kieff ED (1976b) Proteins of Epstein–Barr virus. II. electrophoretic analysis of the polypeptides of the nucleocapsid and the glucosamine- and polysaccharide-containing components of enveloped virus. *Journal of Virology* **18:** 289–297.
Duncan JR, Potter CG, Cappellini MD, Kurtz JB, Anderson MJ & Weatherall DJ (1983) Aplastic crisis due to parvovirus infection in pyruvate kinase deficiency. *Lancet* **ii:** 14–16.
Eamchan P, Nisalak A, Foy HM & Chareonsook OA (1989) Epidemiology and control of dengue virus infections in Thai villages in 1987. *American Journal of Tropical Medicine and Hygiene* **41:** 95–101.
Edelman R, Nimmannitya S, Colman RW, Talamo RC & Top FH Jr (1975) Evaluation of the plasma kinin system in dengue hemorrhagic fever. *Journal of Laboratory and Clinical Medicine* **86:** 410–421.
Ehrenkranz NJ, Ventura AK, Cuadrado RR, Pond WL & Porter JE (1971) Pandemic dengue in Caribbean countries and the southern United States: past, present and potential problems. *New England Journal of Medicine* **285:** 1460–1469.
Ehrlich P (1888) Ueber einen Fall von Anaemie mit Bemerkungen ueber regenerative Veraenderungen des Knochenmarks. *Charité-Annalen*, **13**.
Ellman L, Carvalho A, Jacobson BM et al (1973) Platelet autoantibody in a case of infectious mononucleosis presenting as thrombocytopenic purpura. *American Journal of Medicine* **55:** 723–726.
Epstein M, Achong B & Barr Y (1964) Virus particles in cultured lymphoblasts from Burkitt's lymphoma. *Lancet* **i:** 702–703.
Evans AS (1960) Infectious mononucleosis in University of Wisconsin students: report of a five-year investigation. *American Journal of Hygiene* **71:** 342–362.
Evans AS (1982) The transmission of EB viral infections. In Hooks J & Jordan G (eds) *Viral Infections in Oral Medicine*, pp 211–225. New York: Elsevier/North-Holland.
Fan W, Yu S & Cosgriff TM (1989) The reemergence of dengue in China. *Reviews of Infectious Diseases* **11 (supplement 4):** S847–853.
Fisher-Hoch SP, Mitchell SW, Sasso DR, Lange JV, Ramsey R & McCormick JB (1987) Physiologic and immunologic disturbances associated with shock in Lassa fever in a primate model. *Journal of Infectious Diseases* **155:** 465–474.
Fleisher G, Starr S, Koven N et al (1982) A non-X-linked syndrome with susceptibility to severe Epstein–Barr virus infections. *Journal of Pediatrics* **100:** 727–730.
Fleisher GR, Lennette ET, Henle G et al (1979) Incidence of heterophil-antibody responses in children with infectious mononucleosis. *Journal of Pediatrics* **94:** 723–728.

Fleisher GR, Pasquariello PS, Warren WS et al (1981) Intrafamilial transmission of Epstein–Barr virus infections. *Journal of Pediatrics* **98:** 16–19.

Foon KA, Mitsuyasu RT, Schroff RW et al (1984) Immunologic defects in young male patients with hepatitis-associated aplastic anemia. *Annals of Internal Medicine* **100:** 657–662.

Franciosi RA & Tattersall P (1988) Fetal infection with human parvovirus B19. *Human Pathology* **19:** 489–491.

Frickhofen N & Young NS (1989) Persistent parvovirus B19 infections in humans. *Microbial Pathogenesis* **7:** 319–327.

Frickhofen N, Abkowitz JL, Safford M et al (1990) Persistent B19 infection in patients infected with human immunodeficiency virus type 1 (HIV-1): a treatable cause of anemia in AIDS. *Annals of Internal Medicine* **113:** 926–933.

Gerber P, Walsh JN, Rosenblum EN & Purcell RH (1969) Association of EB-virus infection with the post-perfusion syndrome. *Lancet* **i:** 593–596.

Gerber P, Lucas S, Nonoyama M et al (1972) Oral excretion of Epstein–Barr virus by healthy subjects and patients with infectious mononucleosis. *Lancet* **ii:** 988–989.

Gilbertson WE (1945) Sanitary aspects of the control of the 1943–4 epidemic of dengue fever in Honolulu. *American Journal of Public Health* **35:** 261–270.

Gillespie SM, Cartter ML, Asch S et al (1990) Occupational risk of human parvovirus B19 infection for school and day-care personnel during an outbreak of erythema infectiosum. *Journal of the American Medical Association* **263:** 2061–2065.

Ginsburg CM, Henle G & Henle W (1976) An outbreak of infectious mononucleosis among the personnel of an outpatient clinic. *American Journal of Epidemiology* **104:** 571–575.

Gold D, Bowden R, Sixbey J et al (1990) Chronic fatigue. A prospective clinical and virologic study. *Journal of the American Medical Association* **264:** 48–53.

Golden HD, Chang RS, Prescott W et al (1973) Leukocyte transforming agent: prolonged excretion by patients with mononucleosis and excretion by normal individuals. *Journal of Infectious Diseases* **127:** 471–473.

Golubjatnikov R, Allen VD, Steadman S et al (1973) Prevalence of antibodies to Epstein–Barr virus, cytomegalovirus and toxoplasma in a Mexican highland community. *American Journal of Epidemiology* **97:** 116–124.

Grimstad PR, Barrett CL, Humphrey RL et al (1987) Serologic evidence for widespread infection with LaCrosse and St Louis encephalitis viruses in the Indiana human population. *American Journal of Epidemiology* **119:** 913–930.

Gubler DJ (1987) Current research on dengue. *Current Topics in Vector Research* **3:** 37–56.

Gubler DJ (1988) Dengue. In Monath TP (ed.) *The Arboviruses: Ecology and Epidemiology*, vol. 2, pp 223–260. Boca Raton: CRC Press.

Gubler DJ, Suharyono W, Tan R et al (1981) Viraemia in patients with naturally acquired dengue infection. *Bulletin of the World Health Organization* **59:** 623–630.

Guzman MG, Kouri GP, Bravo J, Soler M, Vazquez S & Morier L (1990) Dengue hemorrhagic fever in Cuba, 1981: a retrospective seroepidemiologic study. *American Journal of Tropical Medicine and Hygiene* **42:** 179–184.

Hagler L, Pastore RA, Bergin JJ & Wrensch MR (1975) Aplastic anemia following viral hepatitis: report of two cases and literature review. *Medicine* **54:** 139–162.

Hahn YS, Galler R, Hunkapillar T, Dalrymple JM, Strauss JH & Strauss EG (1988) Nucleotide sequence of a dengue-2 RNA and comparison of the encoded proteins with those of other flaviviruses. *Virology* **162:** 167–180.

Halstead SB (1972) Dengue: haematologic aspects. *Seminars in Hematology* **19:** 116–131.

Halstead SB (1981) The pathogenesis of dengue. Molecular epidemiology in infectious disease. *American Journal of Epidemiology* **114:** 632–648.

Halstead SB (1988) Pathogenesis of dengue: challenges to molecular biology. *Science* **239:** 476–481.

Halstead SB & O'Rourke EJ (1977a) Antibody-enhanced dengue virus infection in primate leukocytes. *Nature* **265:** 739–741.

Halstead SB & O'Rourke EJ (1977b) Dengue viruses and mononuclear phagocytes. I. Infection enhancement by non-neutralizing antibody. *Journal of Experimental Medicine* **146:** 201–217.

Halstead SB, Scanlon JE, Umpaivit P et al (1969) Dengue and chikungunya virus infection in man in Thailand, 1962–4. IV. Epidemiologic studies in the Bangkok metropolitan area. *American Journal of Tropical Medicine and Hygiene* **18:** 997–1021.

Halstead SB, Udomsakdi S, Simasthien P, Singharaj P, Sukhavachana P & Nisalak A (1970a) Observations related to pathogenesis of dengue hemorrhagic fever. I. Experience with classification of dengue viruses. *Yale Journal of Biology and Medicine* **42:** 261–275.
Halstead SB, Nimmannitya S & Cohen SN (1970b) Observations related to pathogenesis of dengue hemorrhagic fever. IV. Relation of disease severity to antibody response and virus recovered. *Yale Journal of Biology and Medicine* **42:** 311–328.
Hammon WD & Enders JF (1939a) A virus disease of cats, principally characterized by aleucocytosis, enteric lesions and the presence of intra nuclear inclusion bodies. *Journal of Experimental Medicine* **69:** 327–351.
Hammon WD & Enders JF (1939b) Further studies on the blood and haematopoietic tissues in malignant panleucopenia of cats. *Journal of Experimental Medicine* **70:** 557–564.
Hammon WM, Rudnick A, Sather GF et al (1957) Studies on Philippine hemorrhagic fever: relationship to dengue viruses. *Proceedings of the 9th Pacific Scientific Congress*. Bangkok, pp 67–72.
Hamon MD, Newland AC & Anderson MJ (1988) Severe aplastic anaemia after parvovirus infection in the absence of underlying haemolytic anaemia. *Journal of Clinical Pathology* **41:** 1242.
Heath CW, Brodsky AL & Potolsky AI (1972) Infectious mononucleosis in a general population. *American Journal of Epidemiology* **95:** 46–52.
Hellinger WC, Smith TF, Van Scoy RE et al (1988) Chronic fatigue syndrome and the diagnostic utility of antibody to Epstein–Barr virus early antigen. *Journal of the American Medical Association* **260:** 971–973.
Henderson A, Ripley S, Heller M & Kieff E (1983) Human chromosome association of Epstein–Barr virus DNA in a Burkitt tumor cell line and in lymphocytes growth transformed *in vitro*. *Proceedings of the National Academy of Sciences of the USA* **80:** 1987–1991.
Henke CE, Kurland LT & Elveback LR (1973) Infectious mononucleosis in Rochester, Minnesota, 1950 through 1969. *American Journal of Epidemiology* **98:** 483–490.
Henle W, Henle G & Horowitz CA (1974) Epstein–Barr virus-specific diagnostic tests in infectious mononucleosis. *Human Pathology* **5:** 551–565.
Herrman F, Griffin JD, Meuer SG & Buschenfelde KM (1986) Establishment of an interleukin2-dependent T cell line derived from a patient with severe aplastic anemia, which inhibits in vitro haematopoiesis. *Journal of Immunology* **136:** 1629–1634.
Hilkovitz G (1960) Sickle cell disease: the 'aplastic crisis' and erythroid maturation defect occurring simultaneously in three members of a family. *Archives of Internal Medicine* **105:** 76–82.
Hoagland RJ (1955) The transmission of infectious mononucleosis. *American Journal of the Medical Sciences* **229:** 262–272.
Hoagland RJ (1960) The clinical manifestations of infectious mononucleosis: a report of 200 cases. *American Journal of Medicine* **240:** 21–28.
International Agranulocytosis and Aplastic Anemia Study Group (1987) Incidence of aplastic anemia: the relevance of diagnostic criteria. *Blood* **70:** 1718–1721.
Issaragrisil S, Sriratanasatavorn C, Piankijagum A et al (1991) Incidence of aplastic anemia in Bangkok. *Blood* **77:** 2166–2168.
Jain S & Sherlock S (1975) Infectious mononucleosis with jaundice, anaemia and encephalopathy. *British Medical Journal* **3:** 138–139.
Jenkins WJ, Koster HG, March WL et al (1965) Infectious mononucleosis: an unsuspected source of anti-i. *British Journal of Haematology* **11:** 480–483.
Johnson BK, Dhoth F, Tukei PM et al (1990) Dengue-2 virus in Kenya. *Lancet* **336:** 1071.
Jones JF, Ray G, Minnich LL et al (1985) Evidence for active Epstein–Barr virus infection in patients with persistent, unexplained illness: elevated anti-early antigen antibodies. *Annals of Internal Medicine* **102:** 1–7.
Jones PH, Pickett LC, Anderson MJ & Pasvol G (1990) Human parvovirus infection in children and severe anaemia seen in an area endemic for malaria. *Journal of Tropical Medicine and Hygiene* **93:** 67–70.
Kafuko GW, Henderson BE, Kirya BG et al (1972) Epstein–Barr virus antibody levels in children from the West Nile district of Uganda. *Lancet* **i:** 706–709.
Khanna M, Chaturbedi UC, Sharma MC, Pandey VC & Mathur A (1990) Increased capillary permeability mediated by a dengue virus-induced lymphokine. *Immunology* **69:** 449–453.

Kirov SM, Marsden KA & Wongwanich S (1989) Seroepidemiological study of infectious mononucleosis in older patients. *Journal of Clinical Microbiology* **27:** 356–358.

Kitayaporn D, Singhasivanon P & Vasuvat C (1989) Age-adjusted dengue haemorrhagic fever morbidity in Thailand 1983–7. *Southeast Asian Journal of Tropical Medicine and Public Health* **20:** 195–200.

Koch WC & Adler SP (1989) Human parvovirus B19 infections in women of childbearing age and within families. *Pediatric Infectious Disease Journal* **8:** 83–87.

Koopman JS, Prevots DR, Vaca-Marin MA et al (1991) Determinants and predictors of dengue infection in Mexico. *American Journal of Epidemiology* **33:** 1168–1178.

Kouri G, Guzman MG & Bravo J (1986) Hemorrhagic dengue in Cuba: history of an epidemic. *Bulletin of the Pan American Health Organization* **20:** 24–30.

Kuberski TT & Rosen L (1977) A simple method for the detection of dengue antigen in mosquitoes by immuno fluorescence. *American Journal of Tropical Medicine and Hygiene* **26:** 533–537.

Kuberski TT, Rosen L, Reed D & Mataika J (1977) Clinical and laboratory observations on patients with primary and secondary dengue type 1 infections with hemorrhagic manifestations in Fiji. *American Journal of Tropical Medicine and Hygiene* **26:** 775–783.

Kuno G, Gubler DJ, Velez M et al (1985) Comparative sensitivity of three mosquito cell lines for isolation of dengue viruses. *Bulletin of the World Health Organization* **63:** 279–286.

Kurane I, Innis BL, Nisalak A et al (1989) Human T-cell responses to dengue virus antigens. *Journal of Clinical Investigation* **83:** 506–513.

Kurtzman G & Young N (1989) Viruses and bone marrow failure. *Baillière's Clinical Haematology* **2:** 51–68.

Kurtzman GJ, Platanias L, Lustig L, Frickhofen N & Young NS (1981) Feline parvovirus propagates in cat bone marrow cultures and inhibits haematopoietic colony formation in vitro. *Blood* **74:** 71–81.

Kurtzman GJ, Ozawa K, Cohen B, Hanson G, Oseas R & Young NS (1987) Chronic bone marrow failure due to persistent B19 parvovirus infection. *New England Journal of Medicine* **317:** 287–294.

Kurtzman GJ, Cohen B, Meyers P, Amunullah A & Young NS (1988a) Persistent B19 parvovirus infection as a cause of severe chronic anaemia in children with acute lymphocytic leukaemia. *Lancet* **ii:** 1159–1162.

Kurtzman GJ, Gascon P, Caras M, Cohen B & Young NS (1988b) B19 parvovirus replicates in circulating cells of acutely infected patients. *Blood* **71:** 1448–1454.

Kurtzman GJ, Cohen BJ, Field AM, Oseas R, Blaese RM & Young NS (1989a) The immune response to B19 parvovirus and an antibody defect in persistent viral infection. *Journal of Clinical Investigation* **84:** 1114–1123.

Kurtzman G, Frickhofen N, Kimball J, Jenkins DW, Nienhuis AW & Young NS (1989b) Pure red cell aplasia of ten years' duration due to persistent B19 parvovirus infection and its cure with immunoglobulin therapy. *New England Journal of Medicine* **321:** 519–523.

Lang DJ, Garruto RM & Gadjdusek DC (1977) Early acquisition of cytomegalovirus and Epstein–Barr virus antibody in several isolated Melanesian populations. *American Journal of Epidemiology* **105:** 480–487.

Lange JV, Mitchell SW, McCormick JB, Walker DH, Evatt BL & Ramsey RR (1985) Kinetic study of platelets and fibrinogen in Lassa virus-infected monkeys and early pathologic events in Mopeis virus-infected monkeys. *American Journal of Tropical Medicine and Hygiene* **34:** 999–1007.

Lawrence JS & Syverton JT (1938) Spontaneous agranulocytosis in the cat. *Proceedings of the Society for Experimental Biology and Medicine* **38:** 914–918.

Lawrence JS, Syverton JT, Shaw JS & Smith FP (1940) Infectious feline agranulocytosis. *American Journal of Pathology* **16:** 333–354.

Lazarus KM & Baehner RL (1981) Aplastic anemia complicating infectious mononucleosis: a case report and review of the literature. *Pediatrics* **67:** 907–910.

LeDuc JW (1989) Epidemiology of hemorrhagic fever viruses. *Reviews of Infectious Diseases* **11 (supplement 4):** S730–735.

LeFrere JJ, Courouce AM, Bertrand Y, Girot R & Soulier JP (1986a) Human parvovirus and aplastic crisis in chronic hemolytic anemias: a study of 24 observations. *American Journal of Hematology* **23:** 271–275.

LeFrere JJ, Girot R, Courouce AM, Maire-Redelsperger M & Cornu P (1986b) Familial human parvovirus infection associated with anemia in siblings with heterozygous β-thalassemia. *Journal of Infectious Diseases* **153:** 977–979.

Lemon SM, Hutt LM, Shaw JE et al (1977) Replication of EBV in epithelial cells during infectious mononucleosis. *Nature* **268:** 268–270.

Lennette ET, Henle G, Henle W et al (1978) Heterophil antigen in bovine sera detected by immune adherence hemagglutination with infectious mononucleosis sera. *Infection and Immunity* **19:** 923–927.

Liang D, Lin KH, Lin D, Yang C, Hung K & Lin KS (1990) Post-hepatic aplastic anaemia in children in Taiwan, a hepatitis prevalent area. *British Journal of Haematology* **74:** 487–491.

Liu WT, Chen CL, Lee SS et al (1991) Isolation of dengue virus with a human promonocyte cell line. *American Journal of Tropical Medicine and Hygiene* **44:** 494–499.

Lorenz E & Quaisar K (1955) Panmyelopathic nach hepatitis epidemica. *Wiener Medizinische Wochenschrift* **105:** 19–22.

McSweeney PA, Carter JM, Green GJ & Romeril KR (1988) Fatal aplastic anemia associated with hepatitis B viral infection. *American Journal of Medicine* **85:** 255–256.

Maeda H, Shimokawa H, Satoh S, Nakano H & Nunoue T (1988) Nonimmunologic hydrops fetalis resulting from intrauterine human parvovirus B-19 infection: report of two cases. *Obstetrics and Gynecology* **72:** 482–485.

Martin MF (1977) Atypical infectious mononucleosis with bone marrow granulomas and pancytopenia. *British Medical Journal* **5:** 300–301.

Mary JY, Baumelou E, Guiguet M et al (1990) Epidemiology of aplastic anemia in France: a prospective multicentric study. *Blood* **75:** 1646–1653.

Mas P (1979) *Dengue Fever in Cuba in 1977: Some Laboratory Aspects of Dengue in the Caribbean*, PAHO Scientific Publication 375, pp 40–43. Washington DC: PAHO.

Matthews DA, Lane TJ & Manu P (1991) Antibodies to Epstein–Barr virus in patients with chronic fatigue. *Southern Medical Journal* **84:** 832–840.

Mayo DR & Vance DW Jr (1991) Parvovirus B19 as the cause of a syndrome resembling Lyme arthritis in adults. *New England Journal of Medicine* **324:** 419.

Miller G (1990) Epstein–Barr virus. Biology, pathogenesis and medical aspects. In Fields BN, Knipe DM, Channock RM et al (eds) *Virology* 2nd edn, pp 1921–1958. New York: Raven Press.

Miller G, Niederman JC & Andrews L (1973) Prolonged oropharyngeal excretion of Epstein–Barr virus after infectious mononucleosis. *New England Journal of Medicine* **288:** 229–232.

Mir MA & Delamore IW (1973) Aplastic anemia complicating infectious mononucleosis. *Scandinavian Journal of Haematology* **11:** 314–318.

Mitchell SA, Welch JM, Weston-Smith S et al (1990) Parvovirus infection and anaemia in a patient with AIDS: case report. *Genitourinary Medicine* **66:** 95–96.

Monath TP (1987) Yellow fever: a medically neglected disease. Report on a seminar. *Reviews of Infectious Diseases* **9:** 165–175.

Monath TP (1990) Flaviviruses. In Fields BN, Knipe DM et al (eds) *Virology* 2nd edn, pp 763–814. New York: Raven Press.

Monath TP & Tsai TF (1987) St Louis encephalitis: lessons from the last decade. *American Journal of Tropical Medicine and Hygiene* **37:** 40S–59S.

Monath TP, Craven RB, Adjukiewicz A et al (1980) Yellow fever in the Gambia, 1978–9: epidemiologic aspects with observations on the occurrence of Orungo virus infections. *American Journal of Tropical Medicine and Hygiene* **198:** 912–928.

Morens DM, Halstead SB, Repik PM, Putvatana R & Raybourne N (1985) Simplified plaque reduction neutralization assay for dengue viruses by semimicro methods in BHK21 cells: comparison of the BHK suspension test with standard plaque reduction neutralization. *Journal of Clinical Microbiology* **22:** 250–254.

Mortimer PP, Humphries RK, Moore JG et al (1983) A human parvovirus-like virus inhibits haematopoietic colony formation in vitro. *Nature* **302:** 426–429.

Naides SJ, Scharosch LL, Foto F & Howard EJ (1990) Rheumatologic manifestations of human parvovirus B19 infection in adults. *Arthritis and Rheumatism* **33:** 1297–1309.

Nakao S, Lai CJ & Young NS (1989) Dengue virus, a flavivirus, propagates in human bone marrow progenitors and haematopoietic cell lines. *Blood* **7:** 319–327.

Nascimento JP, Buckley MM, Brown KE & Cohen BJ (1990) The prevalence of antibody to human parvovirus B19 in Rio de Janeiro, Brazil. *Revista do Instituto de Medicina Tropical de Sao Paulo* **32:** 41–45.

Neff JM, Morris L, Gonzalez-Alcover R, Coleman PH, Lyss SB & Negron H (1967) Dengue fever in a Puerto Rican community. *American Journal of Epidemiology* **86:** 162–184.

Nimmannitya S, Halstead SB, Cohen SN & Margiotta MR (1969) Dengue and chikungunya virus infections in man in Thailand, 1962–4. I. Observations on hospitalized patients with hemorrhagic fever. *American Journal of Tropical Medicine and Hygiene* **18:** 954–971.

Owren PA (1948) Congenital hemolytic jaundice: the pathogenesis of the 'hemolytic crisis'. *Blood* **3:** 231–248.

Ozawa K, Ayub J, Yu-shu H, Kurtzman G, Shimada T & Young N (1987) Novel transcription map for the B19 (human) pathogenic parvovirus. *Journal of Virology* **61:** 2395–2406.

Ozawa K, Ayub J & Young N (1988a) Functional mapping of the genome of the B19 (human) parvovirus by in vitro translation after negative hybrid selection. *Journal of Virology* **62:** 2508–2511.

Ozawa K, Ayub J, Kajigaya S, Shimada T & Young N (1988b) The gene encoding the nonstructural protein of B19 (human) parvovirus may be lethal in transfected cells. *Journal of Virology* **62:** 2884–2889.

Pan American Health Organization (1990) Dengue hemorrhagic fever in Venezuela. *Epidemiology Bulletin* **11:** 7–9.

Pattison J, Jones S, Hodgson J et al (1981) Parvovirus infections and hypoplastic crisis in sickle cell anemia. *Lancet* **i:** 664–665.

Penman HG (1968) Extreme neutropenia in glandular fever. *Journal of Clinical Pathology* **21:** 48–49.

Pereira MS, Blake JM & Macrae AD (1969) EB virus antibody at different ages. *British Medical Journal* **4:** 526–527.

Perillo RP, Pohl DA, Roodman ST & Tsai CC (1981) Acute non-A, non-B hepatitis with serum sickness-like syndrome and aplastic anemia. *Journal of the American Medical Association* **245:** 494–496.

Phillips MJ, Blendis LM, Pouceli S et al (1991) Syncytial giant-cell hepatitis. *New England Journal of Medicine* **324:** 455–460.

PHLS Working Party on Fifth Disease (1990) Prospective study of human parvovirus (B19) infection in pregnancy. *British Medical Journal* **300:** 1166–1170.

Piazza M, Piccinino F & Matano F (1965) Haematological changes in viral (MHV-3) murine hepatitis. *Nature* **250:** 1034–1035.

Pikis A, Kavaliotis J & Manios S (1988) Incidence of aplastic anemia in viral hepatitis in children. *Scandinavian Journal of Infectious Diseases* **20:** 109–110.

Plummer FA, Hammond GW, Forward K et al (1985) An erythema infectiosum-like illness caused by human parvovirus infection. *New England Journal of Medicine* **313:** 74–79.

Pol S, Driss F, Devergie A, Brechot C, Berthelot P & Gluckman E (1990) Is hepatitis C virus involved in hepatitis-associated aplastic anemia? *Annals of Internal Medicine* **113:** 435–437.

Pope JH, Horne MK & Scott W (1968) Transformation of fetal human leucocytes in vitro by filtrates of a human leukemic cell line containing herpes-like virus. *International Journal of Cancer* **3:** 857–866.

Porter DD, Wimberly I & Benyish-Melnick M (1969) Prevalence of antibodies to EB virus and other herpesviruses. *Journal of the American Medical Association* **208:** 1675–1679.

Potter CG, Potter AC, Hatton CSR et al (1987) Variation of erythroid and myeloid precursors in the marrow and peripheral blood of volunteer subjects infected with human parvovirus (B19). *Journal of Clinical Investigation* **79:** 1486–1492.

Purtilo DT & Grierson HL (1991) Methods of detection of new families with X-linked lymphoproliferative disease. *Cancer Genetics and Cytogenetics* **51:** 143–153.

Purtilo DT, Sakamoto K, Barnabei V et al (1982) Epstein–Barr virus-induced diseases in boys with the X-linked lymphoproliferative syndrome (XLP): update on studies of the registry. *American Journal of Medicine* **73:** 49–56.

Read JT & Hellwig RC (1945) Infectious mononucleosis: an analysis of 300 cases with 3 characterized by rare haematologic findings. *Archives of Internal Medicine* **75:** 376–380.

Resnick L, Herbst JS & Raab-Traub N (1990) Oral hairy leukoplakia. *Journal of the American Academy of Dermatology* **22:** 1278–1282.

Rice CM, Lencues EM, Eddy SR, Shin SJ, Sheets RL & Strauss JH (1985) Nucleotide sequence of yellow fever virus: implications for flavivirus gene expression and evolution. *Science* **229:** 726–733.

Rickinson AB & Gregory CD (1988) Burkitt's lymphoma. *Transactions of the Royal Society for Tropical Medicine and Hygiene* **82:** 657–659.

Rosen L (1977) The emperor's new clothes revisited, or reflections on the pathogenesis of dengue hemorrhagic fever. *American Journal of Tropical Medicine and Hygiene* **26:** 337–343.

Rosen L (1989) Disease exacerbation caused by sequential dengue infections: myth or reality? *Reviews of Infectious Diseases* **11 (supplement 4):** S840–842.

Rudnick A, Marchette NJ & Garcia R (1967) Possible jungle dengue: recent studies and hypotheses. *Japanese Journal of Medical Science and Biology* **20:** 69–74.

Saarinen UA, Chorba TL, Tattersall P et al (1986) Human parvovirus B19-induced epidemic acute red cell aplasia in patients with hereditary hemolytic anemia. *Blood* **67:** 1411–1417.

Sabin AB (1952) Research on dengue during World War II. *American Journal of Tropical Medicine and Hygiene* **1:** 30–50.

Salimans MM, Holsappel S, van de Rijke FM, Jiwa NM, Raap AK & Weiland HT (1989) Rapid detection of human parvovirus B19 DNA by dot-hybridization and the polymerase chain reaction. *Journal of Virological Methods* **23:** 19–28.

Samra JS, Obhrai MS & Constantine G (1989) Parvovirus infection in pregnancy. *Obstetrics and Gynecology* **73:** 832–834.

Samsi TK, Wulur H, Sugianto D et al (1990) Some clinical and epidemiological observations on virologically confirmed dengue hemorrhagic fever. *Paediatrica Indonesiana* **30:** 293–303.

Sangkawibha N, Rojansuphot S, Anandrik S et al (1984) Risk factors in dengue shock syndrome: a prospective epidemiologic study in Rayong Thailand. The 1980 outbreak. *American Journal of Epidemiology* **120:** 653–659.

Sawaka CA, Bessette J, Furie B & Desforges JF (1987) Aplastic anemia complicating infectious mononucleosis. *Canadian Medical Association Journal* **136:** 730–731.

Sawyer RN, Evans AS, Niederman JC et al (1971) Prospective studies of a group of Yale University freshmen. I. Occurrence of infectious mononucleosis. *Journal of Infectious Diseases* **123:** 263–270.

Schmader KE, van der Horst CM & Klotman ME (1989) Epstein–Barr virus and the elderly host. *Reviews of Infectious Diseases* **11:** 64–73.

Schooley RT, Carey RW, Miller G et al (1986) Chronic Epstein–Barr virus infection associated with fever and interstitial pneumonitis. *Annals of Internal Medicine* **104:** 636–643.

Schwarz TF, Roggendorf M, Hottentrager B et al (1988) Human parvovirus B19 infection in pregnancy. *Lancet* **ii:** 566–567.

Schwarz TF, Bruns R, Schroder C, Wiersbitzky S & Roggendorf M (1989a) Human parvovirus B19 infection associated with vascular purpura and vasculitis. *Infection* **17:** 170–171.

Schwarz TF, Gurtler LG, Zoulek G, Deinhardt F & Roggendorf M (1989b) Seroprevalence of human parvovirus B19 in Sao Tome and Principe, Malawi and Mascarene Islands. *International Journal of Medical Microbiology* **271:** 231–236.

Serjeant GR, Topley JM, Mason K et al (1981) Outbreak of aplastic crises in sickle cell anaemia associated with parvovirus-like agent. *Lancet* **ii:** 595–597.

Shadduck RK, Winkelstein A, Ziegler Z et al (1979) Aplastic anemia following infectious mononucleosis: possible immune etiology. *Experimental Haematology* **7:** 264–271.

Shade RO, Blundell MC, Cotmore SF, Tattersall P & Astell CR (1986) Nucleotide sequence and genome organization of human parvovirus B19 isolated from the serum of a child during aplastic crisis. *Journal of Virology* **58:** 921–926.

Shiramizu B, Barriga F, Neequaye J et al (1991) Patterns of chromosomal breakpoint locations in Burkitt's lymphoma: relevance to geography and Epstein–Barr virus association. *Blood* **77:** 1516–1526.

Siegl G, Bates RC, Berns KI et al (1985) Characteristics and taxonomy of *Parvoviridiae*. *Intervirology* **23:** 71–73.

Siler JF, Hall MW & Kitchens AP (1926) Dengue: its history, epidemiology, mechanisms of transmission, etiology, clinical manifestations, immunity and prevention. *Philippine Journal of Science* **29:** 1–304.

Simmons JS, St John JH & Reynolds FHK (1931) Experimental studies of dengue. *Philippine Journal of Science* **44:** 1–251.

Sixbey JW, Nedrud JG, Raab-Traub N, Hanes RA & Pagano JS (1984) Epstein–Barr virus replication in oropharyngeal epithelial cells. *New England Journal of Medicine* **310:** 1225–1230.

Sixbey JW, Lemon SM & Pagano JS (1986) A second site for Epstein–Barr virus shedding: the uterine cervix. *Lancet* **ii:** 1122–1124.
Slosek J (1986) *Aedes aegypti* mosquitoes in the Americas: a review of their interactions with the human population. *Social Science and Medicine* **23:** 249–257.
Smith D, Gribble TJ, Yeager AS et al (1978) Spontaneous resolution of severe aplastic anemia associated with viral hepatitis A in a 6-year-old child. *American Journal of Hematology* **5:** 247–252.
Smith MA, Shah NR, Lobel JS, Cera PJ, Gary GW & Anderson LJ (1988) Severe anemia caused by human parvovirus in a leukemia patient on maintenance chemotherapy. *Clinical Pediatrics* **27:** 383–386.
Socinski MA, Ershler WB, Tosato G & Balese RM (1984) Pure red cell aplasia associated with chronic Epstein–Barr virus infection: evidence for T-cell mediated suppression of erythroid colony units. *Journal of Laboratory and Clinical Medicine* **104:** 995–1006.
Sprunt TP & Evans FA (1920) Mononuclear leukocytosis in reaction to acute infections ('infectious mononucleosis'). *Johns Hopkins Hospital Bulletin* **31:** 410–417.
Srivastava VK, Suri S, Bhasin A, Srivastava L & Bharadwaj M (1990) An epidemic of dengue haemorrhagic fever and dengue shock syndrome in Delhi: a clinical study. *Annals of Tropical Paediatrics* **10:** 329–334.
Stock PG, Steiner ME, Freese D, Sharp H & Ascher NL (1987) Hepatitis-associated aplastic anemia after liver transplantation. *Transplantation* **43:** 595–597.
Straus SE, Tosato G, Armstrong G et al (1985) Persisting illness and fatigue in adults with evidence of Epstein–Barr virus infection. *Annals of Internal Medicine* **102:** 7–16.
Strom J (1960) Infectious mononucleosis: is the incidence increasing? *Acta Medica Scandinavica* **168:** 35–39.
Sudgen B & Mark W (1977) Clonal transformation of adult human leukocytes by Epstein–Barr virus. *Journal of Virology* **23:** 503–508.
Sullivan JL (1984) Case 31-1984, case records of the Massachusetts General Hospital. *New England Journal of Medicine* **311:** 314–322.
Sullivan JL, Byron KS, Brewster FE, Baker SM & Ochs HD (1983) X-linked lymphoproliferative syndrome. Natural history of the immunodeficiency. *Journal of Clinical Investigation* **71:** 1765–1768.
Sumaya CV & Ench Y (1986) Epstein–Barr virus infections in families: the role of children with infectious mononucleosis. *Journal of Infectious Diseases* **154:** 842–850.
Summers J, Jones SE & Anderson MJ (1983) Characterisation of the genome of the agent of erythrocyte aplasia permits its classification as a human parvovirus. *Journal of General Virology* **64:** 2527–2532.
Tosato G & Blaese RM (1985) Epstein-Barr virus infection and immunoregulation in man. *Advances in Immunology* **37:** 99–149.
Tosato G, Magrath I, Koski I, Dooley N & Blaese M (1979) Activation of suppressor T cells during Epstein–Barr-virus-induced infectious mononucleosis. *New England Journal of Medicine* **301:** 1133–1137.
Tuchinda M, Dhorreinintra B & Tuchinda P (1977) Histamine content in 24 hour urine in patients with dengue haemorrhagic fever. *Southeast Asian Journal of Tropical Medicine and Public Health* **8:** 80–83.
Twai WS, Chang MH, Chen JY, Lee CY & Liu YG (1989) Seroepidemiological study of Epstein–Barr virus infection in children in Taipei. *Acta Paediatrica Sinica* **30:** 81–86.
Tzakis AG, Arditi M, Whitington PF et al (1988) Aplastic anemia complicating orthotopic liver transplantation for non-A, non-B hepatitis. *New England Journal of Medicine* **319:** 393–396.
Umenai T, Krzysko R, Bektimirov TA et al (1985) Japanese encephalitis: current worldwide status. *Bulletin of the World Health Organization* **63:** 625–631.
Umene K & Nunoue T (1990) The genome type of human parvovirus B19 strains isolated in Japan during 1981 differs from types detected in 1986 to 1987: a correlation between genome type and prevalence. *Journal of General Virology* **71:** 983–986.
Van Doornik MC, Van'T Veer-Korthof ET & Wierenga H (1978) Fatal aplastic anaemia complicating infectious mononucleosis. *Scandinavian Journal of Haematology* **20:** 52–56.
Van Horn DK, Mortimer PP, Young N & Hason GR (1986) Human parvovirus-associated red cell aplasia in the absence of underlying hemolytic anemia. *American Journal of Pediatric Hematology/Oncology* **8:** 235–239.

Wagner EK, Roizman B, Savage T et al (1970) Characterization of the DNA of herpesviruses associated with Lucke's adenocarcinoma of the frog and Burkitt's lymphoma of man. *Virology* **42:** 257–261.

Wang WC, Herrod HG & Presbury GJ (1986) Lymphocyte subsets in children with aplastic anemia. *American Journal of the Medical Sciences* **291:** 304–309.

Watts DM, Burke DS & Harrison BH (1987) Effect of temperature on the vector efficiency of *Aedes aegypti* for dengue 2 virus. *American Journal of Tropical Medicine* **36:** 143–152.

Weiland HT, Salimans MM, Fibbe WE, Kluin PM & Cohen BJ (1989) Prolonged parvovirus B19 infection with severe anaemia in a bone marrow transplant recipient. *British Journal of Haematology* **79:** 300.

White DG, Woolf AD, Mortimer PP, Cohen BJ, Blake DR & Bacon PA (1985) Human parvovirus arthropathy. *Lancet* **i:** 419–421.

Wilkinson LS, Petz LD & Garraty G (1973) Reappraisal of the role of anti-i in haemolytic anemia in infectious mononucleosis. *British Journal of Haematology* **25:** 715–722.

Woernle CH, Anderson LJ, Tattersall P & Davison JM (1987) Human parvovirus B19 infection during pregnancy. *Journal of Infectious Diseases* **156:** 17–20.

Woolf AD, Campion GV, Chishick A et al (1989) Clinical manifestations of human parvovirus B19 in adults. *Archives of Internal Medicine* **149:** 1153–1156.

Work TH, Rodriquez FR & Bhatt PN (1959) Kyasanur forest disease: virological epidemiology of the 1958 epidemic. *American Journal of Public Health* **49:** 869–874.

World Health Organization (1985) Viral hemorrhagic fevers. Report of a WHO expert committee. *World Health Organization Technical Report Series* **721:** 5–126.

World Health Organization (1986) *Dengue Haemorrhagic Fever: Diagnosis, Treatment and Control*, pp 1–60. London: World Health Organization.

Yadav M, Umamaheswari S & Ablashi DV (1990) Low prevalence of antibody to human herpesvirus-6 (HHV-6) in Kadazans. *Southeast Asian Journal of Tropical Medicine and Public Health* **21:** 259–263.

Yao QY, Rowe M, Martin B, Young LS & Rickerson AB (1991) The Epstein–Barr virus carrier state: dominance of a single growth-transforming isolate in the blood and in the oropharynx of healthy virus carriers. *Journal of General Virology* **72:** 1579–1590.

Young N (1988) Haematologic and haematopoietic consequences of B19 parvovirus infection. *Seminars in Hematology* **25:** 159–172.

Young NS (1990) Flaviviruses and bone marrow failure. *Journal of the American Medical Association* **263:** 3065–3068.

Young N, Harrison M, Moore J, Mortimer P & Humphries RK (1984a) Direct demonstration of the human parvovirus in human erythroid progenitor cells infected in vitro. *Journal of Clinical Investigation* **74:** 2024–2030.

Young NS, Mortimer PP, Moore JG & Humphries RK (1984b) Characterization of a virus that causes transient aplastic crisis. *Journal of Clinical Investigation* **73:** 224–230.

Young NS, Issaragrassil S, Chieh CW & Takaku F (1986) Aplastic anaemia in the Orient. *British Journal of Haematology* **62:** 1–6.

Zeldis JB, Dienstag JL & Gale RP (1983) Aplastic anemia and non-A, non-B hepatitis. *American Journal of Medicine* **74:** 64–68.

Zhu XX, Zeng Y & Wolf H (1986) Detection of IgG and IgA antibodies to Epstein–Barr virus membrane antigen in sera from patients with nasopharyngeal carcinoma and from normal individuals. *International Journal of Cancer* **37:** 689–691.

Zoumbos NZ, Gascón P, Djeu JY, Trost SR & Young NS (1985a) Circulating activated suppressor T lymphocytes in aplastic anemia. *New England Journal of Medicine* **312:** 257–265.

Zoumbos N, Raefsky E & Young N (1985b) Lymphokines and haematopoiesis. *Progress in Haematology* **16:** 201–227.

Zulik R & Bako F (1971) Aplastic anaemia and infectious hepatitis. *Lancet* **i:** 44.

2

Human retroviruses

T. WEBER
G. HUNSMANN
W. STEVENS
A. F. FLEMING

Ellermann and Bang were the first to find a relation between viruses and leukaemia in 1908. Since then numerous retroviruses causing leukaemias as well as solid tumours in animals have been identified. The search for an association of human tumours and leukaemias with retroviruses was frustrating for decades. With the discovery of interleukin 2 (IL-2) (Poiesz et al, 1980a), long-term cultures of human T lymphocytes provided the means for the isolation of the first human retrovirus, human T-cell lymphotropic virus type-1 (HTLV-1) (Poiesz et al, 1980b). This virus was found to be associated with a newly defined type of human leukaemia/lymphoma, namely adult T-cell leukaemia/lymphoma (ATL) (Yoshida et al, 1982). A second human oncovirus, HTLV-2, was isolated from a patient with hairy cell leukaemia (Kalyanramen et al, 1982). In 1981 a cluster of patients with a novel disease of acquired cellular immunodeficiency, later known as the acquired immunodeficiency syndrome (AIDS), was first described in Los Angeles (Centers for Disease Control, 1981). In the following 2 years several groups isolated a retrovirus from patients with AIDS. This virus was called lymphadenopathy-associated virus (LAV), human T-cell/lymphoma virus type 3 (HTLV-3) or AIDS related virus (ARV) (Coffin, 1986). In 1986 these isolates were grouped under the name human immunodeficiency virus (HIV) (Coffin, 1986). Subsequently, Clavel and colleagues (1986) identified another virus, HIV-2, more closely related to the simian immunodeficiency virus (SIVmac) than to HIV-1, but also associated aetiologically with acquired immunodeficiency.

Virus classification and structure

Classification

By differences in their structure retroviruses are classified morphologically into four different types, A to D. The type C viruses HTLV-1 and HTLV-2 are classified with bovine leukaemia virus (BLV) in the BLV HTLV group. With regard to the modes of transmission, *exogenous* retroviruses are

Baillière's Clinical Haematology—
Vol. 5, No. 2, April 1992
ISBN 0–7020–1627–6

transmitted horizontally, whereas *endogenous* retroviruses are integrated into the DNA of all cells of an organism, including chromosomes, spermatocytes and oocytes, and thus are transmitted vertically. *Amphotropic* viruses replicate in cells of both the natural host and heterologous species. *Xenotropic* viruses replicate only in cells of a heterologous species. *Ecotropic* viruses replicate only in cells of the host and closely related species. A further classification of the family retroviridae takes their biological and pathogenic properties into account. Viruses associated with malignancies

Name	Abbreviation	Size	Function	Localization
Surface protein	ENV/SU	gp160/ gp120/gp41	External viral glycoproteins	Plasma membrane, virion envelope
Reverse transcriptase	POL/RT	p66/p51	Viral enzymes	Virion
Integration protein	POL/IN	p32	Viral enzyme	Virion
Precursor protein	GAG	p55	Structural capsid protein	Virion
Capsid protein	GAG/CA	p24	Structural capsid protein	Virion
Matrix protein	GAG/MA	p17	Structural capsid protein	Virion
Nucleocapsid protein	GAG/NC	p7	Structural capsid protein	Virion
Protease	POL/PR	p12	Viral enzyme	

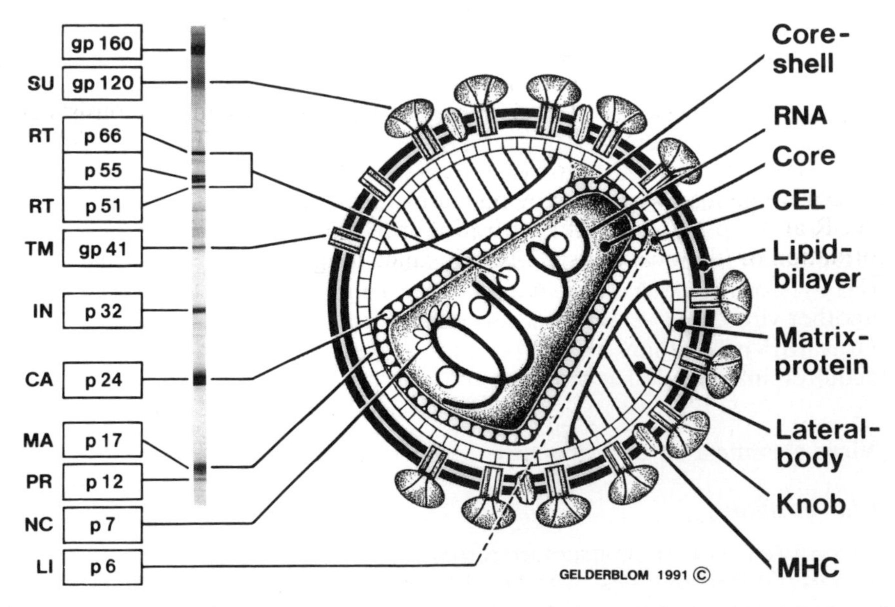

Figure 1. The general structure and distribution of proteins on radioimmunoprecipitation of HIV-1, as an example of the human retroviruses.

are called *oncovirinae*. Those associated with slowly progressive inflammatory and degenerative disorders are named *lentivirinae* and include HIV-1, HIV-2, Visna and Maedi. The third group of *spumavirinae* cause foamy degeneration of cells in culture, but have not yet been associated with disease.

General structure

Retroviruses are rounded particles with an average diameter of about 80 to 130 nm (Figure 1). The electron-dense core, or nucleosid, is composed of a ribonucleoprotein which is surrounded by a protein capsid. Between the capsid and the outer envelope lies the inner core protein. The envelope is a lipid bilayer into which the viral transmembrane glycoprotein, e.g. gp41 of HIV, is anchored. The core proteins of HIV-1 are designated p15 and p24 according to their molecular weight. The p17 molecule is located inside the lipid bilayer. Quantitatively p24 predominates in HIV-1. The major core protein of HIV-2, p26, is somewhat larger than p24 of HIV-1. The major glycoprotein of HIV-1 is gp120 while that of HIV-2 is gp130. The core proteins of HTLVs have similar molecular weights and are designated p15, p17 and p24. In contrast to the HIVs, the size of the cleaved glycoprotein precursor of HTLVs gp68 is much smaller. The outer membrane glycoprotein of HTLVs (gp46) has a molecular weight of 46 000 daltons while the transmembrane protein has a molecular weight of 21 000 daltons.

Genome

The 5′ to 3′ organization of the genome is common to all replication-competent retroviruses (Figure 2). The prototype genome codes for three genes in the 5′ to 3′ order (1) group specific antigen (*gag*), (2) RNA-dependent polymerase (*pol*) and (3) envelope (*env*). The genome consists of two identical ribonucleic acid (RNA) chains (see Figure 1). These are linked together near their 5′ ends by non-covalent bonds. At both ends these replicative genes are flanked by regulatory sequences (R and U5 at 5′, U3 and R at 3′) (Figure 2). After infection, reverse transcription leads to the formation of identical units U3-R-U5, called long terminal repeats (LTR). The *pol* gene codes for four enzyme activities (Varmus, 1988): a protease processes the precursor protein molecules; reverse transcriptase (RT) is an RNA-dependent DNA polymerase; RNAseH removes the template RNA during production of second-strand DNA; endonuclease catalyses the integration of the provirus. The HIVs encode additional proteins called virion infectivity factor (**vif**), transactivator (**tat**), a regulator protein of expression of virion proteins (**rev**) and a negative factor (**nef**) which inhibits the replication of the HIVs. The viral protein **vpu** is found only in HIV-1 while vpx is found only in HIV-2. The overall sequence homology of HTLV-1 and HTLV-2 is about 65%. HTLV-1/-2 have a *rex* and a *tax* gene which encode a p40 and a p27/p21 molecule, respectively. The p40 augments viral RNA expression, while the p27/p21 enhances the expression of viral structural genes. Despite these similarities, the HIVs are classified as

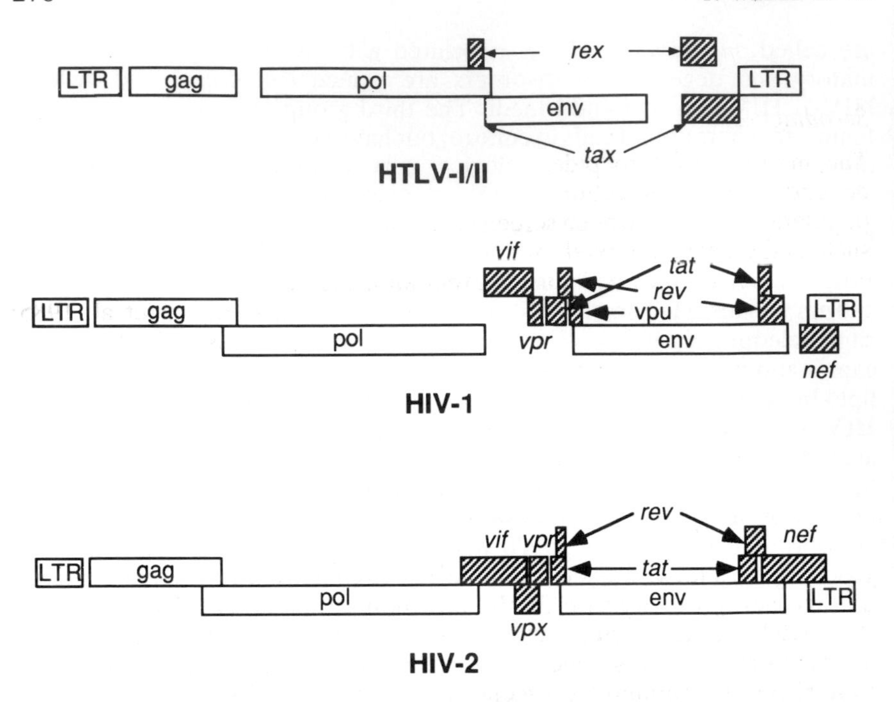

Figure 2. Genomic organization of oncovirinae (HTLV-1/-2) and lentivirinae (HIV-1/-2).

lentiviruses, which are not RNA tumour viruses, while the HTLVs are classified as RNA tumour viruses (Hjelle, 1991).

Replication

The known human retroviruses replicate in lymphocytes, monocyte-derived cells and various tumour cell lines. The virus adsorbs to the host cell membrane via a specific receptor and penetrates into the cytoplasm, where the viral particle is dissolved and the genome RNA is released. In the case of HIVs, the host cell surface receptor is the CD4 protein (Varmus, 1988); in the case of HTLVs the receptors are not yet known. The virus-specific reverse transcriptase transcribes the viral RNA into DNA. The DNA is transported to the cell nucleus and integrated as a provirus into the DNA of the host cell. During replication and integration the LTRs are formed; these contain all of the sequence necessary for its integration and the expression of viral genes. Proviruses are transmitted as chromosomal genes to daughter cells. The mRNA synthesized after proviral transcription activation is used as the viral genome and to produce new virions and non-structural proteins. New viral particles are assembled in the cytoplasm close to the plasma membrane and shed in a budding process (Varmus, 1988).

Seroepidemiology

Serodiagnosis

The majority of seroepidemiological surveys of HIV and HTLV have depended on the detection of virus-specific antibodies in members of the population. Sera have been screened initially by relatively inexpensive tests, such as the enzyme linked immunosorbent assay (ELISA). There may be crossreactivity with antibodies to other antigens, for example HLA class II antigens (Hellings et al, 1987) and malaria antigens (Biggar et al, 1985; Hunsmann et al, 1985a; Wendler et al, 1986) in the case of HIV-1, and possible other related retroviruses (Levine et al, 1988; Yanagihara et al, 1991a) in the case of HTLV-1. These crossreactions necessitate the application of confirmatory tests, such as western blot (WB), indirect immunofluorescence or radioimmunoprecipitation (RIPA), or the identification of proviral DNA by the polymerase chain reaction (PCR). For the HIVs, WB or RIPA are considered positive if there are at least two *env* bands, with or without *pol* and *gag* bands. Positivity for HTLV-1/HTLV-2 requires at least one *env* plus one *gag* band (Anonymous, 1991; Centers for Disease Control, 1991a). Seropositivity to HTLV-1 infection has been reported to become completely negative after 4 years of storage at −70 to −80°C (Aoki et al, 1985). Immunofluorescence assays usually give a higher rate of positives than ELISAs. Immunofluorescence assays detect predominantly HTLV-1-related cellular antigens, including those induced by malignant transformation, while HTLV-ELISAs detect only viral antigens (Aoki et al, 1985).

In the serodiagnosis for HTLV-1, some workers have applied more stringent criteria, especially in Africa. Some defined positivity as sera reactive with at least *gag*-encoded p19 or p24 plus either *env*-encoded antigens (gp46 or gp61/68) or p40 **tax** antigen, with there being at least three virus-encoded specific bands on WB or RIPA (Delaporte et al, 1989a; Verdier et al, 1989). Using even more stringent criteria, sera have been considered positive when they have shown at least four virus-specific bands, including p19, p24 and gp46, on WB (Goubau et al, 1990). Sera reacting with fewer specific bands are indeterminate, and results need to be confirmed by the examination of subsequent blood samples or the application of other assays, for example PCR or virus isolation. Currently ELISAs and WB do not discriminate between HTLV-1 and HTLV-2, but the use of synthetic peptides in ELISAs permits a 100 per cent specific differentiation between HTLV-1 and HTLV-2 (Khabbaz et al, 1992).

The sensitivity and specificity of currently employed HIV-1 ELISA tests are at least 99% (Schwartz et al, 1990). An inexpensive way to reduce the rate of false positives and the number of WBs required, is the application of two anti-HIV-1 screening tests in series (Spielberg et al, 1990; Nick et al, 1991): only sera giving discrepant or doubtful results need be submitted for WB. It is important that the two tests should be based on different principles of antibody detection, for example a competitive ELISA and particle agglutination, and use different sources of antigen (Fleming, 1988).

More information about the power of a diagnostic test can be obtained by calculating the positive predictive value (PPV), which is the likelihood that an individual is truly infected if the test is positive (the percentage of all positive tests which are true positives). If a test has a high specificity, for example 99.9%, the majority of positive results will be false while prevalence remains less than 0.1%. When prevalence rises to 1%, PPV is 91%, and when prevalence is 10%, PPV is 99% (Chin, 1990).

Population sampling

A major problem with seroepidemiology has been selection bias in the population groups studied. Sentinel surveillance is the repeated study of well-defined and accessible population groups. Sentinel groups with high risk behaviours, such as male homosexuals, intravenous drug users (IVDUs), female prostitutes and patients with sexually transmitted diseases (STDs), are of the greatest importance in monitoring the pandemic while prevalence remains low in the general population. Nominal testing, that is when results are linked to the patients, and the need to obtain informed consent before testing, introduce bias due to refusal by those who perceive their own risk but prefer to remain ignorant of their HIV-status. Participation bias is minimized by unlinked anonymous screening (Chin, 1990; Worm and Kvinesdal, 1990). Other sentinel groups have been chosen as being accessible but more representative of the general population. If all patients attending hospital are tested, there will be overestimation of HIV positivity due to the inclusion of patients with conditions associated with transmission (e.g. STD, pelvic inflammatory disease) or with HIV-disease (e.g. *Pneumocystis carinii* pneumonia, tuberculosis) (St Louis et al, 1990). Voluntary potential blood donors are a self-selected group of adults, and may include in one location an over-representation of HIV positives because persons at risk abuse the Blood Transfusion Service as a means to free testing, or under-representation in another location due to self-exclusion. Pregnant women attending antenatal clinics are obviously representative of the sexually active population, except that both involuntary infertility due to STD and deliberate infertility in sex workers are associated with high risk of HIV: unlinked anonymous testing of pregnant women or their newborn infants provides minimally biased data of seroprevalence (Chin, 1990; Peckham et al, 1990). Whole populations can be assessed economically by the methods of lot quality assurance sampling or cluster sampling (Rwandan HIV Seroprevalence Study Group, 1989; Chin, 1990).

HUMAN T-CELL LYMPHOTROPIC VIRUS TYPE 1

Epidemiology

HTLV-1 and HTLV-2 are transmitted by sexual intercourse, from mother to child through breast-feeding, by blood transfusion and by needle sharing of IVDUs. The efficiency of sexual transmission from male to female is higher than the rate of female to male transmission (Murphy et al, 1989). As with HIV-1 and HIV-2, the risk of male infection seems to be increased with concomitant penile ulcers or concurrent syphilis (Kajiyama et al, 1986; Murphy et al, 1989; Verdier et al, 1989). The infection rate of babies born to HTLV-1-positive mothers has been reported to be 16% during the first 18 months and 26% by the age of 4 years (Tajima et al, 1987). Poor housing and hygiene may facilitate vertical transmission (Weber, 1989).

HTLV-1 is associated aetiologically with adult T-cell leukaemia/lymphoma (ATL) (Takatsuki et al, 1985) and with a chronic neurological disorder which has similarities to multiple sclerosis (Gessain et al, 1985; Bhigjee et al, 1990): the condition is called tropical spastic paraparesis (TSP) or HTLV-1 associated myelopathy (HAM), and is usually designated as TSP/HAM. HTLV-1 infection has been reported to be associated with polymyositis in Jamaica (Morgan et al, 1989), and there is some evidence that HTLV-1 infection is associated with infective dermatitis of children in Jamaica (LaGrenade et al, 1990). A recent report (Hattori et al, 1991) suggests that HTLV-1 infection of a double-negative CD4−, CD8− subset of T cells may lead to malignant lymphoma of gastrointestinal/lymphoid tissue.

Higher frequencies of HTLV-1 antibodies have been demonstrated in patients with B-cell chronic lymphatic leukaemia than in the symptom-free population of both Nigeria and Jamaica (for review see Fleming, 1990a). The reason is obscure but, at most, HTLV-1 could be a cofactor in the aetiology of chronic lymphatic leukaemia in not more than 20% of patients.

Japan and far-east Asia

The most detailed information on the seroepidemiology of HTLV-1 is available from Japan, where ATL has been known to be endemic for some time (Table 1) (Uchiyama et al, 1977). The seroprevalence of antibodies to HTLV-1 is high in south-western regions, especially on Kyushu and Shikoku islands, while the prevalence is low on the northern island Hokkaido and in the northern parts of the island of Honshu (Hinuma et al, 1982). In the

Table 1. Epidemiology of HTLV-1 and HTLV-2.

	HTLV-1	HTLV-2
Endemic regions	South-western Japan, Taiwan	
	West and central Africa, Natal (South Africa), Seychelles	Gabon
	Caribbean, south-east USA (Blacks), central-south America (Guaymi and Yanomani Indians)	Central American (Guaymi Indians)
	Australia (Aborigines), Papua New Guinea, Solomon Islands	
	Israel, Iraq, Iran (Jews)	
Epidemic spread	IVDUs, USA, Argentina, Italy	IVDUs USA, Italy

For references, see text.

non-endemic areas, seroprevalence rates among migrants from areas of high mortality for malignant lymphoma, especially Shikoku and Kyushu, were significantly higher than those migrating from a low mortality area (Tajima et al, 1986). The Kagoshima district in Kyushu is highly endemic for HTLV-1. In healthy residents, including blood donors, the seroprevalence of HTLV-1-antibodies was 11.9%. The prevalence of HTLV-1-antibodies has been reported to be 98.3% in ATL patients, 28.9% in other lymphoproliferative disorders and 10.6% in myeloproliferative disorders (Hanada et al, 1989). In this study the prevalence of HTLV-1-antibodies in non-haematological disorders was found to be 29.5% in pulmonary tuberculosis, 28.5% in leprosy, 33.8% in chronic renal failure, 21.9% in autoimmune diseases, and 47.8% in strongyloidiasis. These findings can be explained only partially by transmission via blood transfusion. In haemodialysis patients for instance, the prevalence of HTLV-1 antibodies was significantly higher than in healthy controls, irrespective of the number of blood transfusions received (Hanada et al, 1989). A study from Tsushima island, northwest of Kyushu, has revealed interesting epidemiological data (Tajima et al, 1987): villages with a low prevalence of HTLV-1 neighbour those with a high prevalence, reflecting the very restricted contact between the inhabitants. Findings from the isolated Sado island, in a non-endemic area off the western coast of Honshu island, have shown similar results. Interestingly, the clinical features of ATL on this island differ from those in other endemic areas and are characterized by a much longer incubation period of about 43.1 months, resembling the smouldering variant of ATL. The clinical features are unusual and characterized by various skin lesions like erythema and exfoliative dermatitis (Aoki et al, 1985).

In south-western Japan, the estimated annual incidence rates of ATL per million adults ranges from 0.6 to 26.4 in females and 3.5 to 40.4 in males (Kondo et al, 1989; Tajima, 1990). Among all registered ATL cases in Japan, 51% have been reported from Kyushu and 29% from metropolitan areas (Tajima, 1990). Interestingly most, but not all, patients with ATL in the metropolitan areas had moved from the ATL-endemic areas during adulthood. The overall risk of ATL was 1.5 times as high in males as in females in Kyushu. The age-specific incidence rate increased steeply until the age of 70, and then decreased markedly in both sexes. Of patients with ATL, 26.5% had a family history of cancer, and the incidence of cancer was markedly higher than in the general population (Ono et al, 1989): specifically, of these 12.2% had lymphoma, 9.9% had haematopoietic malignancies and 8.2% had ATL (Tajima, 1990).

Seroprevalence data from eastern Asia, outside Japan, are sparse. Twenty-five Chinese patients, lifetime residents of Taiwan and without Japanese ancestry, have been described with HTLV-1 associated ATL (Shih et al, 1991). The only person found to be HTLV-1 positive from 1059 subjects from Shanghai, China, was a patient with lung cancer who had received multiple blood transfusions (Pan et al, 1991). A study in Singapore found evidence for HTLV-1 infection in three of 63 male (4.8%) and four of 652 female prostitutes (0.6%) (Sng et al, 1991). Two anti-HTLV-1-positive patients have been described in southern India; one a 52-year-old male with

ATL, the other a 12-year-old boy with biphenotypic acute leukaemia (Chandy et al, 1991).

Africa

The interpretation of serological results are more difficult with sera from Africa than from any other continent, due to a large number of indeterminate results: reports have varied from excessively high prevalence where no or low-specificity confirmatory tests have been applied (Saxinger et al, 1984; Biggar et al, 1985; de-Thé et al, 1985; Williams, 1986), to low or no prevalence where the most stringent confirmatory tests have been used (Weiss et al, 1986). Discussion of seroepidemiology in Africa is confined to those surveys which applied appropriate RIPA or WB, with sera identifying at least one *env* and one *gag* product as the least stringent criterion (Anonymous, 1991).

The highest prevalence of anti-HTLV-1 in the general population is reported from Gabon, especially in the Ogooue river valley (Hunsmann et al, 1984; Delaporte et al, 1989a, 1989b, 1991a) (Figure 3). To the east of this focus, a cluster of HTLV-1-associated TSP/HAM has been described at Lisala, a small town on the Zaire (Congo) river in the Equateur Region of Zaire (Figure 3) (Kazadi et al, 1990): in Lisala 28 (14%) of 200 outpatients with acute illnesses and hospital workers, predominantly Mondungas, were HTLV antibody positive (Goubau et al, 1990). The prevalence of HTLV antibodies declines going northwards from the equatorial forests towards the savanna and sahel regions (Figure 3) (Delaporte et al, 1989a; Louis et al, 1990).

In neighbouring Nigeria to the west, anti-HTLV-1 has been found in populations living in all vegetation zones (mangrove, forest, savanna and sahel), but seropositivity in blood donors was reported to be higher (3.6%) in the north of the country (in guinea and wooded savanna) than in the southern rain forests and mangrove swamps (1.8% around Lagos, 0.7% around Calabar) (Fleming et al, 1983, 1986; Okpara et al, 1986, 1988). A similar increase of seroprevalence from the coast (0.3%) to the northern savanna (5.4%) has been reported in the neighbouring country Benin (Dumas et al, 1991). Intermediate prevalence of seropositivity has been reported from populations in the rest of west Africa: for example, 1.8% in Côte d'Ivoire (Verdier et al, 1989), 1.6% in Liberia and 1.2% in Senegal (Hunsmann et al, 1984). In all populations in west and west central Africa, seroprevalence rises with age up to about 50 years. High risk groups have included female prostitutes, for example 7.4% in Côte d'Ivoire, and patients with leprosy (13.7% in Côte d'Ivoire) (Verdier et al, 1989, 1990). The association with leprosy is unexplained, but could reflect sexual transmission within socially isolated communities.

Data from east Africa are scanty, but Hunsmann et al (1983, 1984) found four (1.7%) of 231 Kenyan students in Germany to be seropositive. Earlier reports of high rates of seropositivity in Ethiopia, especially amongst the Falashas, have not been confirmed by specific testing (Karpas et al, 1986; Weiss et al, 1986; Abebe et al, 1991). It is reported recently that HTLV-1 is

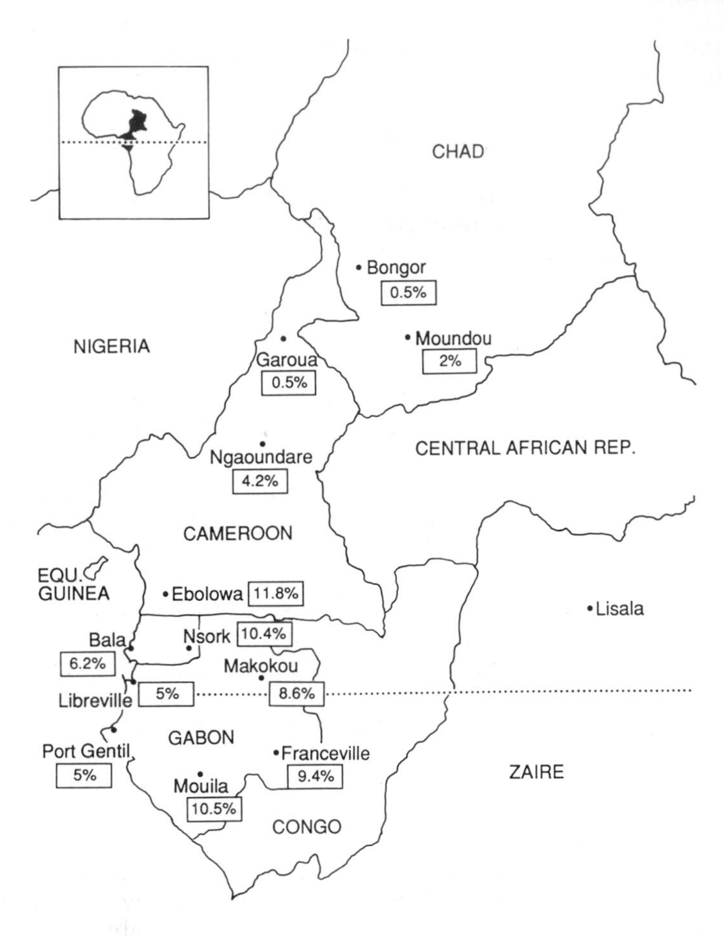

Figure 3. Crude prevalence rates of anti-HTLV-1 antibodies in western central Africa. From Delaporte et al (1989a), with permission of the authors and publishers. Included is the location of Lisala, where Goubau et al (1990) report HTLV seroprevalence of 14% and a high incidence of TSP/HAM.

highly endemic in the Seychelles, at a level comparable to that of Okinawa, Japan (Lavanchy et al, 1991): overall frequency in adults was 6.2%, but was higher in females (7.9%) than males (4.2%), Blacks (7.1%) than Whites (3.7%), and in unskilled (7.7%) than skilled (4.8%). Seroprevalence rose with age to reach 12.7% in women aged 55–64 years. In contrast, HTLV-1 is not endemic on the other Indian Ocean islands of Réunion, Mayotte and Madagascar (Cnudde et al, 1991). The explanation for the striking difference in seroprevalence between the Seychelles and the other Indian Ocean islands lies most likely in the varieties of populations which migrated to these islands, mostly in the nineteenth century.

An early report of one out of 20 black adults from Natal, South Africa, being anti-HTLV-1 positive (Hunsmann et al, 1984) is in agreement with the report of a cluster of HTLV-1 associated myelopathies amongst Zulus (Bhigjee et al, 1990): seroepidemiological surveys are required.

The causative association between TSP/HAM and HTLV-1 in sub-Saharan Africa and the Seychelles is now clear (Verdier et al, 1989; Bhigjee et al, 1990; Kazadi et al, 1990; Lavanchy et al, 1991). However, reports of HTLV-1-positive ATL in Africans remain scanty, probably because laboratory facilities and pathologists are scarce (Fleming et al, 1983, 1986; Hahn et al, 1984; Stewart et al, 1984; Williams et al, 1984; Pagliuca et al, 1988; Delaporte et al, 1989a).

The Americas

The seropositivity rate in Jamaica ranges from 3 to 6% among adults (Murphy et al, 1989). The overall HTLV-1 seroprevalence has been reported to be 5.7% in a group of 1977 patients attending STD clinics in Jamaica. The prevalence increased with age from 5.3% at 14 to 19 years to 14.1% at 30 years and older in women, and from 1.6% at 14 to 19 years to 5.1% at 30 years and older in men (Murphy et al, 1989). Independent risk factors for HTLV-1 in men were penile sores or ulcers and a current diagnosis of syphilis, and in women a history of more than ten lifetime sexual partners. The efficiency of transmission from women to men is lower but may be increased by concurrent penile ulcers or syphilis in men (Murphy et al, 1989). Immigrants from the Caribbean to the UK (Newton et al, 1987) and the USA (Levine et al, 1988; Harrington et al, 1991) are affected as well.

In Panama, 8% of Guaymi Indians were found seropositive for HTLV (Reeves et al, 1990). In an isolated rural area, evidence for household clustering of infection was found, but in contrast no clustering was found among the Indians who lived in the capital of the province. Seropositivity was limited to persons 15 years of age or older. A study in neighbouring Costa Rica found a seroprevalence of less than 1% (Khabbaz et al, 1990). Recently, HTLV-1-positive sera were also found in Venezuelan Amazonian Yanomami Indians (Hunsmann et al, 1990). The virus is also present in some parts of Brazil (Cortes et al, 1989; Costa et al, 1989; Peixinho et al, 1990; Pombo de Oliveira et al, 1990; Takayanagui et al, 1991). All patients in one study were of low socioeconomic class. Patients were of African descent, white or of mixed-race parents, but none was of south American Indian or Japanese inheritance (Pombo de Oliveira et al, 1990). A small seroepidemiological study from Argentina found a prevalence of antibodies to HTLV-1 of 11.6% in 43 HIV-infected IVDUs and 5% in 20 HIV-infected male homosexuals (Bouzas et al, 1990).

A screening programme of blood donors in the USA using ELISA and WB for seroepidemiology found an HTLV-1/-2 seropositivity rate of 0.014 to 0.018% (Centers for Disease Control, 1990); a selected group of 136 HTLV-1/-2 seropositive donors was examined by the PCR technique: about 40% were positive for either HTLV-1 or HTLV-2, while in 15% no viral DNA could be amplified. Prevalence is highest amongst the Black population of the south-eastern states. The viruses are being transmitted to other sections of the population through blood transfusion and IDVU (Hjelle et al, 1990a, 1990b; Lee et al, 1991). A low seroprevalence (0.5%) has been confirmed amongst Eskimos in Alaska (Davidson et al, 1990).

Western Asia

During a systematic survey among Iranian Jews in Israel, a clustering of HTLV-1 infection was found within a cohort of 32 elderly women (Meytes et al, 1990). Though the reasons for this clustering are unclear, a likely explanation may be the high degree of consanguinity among Mashadi Jews. ATL has been reported in four Jews immigrating to Israel from Iran (Sidi et al, 1990). Recent evidence indicates infection of Iranians from Teheran as well, possibly by blood transfusion (B. Kitze et al, unpublished observations).

A family with HTLV-1 infection has also been described in Iraq (Denic et al, 1990): 40 unrelated Iraqi patients with lymphoid malignancies and neurological disorders were HTLV-1 negative.

Australasia and Oceania

In central Australia, an endemic area for HTLV-1 has been found in Aborigines (May et al, 1990). Retrospective analysis of sera from 1977 revealed a seroprevalence of about 16% and this had increased to 34% in 1984/85. No children under the age of 4 years were infected. Others could not confirm these findings and reported a seroprevalence of about 8% in Aborigines (Moody et al, 1990). HTLV-1 is also endemic in Papua New Guinea, as demonstrated by virus isolation from a member of a remote tribe (Yanagihara et al, 1991b): in a small cohort of 37 individuals 14 were HTLV-positive. HTLV-1 infection has also been reported in a single patient from the Solomon Islands (Yanagihara et al, 1991b). Overall the sero prevalence on the Solomon Islands was found to be 2.2% with no over-representation of gender or any specific disease among these patients (Yanagihara et al, 1991a).

Europe

The seroprevalence of antibodies to HTLV-1 in Europe is remarkably low. In Switzerland a seroprevalence of HTLV-1 antibodies has been reported to be 0.69% among 867 HIV-infected individuals (Schüpbach et al, 1988). A similar low percentage of 0.86% HTLV-1 positives has been reported from a cohort of 346 IVDUs from Amsterdam (van den Hoek et al, 1991). Sero-positive cases reported from Belgium, France, England and Spain occurred almost exclusively in immigrants from Africa and the Caribbean (Mowbray et al, 1989; Gessain et al, 1990; Vranckx et al, 1990; Soriano et al, 1991), while in Germany no definite case of HTLV-1 infection could be found in a large survey (Hunsmann et al, 1985b). In contrast, the seroprevalence of HTLV-1 antibodies has been reported to be as high as 4.4% in Italian IVDUs (Gianguglielmo et al, 1991).

From Georgia of the former Soviet Union the first ATL case has been reported in a Caucasian, whose wife and son were also seropositive for HTLV-1, adding support to the notion that HTLV-1 (and HTLV-2) infection may be more widespread than hitherto suspected (Senjuta et al, 1991).

Pathogenesis

HTLV-1 and HTLV-2 can transform lymphocytes in culture, inducing their perpetual growth (Poiesz et al, 1980b; Hjelle, 1991; Yanagihara et al, 1991b). These viruses induce a latent infection of a small subset of cells. Lymphocytes cultured from the peripheral blood of patients with TSP/HAM and of asymptomatic carriers proliferate spontaneously and are predominantly of the CD4 subtype, as are persistently infected T-cell lines. Neither HTLV-1 nor HTLV-2 possess cellular oncogenes, but the regulatory *tax* gene may have oncogenic potentials by inducing high levels of expression of IL-2 and of the α-chain of the IL-2 receptor. As *tax* messenger RNA is not expressed in ATL cell lines, there is no direct evidence of an autocrine stimulation of lymphocyte proliferation leading to malignancy. Transgenic mice carrying the *tax* gene have developed neurofibromatosis, which is further evidence of the oncogenic potential of the *tax* gene (reviewed by Hjelle, 1991). The *tax* gene product has also been shown to down-regulate the expression of a DNA repair enzyme, thus leading to indirect damage of DNA and potentially to chromosomal abnormalities. HTLV-1 induces monoclonal tumours with variable insertion sites. The incubation period from infection or seroconversion to disease has been estimated to be at least 15 years (Newton et al, 1987). Development of ATL in some patients and HAM/TSP in others may be due to malignant transformation of HTLV-1 infected lymphocytes in the former disease and chronic activation in the latter. Sequence comparisons of HTLV-1 isolates from cerebrospinal fluid lymphocytes in TSP/HAM patients to isolates from ATL patients have shown no significant differences (Yoshida et al, 1987).

Adult T-cell leukaemia/lymphoma

Five clinical phases of ATL which are not necessarily temporally related have been suggested (Uchiyama et al, 1977; Takatsuki et al, 1985; Pombo de Oliveira et al, 1990). Asymptomatic carriers are diagnosed either by the demonstration of HTLV-1 antibodies, and/or the detection of proviral DNA in their lymphocytes. Carriers may go on to develop either pre-ATL, smoldering ATL, chronic ATL or acute ATL. The lifetime risk of developing ATL after HTLV-1 infection has been estimated to be about 3% for females and 6.9% for males (Kondo et al, 1989): the reason for a male preponderance of ATL remains unknown. The preleukaemic state or pre-ATL may be diagnosed following the incidental observation of leukocytosis and/or abnormal lymphocytes. In about half of these patients lymphocytosis regresses spontaneously, but it persists in the remaining patients. Some of these go on to develop acute ATL (Table 2). Roughly one-third of HTLV-1 infected patients with clinical manifestations have smoldering or chronic

Table 2. Clinical and laboratory presentations of adult T-cell leukaemia/lymphoma.

Non-Hodgkin's lymphoma
Lymphadenopathy
Skin lesions
Hepatosplenomegaly
Lytic bone lesions
Hypercalcaemia
Pleomorphic cells with convoluted nuclei ('flower' cells, 'cerebriform' cells)
High white blood cell count (30–130 × 10^9/l)
Leukaemic cells are CD4+, IL-2R+, CD8−, terminal deoxynucleotide transferase negative
Survival after diagnosis 6–12 months

From Uchiyama et al (1977), Takatsuki et al (1985) and Tajima (1990).

ATL. Patients with chronic ATL have increased levels of circulating leukocytes. Leukaemias or lymphomas usually involve CD4+ T cells, with the surface phenotype of CD3+, CD8−, CD11+, and interleukin 2 receptor (IL-2R) positive (Uchiyama et al, 1985). Antibodies to HTLV-1 and proviral DNA sequences of HTLV-1 cannot be detected in all cases of ATL (Pombo de Oliveira et al, 1990).

HTLV-1-associated myelopathy

For many years spastic paraparesis without spinal cord compression has been known to occur frequently in tropical and subtropical regions (Roman et al, 1985; Molgaard et al, 1989; Bhigjee et al, 1990; Takayanagui et al, 1991; reviewed in Montgomery, 1989). The association between HTLV-1 infection and TSP in Martinique observed by Gessain et al (1985) was a major discovery of neurology and tropical medicine. Onset is usually between 20 and 50 years of age; women are affected twice as commonly as men. Prevalence of TSP/HAM is high wherever HTLV-1 is endemic; for example it is the most common neurological disorder in Jamaica after stroke. The presenting features are characterized by lumbar back pain as an early complaint, gradual or subacute onset of progressive spasticity and weakness of the legs, frequent sphincter dysfunction, impotence in men and usually mild or insignificant sensory disturbances (Table 3). The tendon

Table 3. Clinical signs of tropical spastic paraparesis/ HTLV-1 associated myelopathy (TSP/HAM).

Pyramidal signs
Progressive spastic paraparesis
Sphincter dysfunction
Mild loss of nerve sensitivity
Slowly progressive course
Occasional atypical lymphocytes in peripheral blood

From Gessain et al (1985), Roman et al (1985), Bhigjee et al (1990) and Goubau et al (1990).

reflexes of the upper extremities may be brisk in up to half of the patients. Cranial nerves, coordination and intellectual functioning remain intact. Within 10 years one-half or more of patients are confined totally to a wheelchair (for review see Montgomery, 1989). Clinically it may be impossible to differentiate TSP/HAM from multiple sclerosis (Newton et al, 1987). There is no effective treatment.

HUMAN T-CELL LYMPHOTROPIC VIRUS TYPE 2

HTLV-2 was isolated in 1982 from a patient with a T-cell variant of hairy cell leukaemia (Kalyanramen et al, 1982). Further isolates have been obtained since then from patients with aplastic anaemia and prolymphocytic leukaemia (reviewed by Hjelle, 1991). The recent report that HTLV-2 may be associated with the chronic fatigue immune dysfunction syndrome (DeFreitas et al, 1991) needs to be confirmed.

Diagnosis and seroepidemiological studies of HTLV-2 infection by ELISA, WB or RIPA have been hampered by the high degree of cross-reactivity between HTLV-1 and HTLV-2, but recently the PCR and synthetic peptide-based ELISA tests permit distinction (Khabbaz et al, 1992).

HTLV-2 has been shown to be present at low levels of endemicity amongst American Indians, including blood donors in New Mexico (HTLV seropositivity 0.72 per 1000, of which nine out of ten were HTLV-2) (Hjelle et al, 1990a) and Guaymis in Panama (Lairmore et al, 1990). HTLV-2 has been demonstrated by PCR in two subjects in Gabon, unexposed to blood transfusion or other risk factors, and prevalence has been estimated to be 0.3% (95% confidence limit 0.1–0.9%) in Libreville (Delaporte et al, 1991a, 1991b).

HTLV-2 is spreading epidemically: an unexpected number of HTLV infections in north American IVDUs have been shown to be due to HTLV-2 (Lee et al, 1989; Biggar et al, 1991). Amongst 3217 IVDUs in eight cities in the USA during 1988 and 1989, HTLV seropositivity ranged from 0.4 to 18%, with the highest rates being in Los Angeles, New Orleans and Seattle (Khabbaz et al, 1992): 69% were classified as having HTLV-2 infection; seroprevalence was highest amongst heroin users, Blacks and other racial minorities and those aged over 40 years. HTLV-2 infection has also been reported in Italian IVDUs (Zella et al, 1990).

HUMAN IMMUNODEFICIENCY VIRUSES

Transmission

HIV-1 and HIV-2 are transmitted by three routes: (1) intimate sexual contact, (2) vertically from mother to fetus or infant, and (3) by the exchange of blood.

Sexual transmission

In the global perspective, heterosexual contact is the predominant mode of transmission and carries with it the heavy impact on the family, society, demography and the economy. However, heterosexual intercourse is a less efficient mechanism of transmission than is penetrative male homosexual intercourse (Cameron et al, 1989; Holmes et al, 1990). There is an apparent twofold difference between the probabilities of male to female than female to male transmission in sub-Saharan Africa; this explains in part the bias in the sex ratio of HIV-1 infection, where the overall adult male to female ratio is 1:1.4 (Anderson et al, 1991). Other reasons for the greater number of African women than men being infected are sociological and related to the lower perceived social value of women, their poorer education, their economic inability to protect themselves from high-risk exposure and their commencement of sexual activity at an earlier age (Anstee, 1989). Seroprevalence peaks in females as early as 15–19 years or 20–24 years, so that the highest incidence of AIDS and mortality coincides with what is normally the most active period of reproductive and productive life. In males, peaks of prevalence and incidence are 5 to 10 years later than in females (Fleming, 1990b; Anderson et al, 1991).

In a study of supposedly stable partnerships in the USA, in which the index had a well established source of risk, 61 (20%) of 307 female partners of HIV-infected males and only one (1%) of 72 male partners of infected females were found to be infected (Padian et al, 1991): this much greater odds of male to female transmission than vice versa is not explained and needs confirmation.

The risk of infection increases with the number of sexual contacts and the numbers of sexual contacts of the partner(s). Transmission is facilitated by other STDs, especially genital ulcers but also by non-ulcerative STDs, including chlamydial infections, gonorrhoea and trichomoniasis (Cameron et al, 1989; Laga et al, 1991). Uncircumcised men appear to be more easily infected than circumcised men. The heterosexual epidemic is being driven largely through (1) a core group of high transmitters, who include long-distance lorry drivers, the military and female prostitutes (Plummer et al, 1991), (2) a high rate of change of sexual partners early in the sexually active age range, (3) the preference of men for female partners 5–10 years younger than themselves and often still in adolescence, and (4) the greater efficiency of transmission from male to female than vice versa (Anderson et al, 1990, 1991).

Insufficient attention has been given to the role of both irregular and regular military forces in the spread of HIV during civil wars, for example in Uganda and Mozambique (reviewed by Fleming, 1990b). In Uganda, the highest incidences of AIDS, outside the capital Kampala, are reported in Rakai and Masaka Districts (in the south) and Gulu District (in the north): this geographical distribution is positively correlated to the ethnic patterns of recruitment of the Ugandan National Liberation Army (UNLA) and the areas of conflict in the civil war in the late 1970s and early 1980s (Smallman-Raynor and Cliff, 1991). It can be foreseen that all present and future political destabilizations will leave a legacy of rural or urban epidemics of HIV and AIDS.

Vertical transmission

There are three times during which transmission of HIV from mother to infant can occur; (1) during pregnancy, (2) at delivery, and (3) after delivery; these span a period of time greater than that defined strictly as perinatal (reviewed by Ryder and Temmerman, 1991).

Transplacental infection makes by far the largest contribution to vertical transmission. HIV infection of fetuses in the first trimester has been demonstrated by several workers, but transmission appears to be most frequent during the third trimester (Ehrnst et al, 1991). HIV-1 seropositive women are more infectious for their infants during the second peak of viraemia associated with clinical disease and advanced immunosuppression, as shown by CD4 $<400 \times 10^6$/l and p24 antigenaemia (Ryder et al, 1989; reviewed in Ryder and Temmerman, 1991). A certain number of infants become infected during passage through the birth canal: first-born twins experience more trauma during delivery and are more often HIV infected than second-born twins (Goedert et al, 1991). Transmission during delivery may be facilitated by the presence of chorioamnionitis (Ryder and Temmerman, 1991).

Apparently infected mothers do not often transmit HIV to their infants post partum, unless they experience the first peak of viraemia, which coincides with seroconversion, while breast-feeding. This can happen when women suffer severe peripartum haemorrhage and subsequently receive a transfusion of HIV contaminated blood, or they become infected later, presumably sexually (Ryder and Temmerman, 1991; Van de Perre et al, 1991). So, paradoxically, infants may be at greater risk of acquiring HIV from mothers who are HIV negative than from mothers who are HIV positive at delivery. Breast-feeding, however, is not a major route of transmission of HIV-1; breast-feeding does decrease morbidity in all children (Ryder et al, 1991) and delays progression to AIDS in HIV-infected children (Tozzi et al, 1990).

Reported rates of transmission from HIV-1 infected mothers to their infants have varied considerably: the European Collaborative Study (1991) reported 13% in 600 infants born to mothers who were mostly symptom free; many African women have more advanced disease, and rates of transmission have been reported generally to be 30 to 40% (reviewed in Ryder and Temmerman, 1991). Vertical transmission of HIV-2 has been documented but the risk appears to be much less than with HIV-1 (Matheron et al, 1990; Morgan et al, 1990).

Transmission to infants cannot be discussed without mention of the related adverse effects on the course and outcome of pregnancy of maternal HIV infection. In Africa, but not in Europe, maternal seropositivity is associated with a history of previous infant death (odds ratio (OR) 2.9), spontaneous abortion (OR 2.5), low birthweight for gestational age (OR 2.3), premature delivery (<38 weeks) (OR 2.1), neonatal death and infant death (Lallement et al, 1989; Ryder et al, 1989; Braddick et al, 1990; Miotti et al, 1990; Temmerman et al, 1990; Lepage et al, 1991; reviewed in Ryder and Temmerman, 1991): of 475 infants born to Zairean women who were HIV-1 seropositive at time of delivery, only 314 (66%) were alive and without AIDS at the end of the first year, compared to 90% of infants born to HIV-1 seronegative women (Ryder et al, 1989).

Transmission by blood

The mean titres of tissue culture infective doses (TCID) in plasma were 30, 3200 and 3500 per ml in people with asymptomatic HIV-1 infection, AIDS related complex (ARC) and AIDS respectively: in peripheral blood mononuclear cells mean titres were respectively 20, 2700 and 2200 TCID per 10^6 cells (Ho et al, 1989). In needlestick simulations, a mean volume of 0.034 μl (range 0.004–0.26 μl) of blood was transmitted by hollow-bore needles (Hoffman et al, 1989). The rate of transmission following accidental needlesticks with HIV infected blood is low, less than 0.5% (Berkley, 1991), the risk being greater, presumably, with blood from symptomatic patients and with larger volumes of blood being injected. In intravenous exposures to simulate IVDU needle-sharing practices, volumes of blood on average 1000 times larger were transmitted (mean 34 μl; range 18–67 μl) (Hoffman et al, 1989), making this the efficient mechanism for infection with HIV which it obviously is. The transfusion of infected blood or blood products carries effectively 100% rate of transmission.

Transfusion of blood and blood products. The transmission of HIV-1 by blood products, for instance factor VIII concentrates, and by blood transfusion was a major problem in the early 1980s in all parts of the world. According to a model calculation the incidence of transfusion-associated HIV-1 infection was about 1.1% per transfused unit of blood in San Francisco in 1982 (Busch et al, 1991a). However, since 1985, transmission by this route has been effectively controlled in developing countries through discouraging the recruitment of paid blood donors, encouraging self-exclusion of potential volunteer donors with high risk behaviour, screening of all units for antibodies against HIV and the inactivation of virus in blood products (Contreras and Barbara, 1990; Madhok and Forbes, 1990). By 1987, the probability of contracting HIV was reduced to 1/153 000 per unit transfused in the USA (Cummings et al, 1989). Even in a high risk metropolitan area, the chances of screened blood donor being HIV-1 infectious has been estimated to be not more than 1 in 61 171, using cocultivation and PCR to identify HIV-DNA (Busch et al, 1991b). However, the tragic consequences of transmission, especially to haemophiliacs, before 1985 remains in the western world.

In contrast, blood transfusion in developing countries, especially in sub-Saharan Africa, still carries a high and even an increasing risk for the recipients of acquiring HIV, besides other blood-borne infections, including hepatitis B and C, malaria and syphilis (Fleming 1990b; Jäger et al, 1991). This is because of: (1) the high frequencies of severe anaemia and exsanguination following haemorrhage from any cause with delays before hospitalization, leading to demands for blood transfusion between three and ten times that per hospital bed in the UK; (2) the high prevalence of HIV infection in potential blood donors (e.g. 20%); (3) the absence of recognizable subgroups of the population (e.g. male homosexuals or IVDUs) who can be excluded from the donor panel; and (4) the absence of screening for anti-HIV in many hospital laboratories. Even when there is effective testing for HIV antibodies, only four out of five infected donors will be detected, the other donors being in the window period, while the epidemic is in the exponential phase of expansion and the doubling time of seropositivity is 9 months.

Subjects commonly at risk of acquiring HIV infection through blood transfusion are: (1) preschool children with malaria and anaemia (Mingiele, 1990); (2) patients with sickle-cell disease in Africa or thalassaemia major in Asia; (3) women with anaemia in pregnancy and/or obstetric haemorrhage; and (4) victims of trauma (Fleming, 1990b).

Intravenous drug users. About one-fourth of all AIDS cases reported in the USA in 1990 had a history of intravenous drug use (Centers for Disease Control, 1991b). The number of cases of AIDS among heterosexual IVDUs in the European Region of WHO increased from 45 in 1984 to 3823 in 1989, a more rapid rise than in any other transmission group (European Centre for Epidemiological Monitoring of AIDS, 1990). Over 80% of cases were in France, Italy and Spain; IVDU is the major route of transmission in southern Europe. This is mirrored on the southern Mediterranean littoral, where in the Eastern Mediterranean Region of WHO seropositivity in IVDUs jumped four-fold from 3.3 to 13.6% in 1988/89 (Wahden, 1989). There have been recent explosive increases of HIV-1 seropositivity in IVDUs to over 50% in a matter of months in Bangkok and Chang Mai, Thailand (Poshyachinda, 1990) and Manipur, India (Naik et al, 1991). There is a zone from the Iberian peninsula to the south-east Asian peninsula where IVDUs have high prevalence of infection with HIV-1, and are likely to infect the general population.

Transmission in the health care setting

Blood-borne transmission of HIV may occur from (1) health care worker to patient, (2) patient to patient, and (3) patient to health care worker (World Health Organization, 1991). Fortunately, transmission by any of these three routes is rare, and from health care worker to patient is rarest of all, there being only one documented instance, from a dentist to patients (Centers for Disease Control, 1991c).

Patient to patient. Medical injections are extremely popular in sub-Saharan Africa due to a strong belief in their especial efficacy. At least 65% of the general population in many countries receive one or more injections in 2–5 years. Reusable syringes and needles are standard equipment and even disposables are reused: sterilization between use is often inadequate, as shown by high frequencies of gluteal abscesses (Berkley, 1991). Although the contribution to the total epidemic is probably small, receiving medical injections (but not immunizations) has been shown to be a risk factor for HIV-1 infection in Zaire (Mann et al, 1986), Congo (Nicholas-Randeggar et al, 1989) and Uganda (Konde-Lule et al, 1989), and for HIV-2 in the Gambia (Wilkins et al, 1989). In other communities, for example Rwanda, an association between medical injections and HIV positivity cannot be demonstrated, possibly because of a local availability of disposables or an ability to sterilize efficiently (Lepage et al, 1986; Lepage and Van de Perre, 1988). Scarification, circumcision and other invasive procedures carried out by traditional healers are in theory able to transmit HIV, but there are few data (reviewed by Berkley, 1991): unqualified practitioners with syringes and needles must represent a far greater hazard.

There have been large nosocomial outbreaks of HIV-1 infection in Romania and in the former Soviet Union, due to failures in sterilization (Pokrovsky and Eramova, 1989; Berkley, 1991; Hannam, 1991). In Romania over 1100 children and in the former Soviet Union at least 260 children have been infected by injections of small amounts of blood with unsterilized needles and syringes because of shortness of equipment (Gromyko, 1991; Hersh et al, 1991).

Patient to health care worker. The risk of infection with HIV for health care workers at the place of work is small; it has been estimated that before immunization became generally available, 12 000 health care workers in the USA were infected each year with hepatitis B virus (HBV), and that 250 die each year of direct or indirect consequences of nosocomial HBV; in comparison there was a total of 24 occupational HIV infections reported up to February 1991, and the worst published estimate is 64 health care workers contacting HIV at work each year (Centers for Disease Control, 1989; Jagger and Pearson, 1991). The most common route of infection is through deep needlestick (see above); injuries with solid suture needles or contamination of the intact skin and mucous membranes carry risks which are immeasurably small (Henderson et al, 1990; Heald, 1991; reviewed by Fleming, 1991a).

Epidemiological patterns

Pattern 1

Epidemiological pattern 1 involves north America, Europe, Australasia and other 'western' communities. It is characterized by male homosexual contact being the predominant mode of transmission, with IVDU making an important contribution. Transmission by blood transfusion is now effectively controlled (Schimpf et al, 1989). The numbers of new infections have levelled off or even declined (Artzrouni, 1990; Holmes et al, 1990). However, the tragic homosexual epidemic is likely to be seen as the prelude to a more slowly progressive but eventually more widespread heterosexual epidemic. There is a steady increase of heterosexual men and women infected in the USA: in fact, women are the fastest growing group of persons infected with HIV (Centers for Disease Control, 1991d; Ellerbrock et al, 1991; Rosser, 1991; Shayne and Kaplan, 1991). There has been also a dramatic increase in the proportion of patients with AIDS who have acknowledged intravenous drug use. Inner-city minority populations are disproportionately highly represented among AIDS patients, and HIV seroprevalence is significantly higher among American Blacks and Hispanics (Centers for Disease Control, 1991b).

Owing to greater freedom of travel following political changes, the AIDS pandemic is likely to spread throughout eastern Europe. The majority of AIDS cases reported in Czechoslovakia and Hungary have been in homo-bisexual men, but in Poland the number of HIV infected IVDUs has increased dramatically and accounts for 71% (975/1373) of all HIV infections detected so far (Gromyko, 1991). In this, Poland resembles southern Europe (European Centre for Epidemiological Monitoring of AIDS, 1990).

Pattern 2

Epidemiological pattern 2 involves sub-Saharan Africa, the Caribbean and, increasingly, Latin America. It is characterized by heterosexual contact being the predominant mode of transmission. As at least half of infected adults are sexually active women, vertical transmission occurs tragically often, and 7% or more of HIV-infected subjects are infants or young children. Transmission by blood transfusion still accounts for about 10% of the epidemic in Africa.

Nowhere is the pandemic worse than in sub-Saharan Africa. HIV-1 is epidemic across a wide belt of central and east Africa, and has spread into west and southern Africa (Figure 4): the highest prevalence is around the great lakes of central Africa, for example in Kigali, Rwanda, where 38% of women attending antenatal clinics and about 90% of female prostitutes are anti-HIV-1 positive. In the extreme west of Africa, in Mauritania, Senegal, the Gambia, Cape Verde, Guinea-Bissau, Guinea and Sierra Leone, HIV-2 predominates (De Cock et al, 1991): in the general adult population, HIV-2 positivity has high prevalence (6–10%) only in Guinea-Bissau, but in this and other countries, such as the Gambia and Senegal, HIV-2 is epidemic in female prostitutes (25–30% seropositivity). HIV-2 occurs also further east, in Côte d'Ivoire, Burkina-Faso and Nigeria, for example, where HIV-1 predominates (Figure 4), and only sporadically so far in east, central and southern Africa.

In the Caribbean and central America, the AIDS pandemic clusters in 'hot spots', which include Bermuda, Bahamas, Turks and Caicos Islands and French Guiana, all of which have reported rates of AIDS in the range 143–318 per 100 000 population (Anonymous, 1992). In San Pedro, Honduras, the reported seroprevalence among prostitutes increased from 19 to 35% between 1989 and 1990 (Kimball et al, 1991). The majority of 1485 AIDS cases reported in the Dominican Republic from 1983 to 1990 has been reported since 1989; more than half had been infected heterosexually

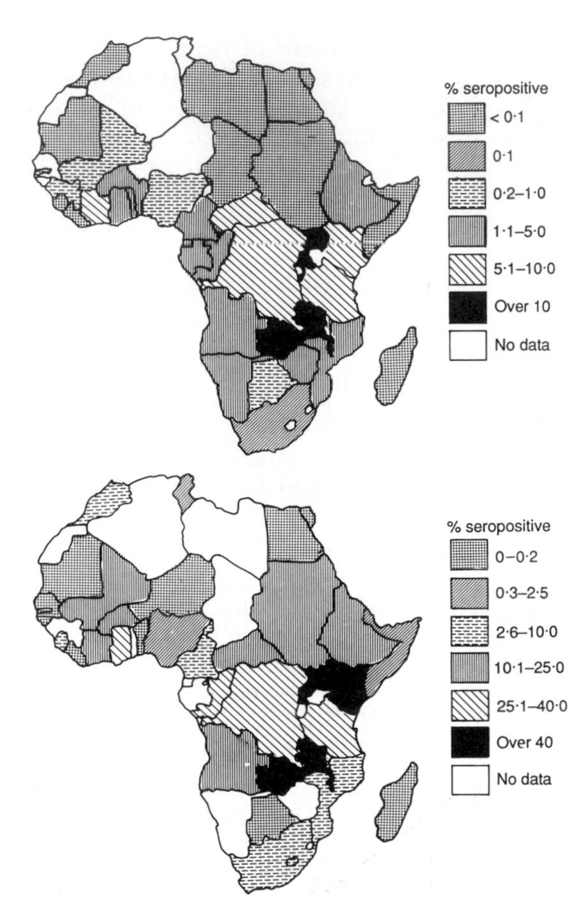

Figure 4. Estimates of recent HIV-1 seroprevalence in low-risk (above) and high-risk (below) urban populations in Africa. Low-risk samples drawn from populations of pregnant women and blood donors; high-risk samples drawn from prostitutes, bar girls, clients of prostitutes and patients attending STD clinics. From Potts et al (1991), with permission of the authors and publishers.

(Garris et al, 1991). In Haiti as many as one in ten pregnant women are HIV infected (Palca, 1991). In Brazil the seroprevalence of HIV-1 infection is as high as 45% in homosexual male prostitutes, 38% in the wives of haemophiliac patients, 28% in bisexual men and 9% in prostitutes from rural areas (Peixinho et al, 1990; Ivo-dos-Santos et al, 1991). Dual infections with HIV-1 and HIV-2 or HTLV-1 are reported not infrequently (Cortes et al, 1989; Peixinho et al, 1990).

In none of these pattern 2 populations has the epidemic stabilized or reached a plateau: further and catastrophic increases are predicted for the next decade.

Pattern 3

Epidemiological pattern 3 covers Asia, the Middle East and north Africa. HIV was not introduced or did not spread extensively until the mid or late 1980s. However, there have been recent explosive increases of HIV-1 seropositivity in IVDUs to more than 40% in Chiang Mai and Bangkok, Thailand (Poshyachinda, 1990) and Manipur, India (Naik et al, 1991). Similar jumps of seroprevalence are reported in female prostitutes and attenders of STD clinics in these cities and in Bombay (Dickman, 1991; Palca, 1991; Potts et al, 1991; Rübsamen-Waigmann et al, 1991; reviewed in Fleming, 1991b). In other parts of Asia, for example South Korea, HIV seroprevalence remains low, with men returning from overseas jobs presenting as the highest risk group (Kyung-Hee et al, 1991). It is predicted that there will be about 3 million HIV-infected individuals in Asia by the year 2000: the pandemic in the vast population of Asia could overshadow even the African epidemic in the next century.

Global perspective

During the past decade, AIDS has become a global health problem with almost half a million cases reported to the World Health Organization (WHO) from 164 countries (Anonymous, 1992), but as in some countries only 5 to 10% of the actual numbers of AIDS cases are reported (Dickman, 1991; Palca, 1991), the true figure of AIDS cases worldwide may be over one million. Over half of all patients in whom AIDS has been diagnosed have already died: for example, of more than 179 000 persons with AIDS recorded in the USA from 1981–1990, over 113 000 (63%) have died (Centers for Disease Control, 1991b). These figures do not reveal the extent of the pandemic: WHO estimates more than 10 million adults and 1 million children are infected worldwide with HIV. Of these, 7 million adults and half a million children are in Africa, 1 million in the north America, 1 million in the Caribbean and Latin America, 500 000 in western Europe and 500 000 in Asia (Figure 5); Oceania and Australasia, eastern Europe with the former Soviet Republics, north Africa with the Middle East are less affected, but each region has 20 000–30 000 infected persons (Palca, 1991). With a mean incubation period from time of infection to the development of AIDS of 8–10 years in adults and 2 years in infants, it is projected that nearly all HIV-1-infected individuals will develop AIDS within the next 15 years (Quinn et al, 1989). By the year 2000, 40 million people may be infected with HIV, of whom more than 90% will live in developing countries; the viruses have already spread from major cities to the rural areas in India and in many African countries (Dickman, 1991).

Clinical staging

A number of different classification schemes for HIV-related illnesses have been proposed. The two most frequently used are the Walter Reed (WR) and the Centers for Disease Control (CDC) classifications. These

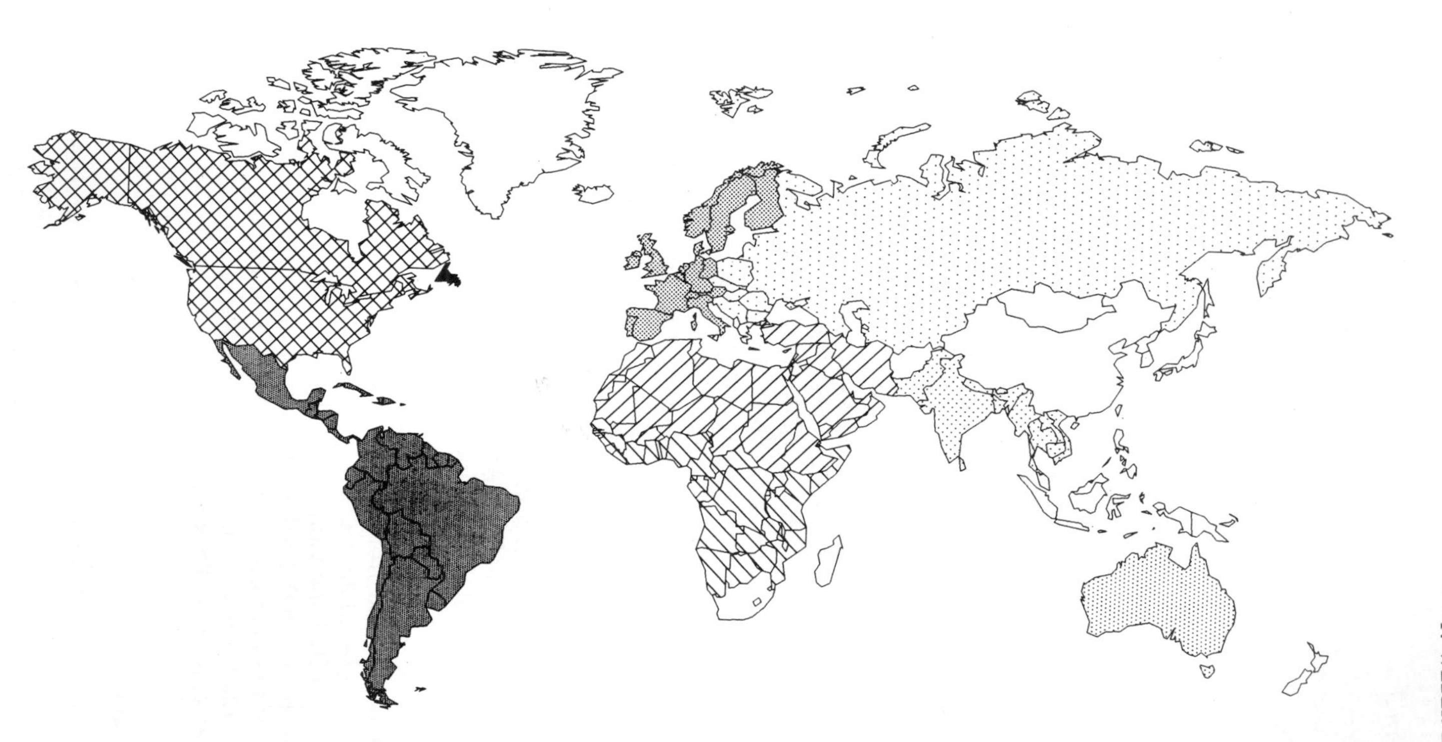

Figure 5. A global perspective of the pandemic HIV. Modified from Palca (1991), with permission of the author and publishers.

North America
1 million infected
m: 1 in 75
f: 1 in 700

The Caribbean and Latin America
about 1 million infected
m: 1 in 125
f: 1 in 500

Western Europe
500 000 infected
m: 1 in 200
f: 1 in 1400

Sub-Saharan Africa without South Africa
about 7 million infected
m: 1 in 50
f: 1 in 4000

North Africa and Middle East
30 000 infected
m: ?
f: ?

Eastern Europe and USSR
20 000 infected
m: 1 in 5000
f: 1 in 30 000

Asia and South-east Asia
500 000 infected
m: 1 in 2500
f: 1 in 3500

Oceania, New Zealand and Australia
30 000 infected
m: 1 in 200
f: 1 in 1400

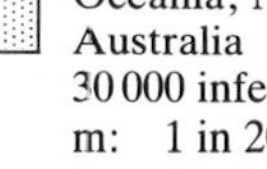

No data

classifications can hardly be applied in developing countries. The World Health Organization has proposed a staging system for HIV infection and disease which is primarily based on clinical criteria and organized into four prognostic categories (Table 4) (Anonymous, 1990).

If available a 'laboratory axis' can be added to the 'clinical axis'. Depending on the absolute CD4 count per microlitre (>500, 500–200, <200), the clinical axis can be subdivided into three strata (A, B, C). In places where

Table 4. World Health Organization proposed clinical staging system of HIV infection and disease.

Clinical stage 1
Asymptomatic
Persistent generalized lymphadenopathy
Performance scale 1: asymptomatic, normal activity
Clinical stage 2
Early (mild) disease
Weight loss <10% of body weight
Minor mucocutaneous manifestations (seborrhoeic dermatitis, prurigo, fungal nail infections, recurrent oral ulcerations, angular cheilitis)
Herpes zoster, within the last 5 years
Recurrent upper respiratory tract infections (i.e. bacterial sinusitis)
And/or Performance scale 2: symptomatic, normal activity
Clinical stage 3
Weight loss >10% body weight
Unexplained chronic diarrhoea >1 month
Unexplained prolonged fever (intermittent or constant) >1 month
Oral candidiasis (thrush)
Oral hairy leukoplakia
Pulmonary tuberculosis, within the past year
Severe bacterial infection (i.e. pneumonia, pyomyositis)
And/or Performance scale 3: bed-ridden <50% of the day during the last month
Clinical stage 4
HIV wasting syndrome (i.e. weight loss >10% of body weight, plus either unexplained chronic diarrhoea >1 month, or chronic weakness and unexplained prolonged fever >1 month)
Pneumocystis carinii pneumonia
Toxoplasmosis of the brain
Cryptosporidiosis with diarrhoea >1 month
Cryptococcosis, extrapulmonary
Cytomegalovirus disease of an organ other than liver, spleen or lymph nodes
Herpes simplex virus infection, mucocutaneous >1 month or visceral any duration
Progressive multifocal leukoencephalopathy
Any disseminated endemic mycosis (i.e. histoplasmosis, coccidioidomycosis)
Candidiasis of the oesophagus, trachea, bronchi or lungs
Atypical mycobacteriosis, disseminated
Non-typhoid *Salmonella* septicaemia
Extrapulmonary tuberculosis
Lymphoma
Kaposi's sarcoma
HIV encephalitis (clinical finding of disabling cognitive and/or motor dysfunction interfering with activities of daily living, progressing over weeks to months, in the absence of a concurrent illness or condition other than HIV infection that could explain the findings)

Anonymous (1990).

the CD4 count cannot be obtained, three different strata can be derived from the absolute lymphocyte count, A >2000 per μl, B 1000–2000 per μl and C <1000 per μl. The prognostic value of this proposed combined clinical and laboratory staging system has yet to be evaluated by longitudinal studies.

Haematological disorders associated with HIV infection

Haematological abnormalities are well recognized in HIV disease and may result from diverse influences on the haematopoietic tissue. In general it appears that the incidence of anaemia and other cytopenias increases with progressive immunological deterioration and in advanced disease states. However, isolated cytopenias, particularly thrombocytopenia, may be the presenting manifestation of HIV infection. Dysregulations of haematopoiesis by alterations in the T-cell subpopulations (Carlo-Stella et al, 1987), production of inhibitory glycoproteins (Liederman et al, 1987), antibody-mediated cytotoxicity (Donahue et al, 1987) and infection of haematopoietic progenitor cells by HIV-1 (Folks et al, 1988) have all been implicated as mechanisms disturbing haematopoiesis.

Anaemia

Anaemia is commonly seen in patients with AIDS, affecting 70–95% at presentation (Frontiera and Myers, 1987; Zon et al, 1987; Spivak et al, 1989). African women with AIDS may present for the first time with anaemia in pregnancy (A. F. Fleming, unpublished observations). The anaemia is typically normochromic, normocytic with an inappropriately low reticulocyte count suggesting a hypoproliferative disorder. Anisopoikilocytosis is a common finding (Perchoka and Rodgers, 1988). The anaemia may reflect a reticuloendothelial iron block (Castella et al, 1985; Gupta et al, 1986), or the effects of treatment with either antiviral, antineoplastic or antimicrobial drugs (see below). Erythroid hypoplasia with severe anaemia has been reported in patients with disseminated *Mycobacterium avium intracellulare* infection (Sadhana et al, 1990). Patients have been described with the combination of aplastic anaemia, HIV infection and additional organisms, including parvovirus B19 and *Leishmania donovani* (Crocchiolo et al, 1988). In contrast, erythrocytosis has been reported on a few occasions, some cases being associated with zidovudine therapy (Willocks et al, 1990; Kennedy et al, 1991).

In a study by Burkes et al (1987), 20% of HIV infected patients had subnormal vitamin B_{12} levels. Beach and colleagues (1989) confirmed this when they found deficiency or borderline deficiency of B_6 and B_{12} in a third of their asymptomatic HIV seropositive patients.

Haemolysis secondary to red cell autoantibodies appears uncommon, although a positive Coombs' test occurs in up to 20% of HIV patients (McGinniss et al, 1986; Bolton-Maggs et al, 1991). These autoantibodies are probably of little clinical importance, but may give rise to problems in grouping and crossmatching for patients requiring blood transfusion.

Leucopenias

Leucopenia is seen in as many as 75% of AIDS patients and appears to be less clearly related to the stage of the disease than is the anaemia. It may result from a lymphopenia, granulocytopenia or both. Mir and colleagues (1988) found a 79% incidence of lymphopenia in 40 patients with AIDS. Neutropenia is a frequent haematological finding, being found in approximately 40% of patients with AIDS (Murphy et al, 1989). The pathogenesis is still poorly understood. It is generally assumed that there is a reduced neutrophil production as a direct consequence of HIV infection (Folks et al, 1988) or from a secondary mechanism, for example the production of an inhibitory glycoprotein (Liedermann et al, 1987). Several independent studies provide evidence that neutrophil-bound immunoglobulin may contribute to the pathogenesis of HIV-associated neutropenia (Klaasen et al, 1991). Monocytopenia was apparent in 8.6% of 925 HIV-positive patients studied by Mir et al (1988). This was found in a higher percentage (35%) of patients in studies in which marrow aspirates were done (Treacy et al, 1987). The peripheral blood smear abnormalities may include atypical lymphocytes, granulocytes with nuclear hyposegmentation, and vacuolated monocytes.

Disorders of haemostasis

Thrombocytopenia occurs with increased frequency in HIV-seropositive patients, and this may be an early manifestation of the AIDS related complex (ARC) (Goldsweig et al, 1986). Several studies have shown that the incidence of thrombocytopenia ranges between 5 and 12% in ARC patients (Abrams et al, 1984; Murphy et al, 1987) and may be as high as 30–70% in patients with full blown AIDS (Murphy et al, 1987). The mechanism remains a topic of controversy. An immune-mediated mechanism, similar to that present in other forms of immune thrombocytopenia, is probably present (Walsh et al, 1986). Other mechanisms which may be involved include impaired thrombopoiesis due to stem cell damage (Donahue et al, 1987), altered regulation of platelet production, reticuloendothelial dysfunction or the toxic effect of ingested medications. Several cases of thrombotic thrombocytopenic purpura and haemolytic uraemic syndrome have been reported in patients with HIV infection (Ezforzado et al, 1991). The pathogenic mechanisms of this association are speculative, but the generation of antibodies and circulating immune complexes against platelet and endothelial receptors may play a role (Olivarria et al, 1989).

Cohen et al (1986) amongst several other workers, have described the presence of a lupus anticoagulant and also anticardiolipin antibodies in patients with HIV disease. These patients have prolonged partial thromboplastin times and prolonged Russell viper venom times. It was postulated that these antibodies were related to opportunistic infections. Deep venous thrombosis and pulmonary embolism have been reported only rarely in these patients. Isolated deficiencies in the prothrombin level, as well as prolonged bleeding times and abnormal platelet aggregation have been demonstrated in some seropositive patients (Bernstein et al, 1987).

Bone marrow

Although bone marrow changes are seen often in HIV disease, few changes appear specific, and in the evaluation of aspirates one must consider the possible haematological effects of various drugs, infectious pathogens and malignancies. The most comprehensive study appears to have been done by Karcher and Frost (1991) on the trephines and aspirates of 216 patients. Marrow cellularity was normal or increased in 53% of specimens. A markedly hypocellular marrow was rare. There did not appear to be any correlation between clinical progression of disease, peripheral counts and the marrow cellularity. Myelodysplasia in marrows from patients with AIDS was first described by Schneider and Picker (1985) and is seen commonly, involving at least one of the three major haematopoietic cell lines. In the study of Karcher and Frost (1991), 69% of the aspirates showed myelodysplasia with dyserythropoiesis being the most common manifestation. The dysplastic erythroid features may include multinucleation, nuclear irregularities and internuclear chromatin bridges. A number of mechanisms for HIV-related myelodysplasia have been proposed: (1) a direct result of the disease; (2) drug toxicity; and (3) secondary effect of opportunistic infections (Schneider and Picker, 1985).

Lymphoid aggregates were common in most series and are thought to represent a reaction to viral insult. There was no association between lymphoid aggregates and the presence of lymphoma. These lymphoid aggregates were of two types: (1) small, well circumscribed and composed of small lymphocytes; or (2) large, poorly circumscribed aggregates. A mild to moderate plasmacytosis was common.

Bone marrow aspirates have shown infiltration with infectious agents such as *Cryptococci*, *Histoplasma*, *P. carinii*, *M. tuberculosis* and *Toxoplasma* (Jaghadha et al, 1985; Namik et al, 1987). Granulomas, with or without necrosis, consisting of histiocytes, lymphocytes and plasma cells may occur in trephine biopsies (Castella et al, 1985). These granulomas are usually ill-formed, loose aggregates that may reveal the organisms mentioned above. Disseminated *M. avium intracellulare* infection results in an increase in bone marrow reticulin, occasional granulomas and, less commonly, pseudo-Gaucher cells. Histiocytic erythrophagocytosis has been observed in numerous marrows, but is probably a non-specific finding, often seen in association with other viral, fungal or bacterial infections and in some lymphoid malignancies (Lortholary et al, 1990).

Other non-specific marrow findings are: (1) anaemia of chronic disorders, as mentioned before, in up to 65% of marrows; (2) reticulin fibrosis, which may be focal or diffuse; (3) serous fat atrophy; and (4) increase in eosinophils, particularly following zidovudine therapy (McWhinney and Nathwani, 1990).

A malignant neoplasm has been identified in up to 9% of marrows (Karcher and Frost, 1991). These are discussed below and in other chapters, and include clinically aggressive B cell lymphomas, Hodgkin's disease, myeloma and Kaposi's sarcoma. Kaposi's sarcoma rarely involves the marrow. Acute non-lymphoid leukaemias or myeloproliferative disorders do not seem to occur more frequently in HIV-infected patients. Peters et al (1990) have reported, however, cases of acute myeloblastic leukaemia (AML) in AIDS patients. In a recent study by Murthy et al (1991), the presence of infected myelomonoblasts raises the possibility of direct or indirect viral transformation. The profound T-cell immunodeficiency of AIDS might contribute to both myelodysplasia and AML, possibly due to defective T-cell control of haematopoiesis or to a failure of immune surveillance (Chikkappa and Phillips, 1984).

Lymphoma

Non-Hodgkin's lymphoma (NHL) is common in patients with advanced AIDS (Knowles et al, 1988; Kaplan, 1990). It is being seen more often and is emerging as a more common cause of death, and this may be related to prolonged survival of patients receiving sophisticated levels of care, including zidovudine: for example in London, median survival of AIDS patients doubled between 1987 and 1989, from 10 to 20 months, and deaths due to lymphoma rose to 16% in 1989 (Peters et al, 1991).

Histologically, HIV-associated lymphomas include intermediate grade categories (large cell) and high grade (small non-cleaved, immunoblastic) categories. Usually they are of B-cell origin. The high frequency of extranodal disease is remarkable and can be as high as 87%. The sites most frequently involved are the gastrointestinal tract (27%), the central nervous system (CNS) (21%), bone marrow (21%) and liver (6%) (Knowles et al, 1988). Between 1973 and 1987 the incidence of NHLs increased over tenfold and Kaposi's sarcoma incidence increased over 5000-fold in single San Francisco men 20 to 49 years of age (Rabkin et al, 1991). Increases in NHLs were restricted to high grade and diffuse large cell (intermediate grade) histological types. In 1987, HIV was associated with 14% of all reported cancers (except non-melanoma skin cancer) in men aged 20 to 49. It has been estimated that 1890 to 2730 excess cases of NHLs and 6490 to 8320 excess cases of Kaposi's sarcoma occurred in the USA in 1990 (Rabkin et al, 1991). A retrospective epidemiological study identified three categories of AIDS-associated lymphomas (Beral et al, 1991). Primary lymphomas of the CNS without specified histological subtype were seen in about 0.5% of patients in all age groups. Systemic lymphomas were either immunoblastic lymphomas or Burkitt's lymphomas. The incidence for the former rose steadily with age to more than 3% for persons aged over 50 years, while the latter had a peak incidence of 1.8% in adolescents and declined to 0.6% for patients older than 30 years. Epstein–Barr virus (EBV) sequences have been detected in about half of these B-cell lymphomas. Recently it has been shown that primary CNS lymphomas in AIDS patients contain short non-protein-coding EBV transcripts (MacMahon et al, 1991).

Iatrogenic changes

A variety of drugs used to treat the infectious complications of AIDS, including ganciclovir, pentamidine, trimethoprim–sulphamethoxazole, pyrimethamine, sulphadiazine, dapsone and amphotericin B, can induce significant myelosuppression in AIDS patients. The haematological effects of these drugs may be worsened when combined with zidovudine (Glatt et al, 1988). The dose-limiting toxicity seen with the administration of zidovudine is myelosuppression. Neutropenia, anaemia and red cell macrocytosis are common (Richman et al, 1987). Zidovudine has been shown to elevate the platelet count initially in a dose-independent fashion (Montaner et al, 1990), but a reduction in platelets may be a late complication. Zon et al (1987) and Frontiera and Myers (1987) have compared bone marrow morphologies of patients who received zidovudine therapy and those who did not, and no striking differences were noted between groups, although numbers studied were small.

Haematological complications in childhood

Children are also infected by HIV, but much less work has been done on the haematological findings in this age group. Thrombocytopenia is a common haematological finding in 10–15% of infected children (Abrahams and Rogers, 1991). Leucopenia is seen also, but the incidence is less well documented. Lymphopenia is seen less frequently in the paediatric population than in adults. Lymphocytosis with neutropenia has also been described, particularly in children with lymphocytic interstitial pneumonia.

Most children develop a normochromic, normocytic anaemia with an inappropriately low reticulocyte count. Several of the children studied by Abrahams and Rogers (1991) developed a macrocytic anaemia with normal vitamin B_{12} and folate levels. Sandhaus and Scudder (1989) described the bone marrow findings in eight children with HIV infection. These aspirates appeared normocellular with lymphoid aggregates, but many of the abnormalities observed in the adult population were not noted in this small series.

Abnormalities of coagulation are not seen commonly in the HIV-infected child.

Human immunodeficiency virus type-2

The main discussion has referred to HIV-1 unless HIV-2 was specified. West African experience of HIV-2, as presented as the VIth International Conference on AIDS in Africa, Dakar, December 1991, has been reviewed by Colebunders (1991). Compared to HIV-1, sexual transmission of HIV-2 is about three times and vertical transmission is about ten times less efficient: HIV-2 causes immunosuppression and AIDS, but compared to HIV-1 viral loads are lower, CD4 lymphocyte counts are less decreased in the asymptomatic, there is less pathogenesis and the rate of development of AIDS was 12-fold lower for infected female prostitutes. The lower pathogenicity explains why the prevalence of HIV-2 increases with age in adults, in contrast to HIV-1 which has peak prevalence at 20–40 years. The lower rate of transmission explains why HIV-1 is now more prevalent in countries, e.g. Côte d'Ivoire, despite HIV-2 being introduced first (see *Epidemiology: Pattern 2*).

SUMMARY

It was only in 1980 that the first human retrovirus, HTLV-1, was isolated. Since then, HTLV-2, HIV-1 and HIV-2 have been identified. All four viruses are transmitted with varying efficiency sexually, vertically from mother to infant, and through blood by transfusion or contamination.

HTLV-1 is endemic in populations in south-west Japan, Taiwan, sub-Saharan Africa, the Caribbean, southern USA, central and south America, Australia, Papua New Guinea, Solomon Islands and western Asia. There is now epidemic spread amongst IVDUs in north and south America and southern Europe. HTLV-1 is the aetiological agent of adult T-cell leukaemia/lymphoma (ATL) and tropical spastic paraparesis/HTLV-1 associated myelopathy (TSP/HAM). Other associations which may be causative are with polymyositis, infective dermatitis, gastrointestinal malignant lymphoma and chronic lymphatic leukaemia. ATL appears to be due to malignant transformation of HTLV-1 infected cells, and TSP/HAM to chronic activation of these cells.

The epidemiology of HTLV-2 is being separated only recently from HTLV-1 through the application of PCR. It has a low level of endemicity in populations of central Africa, and central and south America. It is being spread epidemically amongst IVDUs in north America and southern Europe. Its association with any pathology in man remains uncertain.

HIV-1 is epidemic and spreading rapidly throughout the world. In areas where homosexual contact was the predominant mode of transmission, heterosexual spread is becoming increasingly important. The areas where heterosexual contact is the predominant mode of transmission include the worst affected populations in the world, for example sub-Saharan Africa and some of the Caribbean. There have been recent and explosive increases of HIV-1 seroprevalence in IVDUs and female prostitutes in Asia, especially Thailand and India. Of the diverse pathology following infection, only the haematological consequences are reviewed in detail: these include anaemia, leucopenia, thrombocytopenia, disorders of coagulation and lymphomas.

HIV-2, compared to HIV-1, is less infectious and causes less immunosuppression with more slowly progressive disease. It is prevalent in west Africa, but is spreading, albeit slowly, far beyond.

Acknowledgements

The authors gratefully acknowledge Dr Hans Gelderblom, Robert-Koch-Institut, Nordufer 20, D-1000 Berlin 65, Germany for providing us with Figure 1. Mrs Karin Peinemann, Mrs Sylke Wallbrecht and Miss Feliciti English gave her close attention and hard work in the preparation of the typescript.

REFERENCES

Abebe M, Haimanot RT, Gustafsson A et al (1991) Low HTLV-1 seroprevalence in endemic tropical spastic paraparesis in Ethiopia. *Transactions of the Royal Society of Tropical Medicine and Hygiene* **85:** 109–112.
Abrahams EJ & Rogers M (1991) Paediatric HIV infection. *Baillière's Clinical Haematology* **4:** 333–354.
Abrams DI, Lewis BJ, Beckstead JH et al (1984) Persistent diffuse lymphadenopathy in homosexual men: endpoint or prodrome. *Annals of Internal Medicine* **100:** 801.
Anderson RM, Gupta S & Ng W (1990) The significance of sexual partner contact networks for the transmission dynamics of HIV. *Journal of Acquired Immune Deficiency Syndromes* **3:** 417–429.
Anderson RM, May RM, Boily MC et al (1991) The spread of HIV-1 in Africa: sexual contact patterns and the medical demographic impact of AIDS. *Nature* **352:** 581–589.
Anonymous (1990) Acquired immunodeficiency syndrome (AIDS). Interim proposal for a WHO staging system for HIV infection and disease. *Weekly Epidemiological Record* **65:** 221–224.
Anonymous (1991) AIDS: proposed WHO criteria for interpreting Western blot assay for HIV-1, HIV-2 and HTLV-1/HTLV-2. *Bulletin of the World Health Organization* **69:** 127–130.
Anonymous (1992) Acquired immunodeficiency syndrome (AIDS): data as of 1 January 1992. *Weekly Epidemiological Record* **67:** 9–10.
Anstee M (1989) Women, AIDS and the United Nations. *The Implications of AIDS for Mothers and Children: Acts of the International Conference*, Paris, November 1989, pp 111–117.
Aoki T, Miyakoshi H, Koide H et al (1985) Seroepidemiology of human T-lymphotropic retrovirus type I (HTLV-I) in residents of Niigata prefecture, Japan. Comparative studies by indirect immunofluorescence microscopy and enzyme-linked immunosorbent assay. *International Journal of Cancer* **35:** 301–306.
Artzrouni M (1990) Projections of the HIV/AIDS epidemic for homosexual/bisexual men in France, the Federal Republic of Germany and the United Kingdom. *European Journal of Epidemiology* **6:** 124–135.
Beach R, Mantero-Atrenza E, Van Riel R et al (1989) Nutritional deficiencies in early HIV infection: I plasma vitamin levels. *Abstracts of the Fifth International Conference on AIDS*, Montreal (abstract TH-BU40).
Beral V, Peterman T, Berkelman R & Jaffe H (1991) AIDS-associated non-Hodgkin lymphoma. *Lancet* **337:** 805–809.
Berkley S (1991) Parenteral transmission of HIV in Africa. *AIDS* **5** (supplement 1)**:** S87–S92.
Bernstein L, Cappacino A & Cappacino H (1987) Platelet function and bound antibodies in AIDS-ARC patients with thrombocytopenia. *Blood* **70:** 118a.
Bhigjee AI, Kelbe C, Haribhai HC et al (1990) Myelopathy associated with human T cell lymphotrophic virus type I (HTLV-I) in Natal, South Africa. *Brain* **113:** 1307–1320.
Biggar RJ, Johnson BK, Oster C et al (1985) Regional variation in prevalence of antibody against human T-lymphotropic virus types I and III in Kenya, east Africa. *International Journal of Cancer* **35:** 763–767.
Biggar RJ, Buskell Bales Z, Yakshe PN et al (1991) Antibody to human retroviruses among drug users in three east coast American cities, 1972–1976. *Journal of Infectious Diseases* **163:** 57–63.
Bolton-Maggs PH, Rogan PD, Duguid JKM et al (1991) Cold agglutinins in haemophiliac boys infected with HIV. *Archives of Disease in Childhood* **66:** 732–733.
Bouzas MB, Picchio G, Muchinik G et al (1990) HTLV-I in Argentina. *Journal of Acquired Immune Deficiency Syndromes* **3:** 741–742.
Braddick MR, Kreiss JK, Embree JE et al (1990) Impact of maternal HIV infection on obstetrical and early neonatal outcome. *AIDS* **4:** 1001–1005.
Burkes RL, Cohen H, Krailo M et al (1987) Low serum cobalamin levels occur frequently in the acquired immunodeficiency syndrome and related disorders. *European Journal of Haematology* **38:** 141.

Busch MP, Young MJ, Samson SM et al (1991a) Risk of human immunodeficiency virus (HIV) transmission by blood transfusions before the implementation of HIV-1 antibody screening. The Transfusion Safety Study Group. *Transfusion* **31:** 4–11.
Busch MP, Eble BE, Khayam BH et al (1991b) Evaluation of screened blood donations for human immunodeficiency virus type 1 infection by culture and DNA amplification of pooled cells. *New England Journal of Medicine* **325:** 1–5.
Cameron DW, Simonsen JN, D'Costa LJ et al (1989) Female to male transmission of human immunodeficiency virus type 1: risk factors for seroconversion in men. *Lancet* **ii:** 403–407.
Carlo-Stella C, Ganser A & Hoelzer D (1987) Defective in vitro growth of haemopoietic progenitors in the acquired immunodeficiency syndrome. *Journal of Clinical Investigation* **80:** 286–293.
Castella A, Croxson TS, Mildvan D et al (1985) The bone marrow in AIDS: a histologic, hematologic and microbiologic study. *American Journal of Clinical Pathology* **84:** 425.
Centers for Disease Control (1981) Pneumocystis pneumonia—Los Angeles. *Morbidity and Mortality Weekly Report* **30:** 250.
Centers for Disease Control (1989) Guidelines for prevention of transmission of human immunodeficiency virus and hepatitis B to health-care and public safety workers. *Morbidity and Mortality Weekly Report* **38:** supplement 6.
Centers for Disease Control (1990) Human T-lymphotropic virus type I screening in volunteer blood donors—United States, 1989. *Morbidity and Mortality Weekly Report* **39:** 921–924.
Centers for Disease Control (1991a) Interpretive criteria used to report Western blot results for HIV-1-antibody testing—United States. *Morbidity and Mortality Weekly Report* **40:** 692–695.
Centers for Disease Control (1991b) Update: acquired immunodeficiency syndrome—United States, 1981–1990. *Morbidity and Mortality Weekly Report* **40:** 358–369.
Centers for Disease Control (1991c) Update: transmission of HIV infection during invasive dental procedure—Florida. *Morbidity and Mortality Weekly Report* **40:** 21–27.
Centers for Disease Control (1991d) The HIV/AIDS epidemic: the first 10 years. *Morbidity and Mortality Weekly Report* **40:** 357.
Chandy M, Babu PG, Saraswathy NK et al (1991) HTLV-1 infection in patients with leukaemia in southern India. *Lancet* **338:** 380–381.
Chikkappa G & Phillips PG (1984) Regulation of normal human blood neutrophilic, macrophagic and eosinophilic committed stem cell proliferation by autologous blood T lymphocyte subsets. *Blood* **63:** 356–361.
Chin J (1990) Public health surveillance of AIDS and HIV infections. *Bulletin of the World Health Organization* **68:** 529–536.
Clavel F, Guetard D, Brun-Vézinet F et al (1986) Isolation of a new human retrovirus from West African patients with AIDS. *Science* **233:** 343–346.
Cnudde F, Gessian A, Dandelot JB et al (1991) HTLV-1 in neurological patients from some Indian Ocean islands. *Journal of Acquired Immune Deficiency Syndromes* **4:** 734–735.
Coffin JM (1986) Genetic variation in AIDS viruses. *Cell* **46:** 1–4.
Cohen AJ, Philips TM & Kessler CM (1986) Circulating coagulation inhibitors in the acquired immunodeficiency syndrome. *Annals of Internal Medicine* **104:** 175.
Colebunders RL (1991) After Dakar. *Current AIDS Literature* **4:** 457–458.
Contreras M & Barbara JAJ (1990) Retroviruses and blood transfusion. *Baillière's Clinical Haematology* **3:** 65–77.
Cortes E, Detels R, Aboulafia D et al (1989) HIV-1, HIV-2, and HTLV-I infection in high-risk groups in Brazil. *New England Journal of Medicine* **320:** 953–958.
Costa CM, Salgueiro MR, Carton H et al (1989) Tropical spastic paraparesis in Northeastern Brazil. *Arquivos de Neuropsiquiatria* **47:** 134–138.
Crocchiolo PR, Lizioli A & Leopardi O (1988) HIV and aplastic anaemia. *Lancet* **ii:** 109.
Cummings PC, Wallace EL, Schorr JB & Dodd RY (1989) Exposure of patients to human immunodeficiency virus through transfusion of blood components that test antibody-negative. *New England Journal of Medicine* **321:** 941–946.
Davidson M, Kaplan JE, Hartley TM et al (1990) Prevalence of HTLV-I in Alaska natives. *Journal of Infectious Diseases* **161:** 359–360.
De Cock KM, Brun-Vézinet F & Soro B (1991) HIV-1 infections and AIDS in west Africa. *AIDS* **5** (supplement 1): S21–S28.
DeFreitas E, Hilliard B, Cheney PR et al (1991) Retroviral sequences related to human

T-lymphotropic virus type II in patients with chronic fatigue immune dysfunction syndrome. *Proceedings of the National Academy of Sciences of the USA* **88:** 2922–2926.

Delaporte E, Peeters M, Durand JP et al (1989a) Seroepidemiological survey of HTLV-I infection among randomized populations of western central African countries. *Journal of Acquired Immune Deficiency Syndromes* **2:** 410–413.

Delaporte E, Peeter M, Simoni M & Piot P (1989b) HTLV-I infection in western equatorial Africa. *Lancet* **ii:** 1226.

Delaporte E, Monplaisir N, Louwagie J et al (1991a) Prevalence of HTLV-I and HTLV-II infection in Gabon, Africa: comparison of the serological and PCR results. *International Journal of Cancer* **49:** 373–376.

Delaporte E, Louwagie J, Peeters M et al (1991b) Evidence of HTLV-II infection in central Africa. *AIDS* **5:** 771–772.

Denic S, Nolan P, Doherty J et al (1990) HTLV-I infection in Iraq. *Lancet* **336:** 1135–1136.

de-Thé G, Gazzolo L & Gessian A (1985) Viruses as risk factors or causes of human leukaemias and lymphomas. *Leukemia Research* **9:** 691–696.

Dickman S (1991) AIDS threatens Asia. *Nature* **351:** 682.

Donahue RE, Johnson MM, Zon LI et al (1987) Suppression of in vitro haematopoiesis following human immunodeficiency virus infection. *Nature* **326:** 200.

Dumas M, Houinata D, Verdier M et al (1991) Seroepidemiology of human T-cell lymphotropic virus type I/II in Benin (west Africa). *AIDS Research and Human Retroviruses* **7:** 447–451.

Ehrnst A, Lindgren S, Dictor M et al (1991) HIV in pregnant women and their offspring: evidence for late transmission. *Lancet* **338:** 203–207.

Ellerbrock TV, Bush TJ, Chamberland ME & Oxtoby MJ (1991) Epidemiology of women with AIDS in the United States, 1981 through 1990. A comparison with heterosexual men with AIDS. *Journal of the American Medical Association* **265:** 2971–2975.

European Centre for Epidemiological Monitoring of AIDS (1990) Quarterly report: 30th September 1990. *AIDS Surveillance in Europe* **27:** 5a–8a.

European Collaborative Study (1991) Children born to women with HIV-1 infection: natural history and risk of transmission. *Lancet* **337:** 253–260.

Ezforzado N, Poch E, Almirall J et al (1991) Haemolytic uraemic syndrome associated with HIV infection. *AIDS* **5:** 1041.

Fleming AF (1988) Simplified confirmatory HIV testing. *Lancet* **ii:** 848.

Fleming AF (1990a) Chronic lymphocytic leukaemia in tropical Africa; a review. *Leukemia and Lymphoma* **1:** 169–173.

Fleming AF (1990b) AIDS in Africa. *Baillière's Clinical Haematology* **3:** 177–205.

Fleming AF (1991a) Transmission of HIV and HBV in the health-care setting. *Current AIDS Literature* **4:** 289–291.

Fleming AF (1991b) Epidemiology: editorial comment on papers of outstanding interest. *Current AIDS Literature* **4:** 91–92.

Fleming AF, Yamamoto M, Bhusnurmath SR et al (1983) Antibodies to ATLV (HTLV) in Nigerian blood donors and patients with chronic lymphatic leukaemia or lymphoma. *Lancet* **ii:** 334–335.

Fleming AF, Maharajan R, Abraham M et al (1986) Antibodies to HTLV-1 in Nigerian blood-donors, their relatives and patients with leukaemia, lymphomas and other diseases. *International Journal of Cancer* **38:** 809–813.

Folks TM, Kessler SW, Orenstein JM et al (1988) Infection and replication of HIV-1 in purified progenitor cells of normal human bone marrow. *Science* **242:** 919–922.

Frontiera M & Myers A (1987) Peripheral and blood abnormalities in the acquired immunodeficiency syndrome. *West Journal of Medicine* **147:** 157.

Garris I, Rodriguez EM, de Moya EA et al (1991) Predominance of heterosexual transmission of HIV in Dominican Republic: AIDS surveillance data from 1983–1990. *Abstracts of the VII International Conference on AIDS* **1:** 365.

Gessain A, Barin F, Vernant JC et al (1985) Antibodies to human T-lymphotropic virus type-I in patients with tropical spastic paraparesis. *Lancet* **ii:** 407–410.

Gessain A, Gout O, Saal F et al (1990) Epidemiology and immunovirology of human T-cell leukemia/lymphoma virus type I-associated adult T-cell leukemia and chronic myelopathies as seen in France. *Cancer Research* **50 (supplement):** 5692s–5696s.

Giangugliemo Z, Galli C, Capelli C et al (1991) Prevalence of anti-HTLV-1 among Italian IVDAs and hemophiliacs. *Abstracts of the VII International Conference on AIDS* **1:** 168.

Glatt AE, Chirgwin K & Handesman H (1988) Current concepts: treatment of infections associated with human immunodeficiency virus. *New England Journal of Medicine* **318:** 1439.

Goedert JJ, Duliège AM, Amos CI et al (1991) High risk of HIV-1 infection for first-born twins. *Lancet* **338:** 1471–1475.

Goldsweig HG, Grossmann R & William D (1986) Thrombocytopenia in homosexual men. *American Journal of Hematology* **21:** 243.

Goubau P, Carton H, Kazadi K et al (1990) HTLV seroepidemiology in a central African population with high incidence of tropical spastic paraparesis. *Transactions of the Royal Society of Tropical Medicine and Hygiene* **84:** 577–579.

Gromyko A (1991) The magnitude of HIV/AIDS epidemic in eastern part of Europe. *Abstracts of the VII International Conference on AIDS* **1:** 33.

Gupta S, Inman A & Licorish K (1986) Serum ferritin in acquired immune deficiency syndrome. *Journal of Clinical Laboratory Immunology* **20:** 11.

Hahn BH, Shaw GM, Popovic M et al (1984) Molecular cloning and analysis of a new variant of a human T-cell leukemia virus (HTLV-1b) from an African patient with adult T-cell leukemia-lymphoma. *International Journal of Cancer* **33:** 613–618.

Hanada S, Uematsu T, Iwahashi M et al (1989) The prevalence of human T-cell leukemia virus type I infection in patients with hematologic and nonhematologic diseases in an adult T-cell leukemia-endemic area of Japan. *Cancer* **64:** 1290–1295.

Hannam P (1991) HIV infection and hepatitis B in adopted Romanian children. *British Medical Journal* **302:** 1604.

Harrington WJ, Miller GA, Kemper RR et al (1991) HTLV-I-associated leukemia/lymphoma in South Florida. *Journal of Acquired Immune Deficiency Syndromes* **4:** 284–289.

Hattori T, Asou N, Suzushima H et al (1991) Leukaemia of novel gastrointestinal T-lymphocyte population infected with HTLV-I. *Lancet* **337:** 76–77.

Heald RJ (1991) The dog in the night time. *British Journal of Surgery* **78:** 3–5.

Hellings JA, Theunissen H, Keur W & Siebelink Liauw A (1987) New developments in ELISA verification of anti-HIV screening of blood donors. *Journal of Virological Methods* **17:** 11–17.

Henderson DK, Fahey BJ, Willy M et al (1990) Risk for occupational transmission of human immunodeficiency virus type 1 (HIV-1) associated with clinical exposures. *Annals of Internal Medicine* **113:** 740–746.

Hersh BS, Popovici F, Apetrei RC et al (1991) Acquired immunodeficiency syndrome in Romania. *Lancet* **338:** 645–649.

Hinuma Y, Komoda H, Chosa T et al (1982) Antibodies to adult T-cell leukemia-virus-associated antigen (ATLA) in sera from patients with ATL and controls in Japan: a nation-wide sero-epidemiologic study. *International Journal of Cancer* **29:** 631–635.

Hjelle B (1991) Human T-cell leukemia-lymphoma viruses. Life cycle, pathogenicity, epidemiology, and diagnosis. *Archives of Pathology and Laboratory Medicine* **115:** 440–450.

Hjelle B, Scalf R & Swenson S (1990a) High frequency of human T-cell leukemia-lymphoma virus type II infection in New Mexico blood donors: determination by sequence-specific oligonucleotide hybridization. *Blood* **76:** 450–454.

Hjelle B, Mills R, Mertz G & Swenson S (1990b) Transmission of HTLV-II via blood transfusion. *Vox Sanguinis* **59:** 119–122.

Ho DD, Moudgil T & Alam M (1989) Quantitation of human immunodeficiency virus type 1 in the blood of infected persons. *New England Journal of Medicine* **312:** 1621–1625.

Hoffman PH, Larkin DP & Samuel D (1989) Needlesticks and needleshare—the difference. *Journal of Infectious Diseases* **160:** 546–556.

Holmes KK, Karon JM & Kreiss J (1990) The increasing frequency of heterosexually acquired AIDS in the United States, 1983–88. *American Journal of Public Health* **80:** 858–863.

Hunsmann G, Schneider J, Schmitt J & Yamamoto M (1983) Detection of serum antibodies to adult T-cell leukemia virus in non-human primates and in people from Africa. *International Journal of Cancer* **32:** 329–332.

Hunsmann G, Bayer H, Schneider J et al (1984) Antibodies to ATLV/HTLV-1 in Africa. *Medical Microbiology and Immunology* **173:** 167–170.

Hunsmann G, Schneider J, Wendler I & Fleming AF (1985a) HTLV positivity in Africans. *Lancet* **ii:** 952–953.

Hunsmann G, Schneider J, Bayer H et al (1985b) Antibodies to adult T-cell leukemia virus (ATLV/HTLV-I) in AIDS patients and people at risk of AIDS in Germany. *Medical Microbiology and Immunology* **173:** 241–250.

Hunsmann G, Flügel RM & Walder R (1990) Retroviral antibodies in Indians. *Nature* **345:** 120.

Ivo-dos-Santos J, Couto-Fernandez JC, Santana AJ et al (1991) Prevalence of HIV-1 antibodies in selected groups of a Brazilian city with African sociodemographic characteristics. *Journal of Acquired Immune Deficiency Syndromes* **4:** 448–449.

Jäger H, Jersild C & Emmanuel JC (1991) Safe blood transfusion in Africa. *AIDS* **5** (supplement 1): S163–S168.

Jagger J & Pearson RD (1991) Universal precautions: still missing the point on needlesticks. *Infection Control and Hospital Epidemiology* **12:** 211–213.

Jaghadha V, Aadavolu RH & Hiland CT (1985) Granulomatous inflammation in the acquired immunodeficiency syndrome. *American Journal of Clinical Pathology* **84:** 589–602.

Kajiyama W, Kashiwagi S, Ikematsu H et al (1986) Intrafamilial transmission of adult T-cell leukemia virus. *Journal of Infectious Diseases* **154:** 851–857.

Kalyanramen VS, Sarngadharan MG & Robert-Guroff M (1982) A new subtype of human T-cell leukemia virus (HTLV-II) associated with a T-cell variant of hairy cell leukemia. *Science* **218:** 571–573.

Kaplan LD (1990) AIDS-associated lymphoma. *Baillière's Clinical Haematology* **3:** 139–151.

Karcher DS & Frost AR (1991) The bone marrow in human immunodeficiency virus (HIV)-related disease. *American Journal of Clinical Pathology* **95:** 63–71.

Karpas A, Maayan S & Raz R (1986) Lack of antibodies to adult T-cell leukaemia virus and to AIDS virus in Israeli Falashas. *Nature* **319:** 794.

Kazadi K, Goubau P, Desmeyter J et al (1990) A cluster of HTLV-1 associated tropical spastic paraparesis in Equateur (Zaire): ethnic and familial distribution. *Journal of Neurology, Neurosurgery and Psychiatry* **53:** 4–10.

Kennedy CA, Griffith HS & Mathisen GE (1991) Erythrocytosis after zidovudine for AIDS. *Annals of Internal Medicine* **114:** 250.

Khabbaz RF, Hartley TM, Oberle MW & Rosero-Bixby L (1990) Seroprevalence of human T-lymphotropic virus type I (HTLV-I) in Costa Rica. *AIDS Research and Human Retroviruses* **6:** 959–960.

Khabbaz RF, Onorata IM, Cannon RO et al (1992) Seroprevalence of HTLV-I and HTLV-II among intravenous drug users and persons in clinics for sexually transmitted diseases. *New England Journal of Medicine* **326:** 375–380.

Kimball AM, Gonzales R, Calderon R et al (1991) The AIDS pandemic in the Americas: using surveillance information to reinforce national control programs. *Abstracts of the VII International Conference on AIDS* **1:** 463.

Klaasen RJ, Vlekke ABJ & Von dem Borne AE (1991) Neutrophil bound immunoglobulin in HIV infections is of autoantibody nature. *British Journal of Haematology* **77:** 403–409.

Knowles DM, Chamulak GA & Subar M (1988) Lymphoid neoplasia associated with the acquired immunodeficiency syndrome (AIDS). The New York University Medical Center experience with 105 patients (1981–1986). *Annals of Internal Medicine* **108:** 744–753.

Konde-Lule JK, Berkley SF & Downing R (1989) Knowledge, attitudes and practices concerning AIDS in Ugandans. *AIDS* **3:** 513–518.

Kondo T, Kono H, Miyamoto N et al (1989) Age- and sex-specific cumulative rate and risk of ATLL for HTLV-I carriers. *International Journal of Cancer* **43:** 1061–1064.

Kyung-Hee C, Kim MS, Catania J et al (1991) First HIV seroprevalence in South Korea. *Abstracts of the VII International Conference on AIDS* **1:** 356.

Laga M, Nzila N & Goeman J (1991) The interrelationship of sexually transmitted diseases and HIV infection: implications for the control of both epidemics in Africa. *AIDS* **5** (supplement 1): S55–S63.

LaGrenade L, Hanchard B, Fletcher V et al (1990) Infective dermatitis of Jamaican children: a marker for HTLV-I infection. *Lancet* **336:** 1345–1347.

Lairmore MD, Jacobson S, Gracia F et al (1990) Isolation of human T-cell lymphotropic virus type 2 from Guaymi Indians in Panama. *Proceedings of the National Academy of Sciences of the USA* **87:** 8840–8844.

Lallement M, Lallement-Le-Coeur S, Cheynier D et al (1989) Mother–child transmission of HIV-1 and infant survival in Brazzaville, Congo. *AIDS* **3:** 643–646.
Lavanchy D, Bovet P, Hollanda J et al (1991) High seroprevalence of HTLV-I in the Seychelles. *Lancet* **337:** 248–249.
Lee H, Swanson P, Shorty VS et al (1989) High rate of HTLV-II infection in seropositive i.v. drug abusers in New Orleans. *Science* **244:** 471–475.
Lee HH, Swanson P, Rosenblatt JD et al (1991) Relative seroprevalence and risk factors of HTLV-I and HTLV-II infection in US blood donors. *Lancet* **337:** 1435–1439.
Lepage P & Van de Perre P (1988) Nosocomial transmission of HIV in Africa: what tribute is paid to contaminated blood transfusion and medical injections? *Infection Control and Hospital Epidemiology* **9:** 200–203.
Lepage P, Van de Perre P, Caräel M & Butzler JP (1986) Are medical injections a risk factor for HIV infection in children? *Lancet* **ii:** 1103–1104.
Lepage P, Dabis F, Hitimana D-G et al (1991) Perinatal transmission of HIV-1: lack of impact of maternal HIV infection on characteristics of live births and on neonatal mortality in Kigali, Rwanda. *AIDS* **5:** 295–300.
Levine PH, Blattner WA, Clark J et al (1988) Geographic distribution of HTLV-I and identification of a new high-risk population. *International Journal of Cancer* **42:** 7–12.
Liedermann IZ, Greenberg MI, Adelsberg BR et al (1987) A glycoprotein inhibitor of in vitro granulopoiesis associated with AIDS. *Blood* **70:** 1267–1272.
Lortholary A, Raffi F & Aubertin P (1990) HIV haemophagocytic syndrome. *Lancet* **336:** 1128.
Louis JP, Trebucq A, Hengy C et al (1990) Epidémiologie des infections a rétrovirus VIH1-VIH2 et HTLV1 en République du Tchad. *Bulletin de la Société Pathologie Exotique* **83:** 603–610.
McGinniss MH, Macher AM, Rook AH et al (1986) Red cell autoantibodies in patients with acquired immunodeficiency syndrome. *Transfusion* **26:** 405.
MacMahon EME, Glass JD, Hayward SD et al (1991) Epstein–Barr virus in AIDS-related primary central nervous system lymphoma. *Lancet* **338:** 969–973.
McWhinney P & Nathwani D (1990) Eosinophils, HIV infection and zidovudine. *AIDS* **4:** 817.
Madhok R & Forbes CD (1990) HIV-1 infection in haemophilia. *Baillière's Clinical Haematology* **3:** 79–101.
Mann JM, Francis H, Davachi F et al (1986) Risk factors for human immunodeficiency virus seropositivity among children 1–24 months old in Kinshasa, Zaïre. *Lancet* **ii:** 654–657.
Matheron S, Courpotin C, Simon F et al (1990) Vertical transmission of HIV-2. *Lancet* **335:** 1103–1104.
May JT, Stent G, Bishop F & Schnagl D (1990) Prevalence of antibody to human T-lymphotropic virus type-1 (HTLV-1) in Australian aborigines, and detection in Indonesian sera. *Acta Virologica (Praha)* **34:** 80–84.
Meytes D, Schochat B, Lee H et al (1990) Serological and molecular survey for HTLV-I infection in a high-risk Middle Eastern group. *Lancet* **336:** 1533–1535.
Mingiele M (1990) Le sida chez l'infant, le role de la transfusion sanguine: à propos de 77 observations réalisées à l'hôpital pédiatrique de Kalembe lembe à Kinshasa, Zaïre. *Afrique Médicale* **29:** 466–480.
Miotti PG, Dallabetta G, Ndovi E et al (1990) HIV-1 and pregnant women: associated factors, prevalence, estimate of incidence and role in fetal wastage in central Africa. *AIDS* **4:** 733–736.
Mir N, Costello C, Lukit J et al (1988) HIV disease and bone marrow changes. A study of 60 cases. *European Journal of Haematology* **42:** 339–343.
Molgaard CA, Eisenman PA, Ryden LA & Golbeck AL (1989) Neuroepidemiology of human T-lymphotrophic virus type-I-associated tropical spastic paraparesis. *Neuroepidemiology* **8:** 109–123.
Montaner JG, Fanning M, Gelmon K et al (1990) The effect of zidovudine on platelet counts in HIV infected individuals. *AIDS* **3:** 565–570.
Montgomery RD (1989) HTLV-1 and tropical spastic paraparesis. 1. Clinical features, pathology and epidemiology. *Transactions of the Royal Society of Tropical Medicine and Hygiene* **83:** 724–728.
Moody HR, Thomas MAB, Christiansen K & Bucens MR (1990) Risk of HTLV-1 transmission in renal transplantation among Aborigines. *Medical Journal of Australia* **153:** 564–565.

Morgan G, Wilkins HA, Pepin J et al (1990) AIDS following mother-to-child transmission of HIV-2. *AIDS* **4:** 879–882.
Morgan OS, Rodgers Johnson P, Mora C & Char G (1989) HTLV-1 and polymyositis in Jamaica. *Lancet* **ii:** 1184–1187.
Mowbray J, Mawson S, Chawira A et al (1989) Epidemiology of human T-cell leukaemia/lymphoma virus type 1 (HTLV-1) infections in a subpopulation of Afro-Caribbean origin in England. *Journal of Medical Virology* **29:** 289–295.
Murphy EL, Figueroa JP, Gibbs WN et al (1989) Sexual transmission of human T-lymphotropic virus type I (HTLV-I). *Annals of Internal Medicine* **111:** 555–560.
Murphy MF, Metcalf P, Waters AH et al (1987) Incidence and mechanism of neutropenia and thrombocytopenia in patients with human immunodeficiency virus infection. *British Journal of Haematology* **66:** 337–340.
Murthy A, Ho D & Goetz MB (1991) Relationship between acute myelomonoblastic leukaemia and infection due to human immunodeficiency virus. *Reviews of Infectious Diseases* **13:** 254–256.
Naik TN, Sarkar S, Singh HL et al (1991) Intravenous drug users—a new high-risk group for HIV infection in India. *AIDS* **5:** 117–118.
Namik TS, Boone DC & Meyer PR (1987) A comparison of bone marrow findings in patients with acquired immunodeficiency syndrome (AIDS and AIDS related conditions). *Hematology/Oncology Clinics of North America* **5:** 99–106.
Newton M, Cruickshank K, Miller D et al (1987) Antibody to human T-lymphotropic virus type 1 in West-Indian born UK residents with spastic paraparesis. *Lancet* **i:** 415–416.
Nicholas-Randeggar J, Brunet L, Wilson A et al (1989) Modes de contamination des enfants à Pointe Noire (Congo). *Abstracts of the IV International Conference on AIDS and Associated Cancers in Africa*, Marseille, 82.
Nick S, Chimfuembe E, Hunsmann G & Fleming AF (1991) Simple and inexpensive detection and confirmation of anti HIV-1 in sera in Africa. *AIDS* **5:** 232–233.
Okpara RA, Williams EE, Schneider J et al (1986) Antibodies to human T-cell leukemia virus types I and III in blood donors from Calabar, Nigeria. *Annals of Internal Medicine* **104:** 132.
Okpara RA, Williams EE, Schneider J et al (1988) HTLV-I antibodies in blood donors, patients with leukaemia, acute malaria and multiple blood transfusion recipients in the Cross River State of Nigeria. *East African Medical Journal* **65:** 495–502.
Olivarria F, Mezzano S, Ardiles L et al (1989) Presence of circulating immune complexes in the classic form of haemolytic uraemic syndrome: a constant finding. *Nephron* **52:** 313–316.
Ono K, Shimamoto Y, Suga K et al (1989) Cancer superimposed on adult T-cell leukaemia. *Cancer* **64:** 635–640.
Padian NS, Shiboski SC & Jewell NP (1991) Female-to-male transmission of human immunodeficiency virus. *Journal of the American Medical Association* **266:** 1664–1667.
Pagliuca A, Layton DM, Allen S & Mufti GJ (1988) Hyperinfection with strongyloides after treatment for adult T-cell leukaemia-lymphoma in an African immigrant. *British Medical Journal* **297:** 1456–1457.
Palca J (1991) The sobering geography of AIDS. *Science* **252:** 372–373.
Pan X-Z, Qiu Z-D, Chein N et al (1991) A seroepidemiological survey of HTLV-I infection in Shanghai and Chongqing cities in China. *AIDS* **5:** 782–783.
Peckham CS, Tedder RS, Briggs M et al (1990) Prevalence of maternal HIV infection based on unlinked anonymous testing of newborn babies. *Lancet* **335:** 516–519.
Peixinho ZF, Mendes NF, Longo IM et al (1990) Seroepidemiological studies of HIV-1 infection in large Brazilian cities. *Natural Immunity Cell Growth Regulation* **9:** 133–136.
Perchoka LA & Rodgers GM (1988) Hematological aspects of human immunodeficiency virus infection: laboratory and clinical considerations. *American Journal of Hematology* **29:** 94.
Peters BS, Mathews J, Gompels M et al (1990) Acute myeloblastic leukaemia in AIDS. *AIDS* **4:** 367.
Peters BS, Beck EJ, Coleman DG et al (1991) Changing disease patterns in patients with AIDS in a referral centre in the United Kingdom: the changing face of AIDS. *British Medical Journal* **302:** 203–207.
Plummer FA, Nagelkerke NJD, Moses S et al (1991) The importance of core groups is the epidemiology and control of HIV-1 infection. *AIDS* **5** (supplement 1): S169–S176.

Poiesz BJ, Ruscetti FW, Gadzar AF et al (1980a) Detection and isolation of type C retrovirus particles from fresh and cultured lymphocytes of a patient with cutaneous T cell lymphoma. *Proceedings of the National Academy of Sciences of the USA* **77:** 7415–7419.

Poiesz BJ, Ruscetti FW, Mier JW et al (1980b) T-cell lines established from human T-lymphocyte neoplasias by direct response to T-cell growth factor. *Proceedings of the National Academy of Sciences of the USA* **77:** 6815–6819.

Pokrovsky VV & Eramova EU (1989) Nosocomial outbreak of HIV infection in Elista, USSR. *Abstracts of the V International Conference on AIDS, Montreal*, WA 05.

Pombo de Oliveira MS, Matutes E, Famadas LC et al (1990) Adult T-cell leukaemia/lymphoma in Brazil and its relation to HTLV-I. *Lancet* **336:** 987–990.

Poshyachinda V (1990) *Overview of human immunodeficiency virus infection in Thailand: a concise review of status and epidemiology*. Bangkok Institute of Health and Research, Chulalongkorn University.

Potts M, Anderson R & Boily M-C (1991) Slowing the spread of human immunodeficiency virus in developing countries. *Lancet* **338:** 608–613.

Quinn TC, Zacarias FRK & St. John RK (1989) HIV and HTLV-I infections in the Americas: a regional perspective. *Medicine* **68:** 189–209.

Rabkin CS, Biggar RJ & Horm JW (1991) Increasing incidence of cancers associated with the human immunodeficiency virus epidemic. *International Journal of Cancer* **47:** 692–696.

Reeves WC, Levine PH, Cuevas M et al (1990) Seroepidemiology of human T cell lymphotropic virus in the Republic of Panama. *American Journal of Tropical Medicine and Hygiene* **42:** 374–379.

Richman DD, Fischl MA, Grieco MH et al (1987) The toxicity of AZT in the treatment of patients with AIDS and AIDS related complex. *New England Journal of Medicine* **317:** 192.

Roman GC, Roman LN, Spencer PS & Schoenberg BS (1985) Tropical spastic paraparesis: a neuroepidemiological study in Colombia. *Annals of Neurology* **17:** 361–365.

Rosser SV (1991) AIDS and women. *AIDS Education and Prevention* **3:** 230–240.

Rübsamen-Waigmann H, Briesen HV, Maniar JK et al (1991) Spread of HIV-2 in India. *Lancet* **337:** 550–551.

Rwandan HIV Seroprevalence Study Group (1989) Nationwide community based serological survey of HIV-1 and other human retrovirus infections in a Central African country. *Lancet* **i:** 941–943.

Ryder RW & Temmerman M (1991) The effect of HIV-1 infection during pregnancy and the perinatal period on maternal and child-health in Africa. *AIDS* **5** (supplement 1)**:** S75–S85.

Ryder RW, Nsa W, Hassig SE et al (1989) Perinatal transmission of the human immunodeficiency virus type 1 to infants of seropositive women in Zaïre. *New England Journal of Medicine* **320:** 1637–1642.

Ryder RW, Manzila T, Baende E et al (1991) Evidence from Zaïre that breast-feeding by HIV-1-seropositive mothers is not a major route for perinatal HIV-1 transmission but does decrease morbidity. *AIDS* **5:** 709–714.

Sadhana S, Sathe, Gascone P, Lo W et al (1990) Severe anemia is an important negative predictor for survival with disseminated MAI in acquired immunodeficiency syndrome. *American Review of Respiratory Disease* **142:** 1307–1311.

St Louis ME, Rauch KJ, Petersen LR et al (1990) Seroprevalence rates of human immunodeficiency virus infection at sentinel hospitals in the United States. The Sentinel Hospital Surveillance Group. *New England Journal of Medicine* **323:** 213–218.

Sandhaus LM & Scudder R (1989) Haematologic and bone marrow abnormalities in paediatric patients with HIV infection. *Paediatric Pathology* **9:** 277–288.

Saxinger W, Blattner WA, Levine PH et al (1984) Human T-cell leukemia virus (HTLV-I) antibodies in Africa. *Science* **225:** 1473–1476.

Schimpf K, Brackmann HH, Kreuz W et al (1989) Absence of anti-human immunodeficiency virus types 1 and 2 seroconversion after the treatment of hemophilia A or von Willebrand's disease with pasteurized factor VIII concentrate. *New England Journal of Medicine* **321:** 1148–1152.

Schneider DR & Picker LJ (1985) Myelodysplasia in the acquired immunodeficiency syndrome. *American Journal of Clinical Pathology* **84:** 144–152.

Schüpbach J, Baumgartner A & Tomasik Z (1988) HTLV-1 in Switzerland: low prevalence of specific antibodies in HIV risk groups, high prevalence of cross-reactive antibodies in normal blood donors. *International Journal of Cancer* **42:** 857–862.

Schwartz JS, Kinosian BP, Pierskalla WP & Lee H (1990) Strategies for screening blood for human immunodeficiency virus antibody. Use of a decision support system. *Journal of the American Medical Association* **264:** 1704–1710.

Senjuta N, Pavlish O & Gurtsevitch V (1991) Case of adult T-cell leukaemia in HTLV-I infected family in Georgia, USSR. *Lancet* **338:** 1394.

Shayne VT & Kaplan BJ (1991) Double victims: poor women and AIDS. *Women's Health* **17:** 21–37.

Shih LY, Kuo TT, Dunn P & Liaw SJ (1991) Human T-cell lymphotropic virus type I associated with adult T-cell leukaemia/lymphoma in Taiwan Chinese. *British Journal of Haematology* **79:** 156–161.

Sidi Y, Meytes D, Shohat B et al (1990) Adult T-cell lymphoma in Israeli patients of Iranian origin. *Cancer* **65:** 590–593.

Smallman-Raynor MR & Cliff AD (1991) Civil war and the spread of AIDS in Central Africa. *Epidemiology and Infection* **107:** 69–80.

Sng EH, Thirumoorthy T, Levin A et al (1991) Evidence for HTLV-I infection in Singapore prostitutes. *International Journal of Sexually Transmitted Diseases and AIDS* **2:** 172–175.

Soriano V, Leon-Manzon M, Tor J et al (1991) HTLV-I and HTLV-II in Spain. *Abstracts of the VII International Conference on AIDS* **1:** 164.

Spielberg F, Kabeya CM, Quinn TC et al (1990) Performance and cost-effectiveness of a dual rapid assay system for screening and confirmation of human immunodeficiency virus type 1 seropositivity. *Journal of Clinical Microbiology* **28:** 303–306.

Spivak JL, Barnes DC, Fuchs E et al (1989) Serum immunoreactive erythropoietin in HIV infected patients. *Journal of the American Medical Association* **261:** 3104–3107.

Stewart JSW, Matutes E, Lampert IA et al (1984) HTLV-1 positive T-cell lymphoma/leukaemia in an African resident in UK. *Lancet* **ii:** 984–985.

Tajima K (1990) The 4th nation-wide study of adult T-cell leukaemia/lymphoma (ATL) in Japan: estimates of risk of ATL and its geographical and clinical features. The T- and B-cell Malignancy Study Group. *International Journal of Cancer* **45:** 237–243.

Tajima K, Tominaga S, Suchi T et al (1986) HTLV-I carriers among migrants from an ATL-endemic area to ATL non-endemic metropolitan areas in Japan. *International Journal of Cancer* **37:** 383–387.

Tajima K, Kamura S, Ito S-I et al (1987) Epidemiological features of HTLV-I carriers and incidence of ATL in an ATL-endemic island: a report of the community-based co-operative study in Tsushima, Japan. *International Journal of Cancer* **40:** 741–746.

Takatsuki K, Yamaguchi K, Kawano F et al (1985) Clinical aspects of adult T-cell leukaemia-lymphoma. *Current Topics in Microbiology and Immunology* **115:** 89–97.

Takayanagui OM, Cantos JLS & Jardim E (1991) Tropical spastic paraparesis in Brazil. *Lancet* **337:** 309.

Temmerman M, Plummer FA, Mirza NB et al (1990) Infection with HIV as a risk factor for adverse obstetrical outcome. *AIDS* **4:** 1087–1093.

Tozzi A, Pezzotti P & Greco D (1990) Does breast-feeding delay progression to AIDS in HIV-infected children? *AIDS* **4:** 1293–1304.

Treacy M, Lai L, Costello C et al (1987) Peripheral blood and bone marrow abnormalities in patients with HIV related disease. *British Journal of Haematology* **65:** 289–294.

Uchiyama T, Yodoi J, Sagawa K et al (1977) Adult T-cell leukemia: clinical and hematologic features of 16 cases. *Blood* **50:** 482–492.

Uchiyama T, Hori T, Tsudo M et al (1985) Interleukin-2 receptor (Tac antigen) expressed on adult T cell leukaemia cells. *Journal of Clinical Investigation* **76:** 446–453.

van den Hoek JAR, Al EJM, Huisman JG et al (1991) Low prevalence of human T-cell leukaemia virus-I and -II infection among drug users in Amsterdam, The Netherlands. *Journal of Medical Virology* **34:** 100–103.

Van de Perre P, Simonon A, Msellatin P et al (1991) Postnatal transmission of human immunodeficiency virus type 1 from mother to infant. *New England Journal of Medicine* **325:** 593–598.

Varmus H (1988) Retroviruses. *Science* **240:** 1427–1435.

Verdier M, Denis F, Sangare A et al (1989) Prevalence of antibody to human T cell leukaemia virus type 1 (HTLV-1) in populations of Ivory Coast, West Africa. *Journal of Infectious Diseases* **160:** 363–370.

Verdier M, Denis F, Sangara A et al (1990) Antibodies to human T lymphotropic virus type 1 in

patients with leprosy in tropical areas. *Journal of Infectious Diseases* **161:** 1309–1310.
Vranckx R, Coenjaert A & Muylle LA (1990) Seroepidemiological survey of HTLV-I/HTLV-II in selected Belgian populations. *AIDS Research and Human Retroviruses* **6:** 827–830.
Wahden MH (1989) The evolving epidemiology of AIDS and HIV infection in the Eastern Mediterranean Region WHO. *Eastern Mediterranean Region Epidemiology Bulletin* **15:** 6–13.
Walsh CM, Nardi NA & Karpatkin S (1986) One of the mechanisms of thrombocytopenic purpura in homosexual men. *New England Journal of Medicine* **104:** 47.
Weber J (1989) HTLV-1 and tropical spastic paraparesis. 2. The human T-cell lymphotropic virus type 1. *Transactions of the Royal Society of Tropical Medicine and Hygiene* **83:** 729–731.
Weiss R, Cheinsong-Popov R, Clayden S et al (1986) Lack of HTLV-1 antibodies in Africans. *Nature* **319:** 794–795.
Wendler I, Schneider J, Gras B et al (1986) Seroepidemiology of human immunodeficiency virus in Africa. *British Medical Journal* **293:** 782–783.
Wilkins HA, Chan K, Hayes RJ et al (1989) Risk factors for HIV-2 infection in the Gambia. *Abstracts of the IV International Conference on AIDS and Associated Cancers in Africa*, Marseille, 4.
Williams CKO (1986) AIDS and cancer in Nigerians. *Lancet* **i:** 36–37.
Williams CKO, Alabi GO, Junaid TA et al (1984) Human T-cell leukaemia virus associated lymphoproliferative disease: report of two cases in Nigeria. *British Medical Journal* **288:** 1495–1496.
Willocks L, Ludlam CA & Welsby PD (1990) Polycythaemia and HIV infection. *Lancet* **336:** 812.
World Health Organization (1991) Global programme on AIDS: HIV and HBV transmission in the health care setting. *Weekly Epidemiology Record* **66:** 189–191.
Worm AM & Kvinesdal B (1990) Human immunodeficiency virus surveillance at a sexually transmitted disease clinic in Copenhagen. *International Journal of Sexually Transmitted Diseases and AIDS* **1:** 107–109.
Yanagihara R, Ajdukiewicz AB, Garruto RM et al (1991a) Human T-lymphotropic virus type I infection in the Solomon Islands. *American Journal of Tropical Medicine and Hygiene* **44:** 122–130.
Yanagihara R, Nerurkar VR & Ajdukiewicz AB (1991b) Comparison between strains of human T lymphotropic virus type I isolated from inhabitants of the Solomon Islands and Papua New Guinea. *Journal of Infectious Diseases* **164:** 443–449.
Yoshida M, Miyoshi I & Hinuma Y (1982) Isolation and characterization of retrovirus from cell lines of human adult-T-cell leukemia and its implication in the disease. *Proceedings of the National Academy of Sciences of the USA* **79:** 2031–2035.
Yoshida M, Osame M, Usuhku K et al (1987) Viruses detected in HTLV-I associated myelopathy and adult T-cell leukaemia are identical on DNA blotting. *Lancet* **i:** 1085–1086.
Zella D, Mori L, Sala M et al (1990) HTLV-II infection in Italian drug abusers. *Lancet* **336:** 575–576.
Zon LI, Arkin C & Groopman J (1987) Haematological manifestations of the human immunodeficiency virus (HIV). *British Journal of Haematology* **66:** 251.

3

Anaemia of *Plasmodium falciparum* malaria

RODNEY E. PHILLIPS
GEOFFREY PASVOL

Malaria remains a disease of major health and economic importance in many parts of the world. Unfortunately, estimates of mortality and morbidity caused by the disease are incomplete, largely because of the difficulty in attributing death or illness to malaria in a population where multiple pathology is common, and where a large proportion may harbour malarial parasites and yet remain asymptomatic. As a result, estimates that there are over 250 million clinical cases of malaria worldwide each year, and that over 1 million children die of the disease each year in Africa may well be inaccurate. Mortality from malaria is largely due to *Plasmodium falciparum* and therefore the anaemia caused by this parasite will dominate the discussion.

THE IMPORTANCE OF THE ANAEMIA OF MALARIA

The clinical manifestations of malaria vary from a mild flu-like illness to unrousable coma. In cerebral malaria, which is often heralded by convulsions, there is a rapid deterioration in conscious level, leading to coma. Such a clinical presentation is reasonably characteristic, although it can be mimicked by meningoencephalitis, drug overdose and head injury. However, other manifestations of severe malaria, such as anaemia, are less dramatic, and, while severe anaemia may be recognized clinically, it is not often ascribed to malaria. In many cases, by the time the patient has developed anaemia the peripheral parasitaemia may be scanty, and in some cases absent. Moreover, the clinical picture may be complicated when cardiac failure supervenes. For example we have observed a number of children in Africa, who have died shortly after admission to hospital, in whom a clinical diagnosis of 'pneumonia' has been made but in whom haemoglobin estimation and a blood film have indicated that malarial anaemia leading to cardiac failure was a far more likely cause of death. These anecdotal observations require confirmation but emphasise the potential for misdiagnosis of malarial anaemia.

Mortality

There is little formal documentation of the lethal potential of acute malarial

Baillière's Clinical Haematology—
Vol. 5, No. 2, April 1992
ISBN 0-7020-1627-6

anaemia. In this context it is probably useful to quote figures from the Garki project in northern Nigeria where antimalarial measures, which consisted of mass drug administration, spraying with insecticide and the use of larvicide, resulted in an infant mortality rate of 55 per 1000 per year in the protected villages as compared with a rate of 135 per 1000 per year in the unprotected villages (a reduction of about 60%). In the 1–4 year age group, the mortality rate was also reduced by 60% (from 154 to 61 per 1000 per year) (Molineaux and Gramiccia, 1980). Whilst these figures are dramatic, they unfortunately do not indicate the reduction due to the prevention of malarial anaemia.

Anaemia in malarial areas is often multifactorial, with the different causes interacting in a vicious cycle of nutritional deficiencies, including those of iron and folate, infections such as pneumonia and gastroenteritis, and inherited red cell disorders. A severe attack of malaria may itself prove fatal and anaemia may be the principal cause of death. Statistics from Nigeria (Bruce-Chwatt, 1952) and the Gambia (Greenwood et al, 1987) emphasize the importance of malaria as a cause of childhood mortality, but neither specify the relative role of malarial anaemia. Malaria as a cause of death was found in 9.9% of all autopsies in children under 15 years old between 1933 and 1950 in Lagos, Nigeria (Bruce-Chwatt, 1952). In Uganda, 16% of deaths in infants were attributed to malarial anaemia (Davies, 1948).

Severe falciparum malaria in patients of all ages is frequently accompanied by a life-threatening fall in haematocrit which necessitates treatment with transfusion (Phillips et al, 1986; Warrell et al, 1990). In children, the cause of death during an attack of malaria is often unclear, although anaemia is almost invariably present (Molyneux et al, 1989). Although falciparum malaria is recognized as an important cause of death in endemic areas, the contribution of anaemia to malaria mortality has not as yet been fully assessed.

Morbidity

Morbidity caused by malarial anaemia is considerable. In the Gambia many children aged 1–4 years had anaemia which was primarily associated with malaria parasitaemia (McGregor et al, 1966; Greenwood et al, 1987). The association of asexual parasitaemia, a fall in haemoglobin (Hb) coincident with the rainy season, and the lower Hb levels observed in children with splenic enlargement, implicate malaria as an important cause of anaemia in this part of the world.

In our continuing study of severe malaria in children at Kilifi on the coast of Kenya, 109 (25%) of the 452 paediatric patients admitted to the ward with the primary diagnosis of falciparum malaria had an Hb of less than 50 g/l. Only 52 (12%) patients had case-definition cerebral malaria (unrousable coma with peripheral parasitaemia in which other causes of coma have been excluded). Thus in east Africa there were twice as many admissions with malarial anaemia compared with cerebral malaria. In contrast, in a study of 650 children with severe malaria in west Africa in the Gambia, 66% had cerebral malaria and the rest had severe malarial anaemia (Hb <50 g/l), i.e. the ratio of cerebral malaria to severe malarial anaemia was reversed (Hill et al, 1991). In a further study carried out in Maputo, Mozambique, 32% of the 419 patients under the age of 8 admitted over a 10 day period had cerebral malaria and 28% had severe malarial anaemia (T. Solomon et al, unpublished observations). Whilst there may be many simple explanations for the differences in the ratios of cerebral to anaemic cases, such as the referral patterns to hospital, these figures highlight the relative importance of severe anaemia due to malaria, especially in situations where the more dramatic presentation of cerebral malaria might overshadow its presence. One tantalizing explanation for the inverse relationship between cerebral malaria and anaemia is the possibility that a low Hb level might protect against the development of cerebral malaria. Patients with packed cell volumes <0.20 had a significantly lower chance of having convulsions than those with packed cell volumes of >0.30 (Hendrickse et al, 1971). Alternatively, the pathogenesis of the two conditions might be quite different.

THE NATURAL HISTORY OF MALARIAL ANAEMIA

The course of anaemia caused by malaria is variable but two major clinical patterns emerge. In the first, patients suffering severe acute attacks of malaria and who are seen early after the onset of the clinical symptoms are not anaemic. However, anaemia develops during the course of the infection, its complications and its aftermath (Phillips et al, 1986). It has become clear that the causes of anaemia in malaria, even in these acute episodes, are multifactorial and that they might differ according to the stage of the malarial infection. In a study of uncomplicated falciparum malaria, patients seen within 24 to 48 hours of the onset of fever were usually not anaemic, but there was a steady fall in haematocrit over the next 4–5 days, and this continued well after the peripheral blood parasitaemia had been cleared (Phillips et al, 1986). Uninfected red cells were of normal shape, size and colour, without evidence of fragmentation or spherocytosis. The reticulocyte response to this rapidly developing anaemia was usually brisk, but only once the parasites had been cleared. If the parasite clearance was delayed, the reticulocyte count did not rise despite a severe progressive fall in haematocrit. This delay in reticulocyte response associated with persistent parasitaemia would suggest that the parasites themselves are in some way responsible for the inhibition of erythropoiesis or for suppression of the release of new red cells into the peripheral circulation. Three phases in which the haematocrit falls during treatment have been identified, the first as a result of rehydration, the second correlating with the fall in parasitaemia, and the third indicating a loss of uninfected cells (Davis et al, 1990). The marked persistence of anaemia in this setting has been related to shortened red blood survival of uninfected cells (Weatherall et al, 1983) and to bone marrow suppression following repeated attacks of malaria (Abdalla et al, 1980).

The second pattern in the clinical evolution of anaemia in the context of malaria occurs particularly in an endemic area. Patients are usually children and are clearly anaemic when first seen. The history is usually one of intermittent fevers and general symptoms of ill health occurring insidiously over weeks rather than days. Splenomegaly of varying degree is present on examination and the peripheral blood film shows scanty asexual parasitaemia. In many cases gametocytaemia and malarial pigment in phagocytic cells are seen. Attributing the cause of this anaemia is often difficult, and some sources have included a maximum arbitrary Hb and minimum parasitaemia (Hb <50 g/l in the presence of parasitaemia more than 10 000/μl) to define malarial anaemia (Warrell et al, 1990). This should, however, be regarded rather as a strict research definition.

Sequential studies have emphasized the difficulty of analysing the various mechanisms that contribute to the development of the anaemia of malaria. There is still no comprehensive understanding of the relative contributions made by intravascular haemolysis, extravascular clearance of red blood cells and marrow dysfunction, but a clearer picture is beginning to emerge.

PATHOPHYSIOLOGY

In this section we will review mechanisms which have been described as causing or contributing to the anaemia associated with human falciparum malaria. In the simplest terms anaemia occurs when red cells are destroyed more rapidly than they can be replaced, or when red cell production falls below the minimal level required to maintain the steady state. In malaria both processes are involved, although the relative importance of these mechanisms seems to vary in different clinical situations.

Increased red blood cell destruction

Non-immune mediated haemolysis

Invasion of red cells by parasites, followed by rupture or clearance of these cells by the reticuloendothelial system (RES), inevitably shortens their life span. Whilst there is often correlation between parasitaemia on admission and the severity of anaemia that develops subsequently in both adults (Phillips et al, 1986) and children (Molyneux et al, 1989) with cerebral malaria, in many cases where the onset is insidious there is no correlation between the degree of anaemia and the peripheral parasitaemia.

Parasite destruction of red cells in deep vascular beds may cause losses that are not apparent in studies confined to the peripheral blood (Clark and Tomlinson, 1949; Davis et al, 1990). Weiss (1983) has shown that, in *P. berghei* infections, parasite cycling in the vascular sinuses rather than in the haemopoietic tissue of the bone marrow of A/J mice helps to propagate the infection, particularly as it leads to the juxtaposition of schizont and uninfected red cell (usually a reticulocyte). In addition, there was evidence of phagocytosis by macrophages of parasitized red cells, parasites and uninfected cells.

A similar process appears to occur in malaria in humans, with evidence of macrophage-mediated destruction of parasitized red blood cells (PRBC) in bone marrow. Histological studies of the marrow in falciparum malaria showed large numbers of parasitized cells in the sinusoids where reinvasion of newly released red blood cells would be likely to occur (Wickramasinghe et al, 1987), although in another study very few schizonts were detected in bone marrow aspirates (Smalley et al, 1980). Obstruction of the microvasculature may lead to marrow hypoxia and interfere with the release of reticulocytes, accounting for their absence in the peripheral blood during acute malarial attack. Electronmicroscopic studies of the spleen in patients who died with severe malaria showed extensive phagocytosis of PRBC; most available evidence implicates the spleen and the bone marrow as favoured sites for PRBC destruction (Spitz, 1946; Clark and Tomlinson, 1949; Abdalla et al, 1980; N. Francis, personal communication).

It has been argued for many years that non-parasitized red blood cells (NPRBC) are also removed prematurely from the circulation in malaria (Zuckerman, 1964; Adner et al, 1968). This concept was supported by studies in *P. berghei* infections, where clearance of NPRBC transfused into uninfected mice was more rapid than the clearance of their own red cells (Howard and Mitchell, 1979), suggesting an *intrinsic* red cell defect. Red cell survival studies in man also suggested accelerated removal (Rosenberg et al, 1973), and this has been confirmed in cross-transfusion experiments in patients recovering from *P. falciparum* infection (Looareesuwan et al, 1987a). In these studies, patients, most of whom had had uncomplicated malaria, had a modest reduction in survival of chromium-labelled autologous cells. When labelled compatible cells taken from an *uninfected* donor were transfused into patients convalescing from malaria, the survival of these cells was even shorter than that of autologous cells (Looareesuwan et al, 1987a). These studies therefore, in contrast to those in mice, suggest a defect *extrinsic* to red cells, such as hypersplenism. However, they do not exclude the possibility of opsonization or changes in surface charge of these NPRBC, which could occur shortly after transfusion. Certainly the increased rate of vascular clearance of injected particles, such as colloidal carbon, in infected animals with malaria (Cantrell et al, 1970), and of ^{125}I-labelled microaggregated serum albumin in patients with malaria (Sheagren et al, 1970), would suggest RES hyperactivity.

Phospholipid asymmetry in the lipid bilayer of the membrane is also thought to occur in malaria (Gupta et al, 1982) and exposure of phosphatidylserine in the outer leaflet may lead to recognition and phagocytosis by macrophages. The postulated mechanisms by which uninfected red cells may be recognized and removed from the circulation are shown in Table 1.

Immune-mediated haemolysis

Considerable effort has been expended in searching for an immune basis for the haemolysis observed in malaria. In 1908, Christophers and Bentley contrasted the extraordinary degree of haemolysis despite the paucity of malaria parasites in the blood of patients with blackwater fever. This raised the possibility that an autoimmune process might be involved which could account for the accelerated destruction of uninfected cells. However, early

Table 1. Proposed mechanisms of removal of uninfected cells in *P. falciparum* malaria.

Antibody sensitization
- Autoantibodies
- Antibodies to adsorbed antigens, e.g. EBA 175 (Camus and Hadley, 1985)
- Antibodies within immune complexes binding via C3b receptors (Facer et al, 1979)

Other mechanisms
Intrinsic
- Sodium pump changes (Dunn, 1969)
- Modified plasma membrane phospholipid changes (Gupta et al, 1982)
- Modification in cholesterol content (Vial and Phillippot, 1984)

Extrinsic
- Macrophage activation
- Hypersplenism

efforts failed to detect circulating haemolysins in malaria (Dudgeon and Clark, 1918; Fairley and Bromfield, 1934). Although serum haemolytic activity was not considered an essential pathological marker or a factor in autoimmune anaemia (Dacie and Worlledge, 1969), more precise investigation required reagents capable of detecting putative opsonins on the surface of red cells.

Most studies agree that there is a correlation between malarial infection and the development of a positive direct Coombs' antiglobulin test (DAT) (Table 2), but no one has been able to show conclusively that a positive DAT

Table 2. Sensitization of red cells in *P. falciparum* malaria.

Specificity	Reference
Not specified	Topley (1968)
IgM	Rosenberg et al (1973)
C3b	Greenwood et al (1978)
C3d/IgG	Facer et al (1979)
C3/IgG & C3	Abdalla and Weatherall (1982)
IgG	Jeje et al (1983)
IgG1	Merry et al (1986)

causes the anaemia. Over the last 20 years immunoglobulin (Ig) G and complement C3 have been detected on the surface of erythrocytes in children recovering from falciparum malaria (Topley et al, 1973; Greenwood et al, 1978; Facer et al, 1979, Abdalla et al, 1980; Abdalla and Weatherall, 1982; Jeje et al, 1983). The discovery of a high frequency ($\pm$ 50%) of positive DATs in African children gave some support to the autoimmune hypothesis (Abdalla and Weatherall, 1982), although Abdalla failed to find any correlation between a positive DAT and anaemia.

Facer has argued strongly that immune sensitization accelerates haemolysis in Gambian children with malaria (Facer et al, 1979; Facer, 1980). Quantitative studies have shown, however, that small increases in the IgG coating on red cell surfaces can produce a positive DAT without decreasing red cell survival (Merry and Thompson, 1984). In controlled studies in Thailand, Merry et al (1986) found that the incidence of a positive DAT in uncomplicated malaria (16.4%) was considerably higher than that found in normal Europeans (0.007–0.01%) and in healthy Thai controls (4.5%), but the serological reactions were weak. Furthermore, when the number of molecules of IgG bound per cell were compared there was no significant difference between those with uncomplicated malaria and controls. These low levels of coating are most unlikely to have caused accelerated destruction by the RES (Van der Meulen et al, 1980; Merry and Thompson, 1984). For example, in the study by Jeje et al (1983), the number of molecules of red cell-associated IgG in patients with and without malaria was 629 compared with 395. Whilst these figures might be statistically significant, the difference is unlikely to influence red cell survival.

It remains possible that complement activation could cause haemolysis and yet be undetected by crude antibodies, particularly if a sensitized subpopulation of cells were removed from the circulation before the assay was performed. Using well-characterized reagents, we were unable to detect red cell membrane-bound complement in both severe malaria and blackwater fever in patients from Thailand (A.H. Merry, R.E. Phillips, et al, unpublished observations).

Thus there is a dearth of convincing evidence that antibody-mediated autoimmunity plays an important role in the anaemia of falciparum malaria. In many malarious populations, a positive DAT is common, as are other tests for autoantibodies such as antinuclear and anti-single-stranded DNA (Adu et al, 1982), but this should not be construed to be adequate evidence for autoimmune haemolytic anaemia. Antibody could also be directed against parasite antigen specifically adsorbed onto the surface of the infected cells, as is the case with the 175 kDa erythrocyte binding antigen (EBA) (Camus and Hadley, 1985). Alternatively, malaria antigen–antibody complexes containing complement may bind to the surface of uninfected cells via the C3b receptor (Facer et al, 1979). The failure of corticosteroids to alter red cell survival in acute falciparum malaria is a further pointer that explanations for haemolysis in patients must be sought elsewhere (Charoenlarp et al, 1979).

Heat-damaged red cells and red cells deliberately coated with IgG were removed more rapidly from the circulation of malaria patients than controls (Looareesuwan et al, 1987b; Lee et al, 1989). In these experiments the red cell changes were contrived, but normal donor red cells were also rapidly cleared in similar patients (Looareesuwan et al, 1987b). Even this last experiment cannot be definitive, as conventional cross-matching techniques may fail to detect minor incompatibility, but there is much which points to enhanced clearance by the RES. Whether this is partly mechanical (filtration by a large spleen) or much more subtly mediated by specific red cell–macrophage interactions is unclear.

Decreased red cell production

Morphological bone marrow abnormalities

After repeated attacks of malaria, the bone marrow may be slate grey or black because of the accumulation of malaria pigment (Maegraith, 1948).

Microscopic abnormalities in the marrow which have been reported include aberrations of erythroblast morphology and macrophage hyperplasia (Knuttgen, 1963), erythroid hypoplasia (Srichaikul et al, 1969), failure of reticulocyte release, macrophage hyperplasia (Knuttgen, 1963) and lymphoid hyperplasia (Taliaferro and Mulligan, 1937). Parasites were not found within erythroblasts, presumably reflecting the physical separation of haemopoietic and intravascular compartments; nucleated erythroid precursors can be easily infected *in vitro* (Pasvol and Jungery, 1983).

Dyserythropoiesis

Recent studies of the bone marrow in malaria have identified morphological abnormalities in the erythroid series, collectively termed 'dyserythropoiesis'. These changes are thought to contribute to both the slow recovery observed after a single attack of malaria and the persistent anaemia in individuals subject to prolonged parasitaemia (Abdalla et al, 1980). However, it should be remembered that dyserythropoiesis is not specific for malaria and may occur in other conditions such as vitamin B_{12} and folate deficiency.

Dyserythropoiesis was common in patients with cerebral malaria (Wickramasinghe et al, 1987). The most frequent abnormalities were irregularly shaped nuclei and karyorrhexis. There were also substantial increases in eosinophil granulocytes, plasma cells and especially macrophages (Wickramasinghe et al, 1987). Macrophages frequently contained parasitized red blood cells. Startling changes were also seen in the marrow sinusoids; a high proportion of red cells were parasitized and these cells were tightly packed. Intravascular PRBC usually showed many knobs and these were in close contact with sinusoidal endothelial cells. Some PRBC showed complex interdigitations with adjacent endothelial cells. Thus marrow destruction of erythroid precursors in cerebral malaria may result from dyserythropoiesis and from extensive sequestration of PRBC. Sinusoids were so tightly packed that slowing of blood flow could well lead to hypoxia within the marrow spaces.

While dyserythropoiesis is more common and more extensive in patients with *P. falciparum* infections (Abdalla et al, 1980; Dormer et al, 1983; Phillips et al, 1986), it may occur also in the marrow of patients with *P. vivax* malaria, in which sequestration is said not to occur (Knuttgen, 1987; Wickramasinghe et al, 1989). The main morphological changes include multinuclearity of the normoblasts, intercytoplasmic bridging, karyorrhexis and incomplete and unequal mitotic nuclear divisions. Erythroblast nuclei may be grossly distorted, appearances which suggest severe disturbances of nuclear maturation and division (Knuttgen, 1987). In Thai patients these changes have been observed up to 25 days after commencing treatment for malaria (Phillips et al, 1986). Studies of marrow function strongly suggested that dyserythropoiesis reflects ineffective red cell production (Dormer et al, 1983). Gambian children whose marrows showed dyserythropoietic changes had an increased proportion of red cell precursors in G_2, with an arrest during the progress of cell division through the S phase (Wickramasinghe et al, 1982). These marrow abnormalities contrast with Fleming's description of florid megaloblastic erythropoiesis in the African women who have been severely anaemic with malaria, pregnancy and folate deficiency (Fleming and Allan, 1969). Most studies in Thailand and the Gambia did not find evidence of haematinic deficiency in malaria patients, although changes in iron metabolism were detected (Abdalla et al, 1980; Phillips et al, 1986). It is difficult to assess the contribution dyserythropoiesis makes to the anaemia of malaria. Abdalla et al (1980) linked dyserythropoiesis to persistent anaemia in Gambian children, and speculated that repeated attacks of malaria caused chronic marrow damage. However, the same morphological changes have been seen in acute, uncomplicated falciparum malaria (Phillips et al, 1986) and in *P. vivax* infections where anaemia is usually not severe (Wickramasinghe et al, 1989). The mechanism which damages the marrow is unknown. Injected tumour necrosis factor (TNF) can produce changes resembling dyserythropoiesis in an experimental animal-infected model (Clark and Chaudhri, 1988), and the anaemia of mouse malaria has been inhibited by administering neutralizing antibody specific to mouse TNF. Although there is an association between high TNF concentrations and severe malaria, no causal link has been established. In addition, in animal models at least, there does not appear to be any defect in erythropoietin production (Villeval et al, 1990). During the anaemic phase of malaria in mice, plasma levels of erythropoietin were raised equally in both fatal and non-fatal infections.

Malarial anaemia and parvovirus infection

Whilst the predominant bone marrow findings in malaria are those of dyserythropoiesis, marrow aplasia or hypoplasia has been demonstrated in some cases (Srichaikul et al, 1967; Abdalla et al, 1980). These have occurred largely in acute cases, and have been assumed to be due to the malarial infection itself, although other causes have not been excluded. Recent evidence has focused on the temporary cessation (about 7–10 days) of haematopoiesis caused by human parvovirus B19, which has been shown to be cytotoxic for erythroid progenitor cells (Thorn, 1988). Whilst in most cases in the absence of haemolysis, such short-lived hypoplasia produces only minor falls in Hb level (<10 g/l), in patients with inherited haemolytic anaemias (such as sickle-cell disease, pyruvate kinase deficiency, thalassaemia and hereditary spherocytosis or elliptocytosis) it may cause a dramatic fall. Thus there is no reason why the haemolysis of a common acquired condition, such as malaria, may not result in a particularly severe anaemia in the face of B19 infection. In a pilot study of 24 anaemia patients (haematocrit <0.20) in west Africa, 13 (54%) showed evidence of recent parvovirus B19 infection; of these, seven had positive malarial blood films (Jones et al, 1990). Unfortunately, a non-anaemic control group was not included. During a second visit in the dry season very little anaemia or recent parvovirus B19 infection was detected. However, amongst 81 non-anaemic patients, more than 90% by the age of 2 years showed evidence of past parvovirus B19 infection as evidenced by a positive B19 IgG. On the basis of these data, we postulated that parvovirus B19 may be contributory to a proportion of the severe anaemias seen in young children in Africa. However data from our study in Kilifi in Kenya have not confirmed these findings to date (G. Pasvol, unpublished observations) and only minimal evidence of parvovirus B19 infection has been found in the study population. In any event, parvovirus B19 infection is known to occur in epidemics and the occurrence of such an epidemic in the west African study remains a possibility.

Iron metabolism and malaria

Ferrokinetic studies in malaria have shown decreased iron incorporation into erythroid precursors during acute infection (Srichaikul et al, 1969). During the asexual parasitaemia the serum iron was low and the total iron binding capacity was normal (Abdalla et al, 1980; Phillips et al, 1986). In a study of adults, these changes were found together with stainable iron in the marrow storage elements but not in erythroblasts (Phillips et al, 1986). This picture has been documented in other infections when acute phase reactants are circulating (Esan, 1975). Thus it is possible that a poor marrow response in acute malaria might occur because of the immobilization of iron. Where partial iron deficiency coexists with malaria, especially in areas where hookworm infection is common, iron supply may become inadequate during antimalarial treatment and expansion of the circulating haemoglobin mass.

High serum ferritin concentrations have been found in Asian, African and Melanesian patients with malaria (Oppenheimer et al, 1984; Phillips et al, 1986). The mechanism causing these high levels is likely to be complex. The acute phase response, haemolysis, hepatic damage and possible defective ferritin clearance may all contribute. It is not clear whether this disturbance plays any part in the anaemia of malaria, but it does mean that serum ferritin concentrations must be interpreted carefully in malarious regions.

CHILDHOOD MALARIA AND ANAEMIA

Surveys in the Gambia have shown that children aged 1–4 years have anaemia which becomes worse during the rainy season (Topley, 1968; Greenwood et al, 1987). Haematocrits were lowest in children with detectable parasites, and the strong implication of this work is that control of malaria would considerably alleviate childhood anaemia in the Gambia (Greenwood et al, 1987).

One particularly interesting aspect of severe malarial anaemia in childhood is that the peak age for this complication seems to antedate that of cerebral malaria. Thus, whilst the peak age for malarial anaemia in west Africa was 2 years, the peak incidence for cerebral malaria was 3 years (Brewster et al, 1990). Likewise in east Africa, the mean (SEM) age of 108 patients with severe malarial anaemia was 1.9(0.2) years, whereas for 52 with cerebral malaria it was 3.3(0.3) years (G. Pasvol et al, unpublished observations). The explanations for this are unclear, although in normal development Hb levels are known to reach a nadir by about 1 year of age. It is not known whether those who suffer severe malarial anaemia in early life are the same as those who are more likely to develop cerebral malaria later on, or whether it is this group who are protected from developing cerebral manifestations. It is this sort of important question which the Kilifi project may well answer.

PREGNANCY AND MALARIAL ANAEMIA

Severe anaemia in pregnancy is usually due to multiple aetiology, such as folate deficiency, iron deficiency, haemoglobinopathy and acquired immune deficiency syndrome (AIDS), but falciparum malaria plays a major role in endemic areas (Fleming, 1989).

In parts of the world where malarial transmission is sporadic (i.e. unstable), falciparum infections in all pregnant women, but especially in primigravidae, can produce a dramatic clinical syndrome characterized by coma, hypoglycaemia, pulmonary oedema, anaemia and very high mortality (Warrell et al, 1982, Looareesuwan et al, 1985).

In parts of the world where malarial transmission is intense and levels of acquired immunity high, protective immunity appears to be reduced in pregnancy, especially in primigravidae. Moreover, parasite rates (i.e. the proportion of those with parasitaemia) and densities increase to a maximum in the midtrimester. Demand for folate is high in this situation and folate deficiency is a common complication of malaria during pregnancy; it would seem that the morphological appearances of dyserythropoiesis are unusual (Fleming, 1989). In places such as West Africa, haemolytic anaemia is the predominant clinical finding (Fleming and Allan, 1969). Other manifestations of severe malaria are generally infrequent and malarial parasites may be hard to detect in the blood. Much epidemiological data links this anaemia to malaria (reviewed in Fleming et al, 1986; Fleming, 1989), and effective antimalarial prophylaxis virtually prevents the otherwise inevitable fall in haemocrit (Gilles et al, 1969). In Gilles's study from Ibadan, Nigeria, 63% of untreated women became anaemic (haematocrit <0.28), invariably between the 16th and 24th week of gestation. All anaemic patients had reduced red cell survival, and surface counting studies showed a gradual increase in excess counts over the liver and spleen. Primigravidae are particularly susceptible to anaemia, perhaps because parasitaemias are higher (Gilles et al, 1969). Unchecked, the haemolysis can be severe and life threatening (Fleming and Allan, 1969). When the haematocrit falls below 0.13 and heart failure develops, mortality approaches 50% (Fullerton and Turner, 1962). Lesser degrees of anaemia are associated with placental changes (McGregor et al, 1983) and low fetal birthweight, and in the mother a diminished capacity for work.

GENETIC POLYMORPHISMS AND PROTECTION AGAINST MALARIAL ANAEMIA

Many red cell polymorphisms, such as the sickle-cell trait, thalassaemias, glucose-6-phosphate dehydrogenase deficiency and Melanesian ovalocytosis, are common in areas which are or have been endemic for malaria, and much epidemiological and cellular evidence has accrued over the years to support the hypothesis that these variants are protective against malaria. Supportive data has focused largely on parasite rates, densities and patient mortality, but none of these studies have examined the relationship of these variants and the development of anaemia, one of the two major complications of the disease. Most recently in a large case-control study of 600 cases of severe malaria in the Gambia in west Africa, Hill has shown that a common west African HLA class I antigen (Bw53) is associated with protection (of the order of 40%) against both malarial anaemia and cerebral malaria (Hill et al, 1991). A novel class II haplotype (DRB1*1302–DQB1*0501) was found to provide approximately 55% protection against severe malarial anaemia but not against cerebral malaria. Both the class I and II types were found more frequently in Gambians compared with other racial groups, observations which would further argue that natural selection by malaria has been responsible. The mechanism by which these polymorphisms protect remains to be worked out. One would presume that since red cells express minimal HLA class I molecules on their surface, protection by class I is probably against the liver stage parasites, whereas for class II it would reside with the ability to present blood stage antigen(s) to helper T cells.

SUMMARY

The pathophysiology of the anaemia of falciparum malaria is both complex and multifactorial, and results in a condition which is a major cause of mortality and morbidity in patients, especially children and pregnant women, living in malarial endemic areas. The importance of anaemia as a cause of death in malaria may well be underestimated because of difficulty in diagnosis, especially where parasitaemia may be low and the clinical picture may be confused with other causes of anaemia. Two clinical presentations predominate: severe acute malaria in which anaemia supervenes, and severe anaemia in patients in whom there have been repeated attacks of malaria. The major mechanisms are those of red cell destruction and decreased red cell production. Potential causes of haemolysis include loss of infected cells by rupture or phagocytosis, removal of uninfected cells due to antibody sensitization or other physicochemical membrane changes, and increased reticuloendothelial activity, particularly in organs such as the spleen. Decreased production results from marrow hypoplasia seen in acute infections, and dyserythropoiesis, a morphological appearance, which in functional terms results in ineffective erythropoiesis. The role of parvovirus B19 as a possible cause of bone marrow aplasia in a few cases is postulated.

Finally, there is now evidence which points to genetic factors, HLA associated, which may protect against the development of malarial anaemia and which has become common in areas endemic for malaria.

Acknowledgements

We would like to thank Dina Shah for typing the manuscript and Drs Anthony Scott, Ian Clark, Jan Carlsson, Mary Coates and Barbara Clough for their critical comments. R.E.P. is a Wellcome Trust Senior Clinical Fellow.

REFERENCES

Abdalla S & Weatherall D (1982) The direct antiglobulin test in *P. falciparum* malaria. *British Journal of Haematology* **51:** 415–425.

Abdalla S, Weatherall D, Wickramasinghe S & Hughes M (1980) The anaemia of *P. falciparum* malaria. *British Journal of Haematology* **46:** 171–183.

Adner M, Alstatt L & Conrad M (1968) Coombs-positive haemolytic disease in malaria. *Annals of Internal Medicine* **68:** 33–38.

Adu D, Gwyn Williams D, Quakyi I et al (1982) Anti-ssDNA and antinuclear antibodies in human malaria. *Clinical and Experimental Immunology* **49:** 310–316.

Brewster D, Kwiatkowski D & White N (1990) Neurological sequelae of cerebral malaria in children. *Lancet* **ii:** 1039–1043.

Bruce-Chwatt L (1952) Malaria in African infants and children in southern Nigeria. *Annals of Tropical Medicine* **46:** 173–200.

Camus D & Hadley T (1985) A *Plasmodium falciparum* antigen that binds to host erythrocytes and merozoites. *Science* **230:** 553–556.

Cantrell W, Elko EE & Hopff BM (1970), *Plasmodium berghei:* phagocytic hyperactivity of infected rats. *Experimental Parasitology* **28:** 291–297.

Charoenlarp P, Vanijanonta S & Chantpanyaporn P (1979) The effect of prednisolone on red cell survival in patients with falciparum malaria. *South East Asian Journal of Tropical Medicine and Public Health* **10:** 127–131.

Clark H & Tomlinson W (1949) The pathologic anatomy of malaria. In Boyd MF (ed.) *Malariology*, pp 874–903. Philadelphia: WB Saunders.

Clark I & Chaudhri G (1988) Tumour necrosis factor may contribute to the anaemia of malaria by causing dyserythropoiesis and erythrophagocytosis. *British Journal of Haematology* **70:** 99–103.

Dacie J & Worlledge S (1969) Autoimmune haemolytic anaemic. *Progress in Haematology* **6:** 82–120.

Davies JNP (1948) Pathology of Central African natives: Mulago Hospital post mortem studies. VII: causes of death in African children. *East African Medical Journal* **25:** 228–235.

Davis T, Krishna S, Looareesuwan S et al (1990) Erythrocyte sequestration and anaemia in severe falciparum malaria. Analysis of acute changes in venous hematocrit using a simple mathematical model. *Journal of Clinical Investigation* **86:** 793–800.

Dormer P, Dietrich M, Kern P & Horstmann R (1983) Ineffective erythropoiesis in acute human *P. falciparum* malaria. *Blut* **46:** 279–288.

Dudgeon L & Clarke C (1918) Investigation of fatal cases of pernicious malaria caused by *P. falciparum. Quarterly Journal of Medicine* **12:** 372–390.

Dunn M (1969) Alterations in red cell sodium transport during malarial infection. *Journal of Clinical Investigation* **48:** 674–684.

Esan GJF (1975) Haematological aspects of malaria. *Clinics in Haematology* **4:** 247–256.

Facer C (1980) Direct Coombs antiglobulin reactions in Gambian children with *Plasmodium falciparum* malaria. II. Specificity of erythrocyte-bound IgG. *Clinical and Experimental Immunology* **39:** 279–288.

Facer C, Bray R & Brown J (1979) Direct Coombs antiglobulin reactions in Gambian children with *Plasmodium falciparum* malaria. I. Incidence and class specificity. *Clinical and Experimental Immunology* **35:** 119–127.
Fairley N & Bromfield R (1934) Laboratory studies in malaria and blackwater fever. Part III. A new blood pigment in blackwater fever and other biochemical observations. *Transactions of the Royal Society of Tropical Medicine and Hygiene* **28:** 307–334.
Fleming AF (1989) Tropical obstetrics and gynaecology. 1. Anaemia in pregnancy in tropical Africa. *Transactions of the Royal Society of Tropical Medicine and Hygiene* **83:** 441–448.
Fleming AF & Allan N (1969) Severe haemolytic anaemia in pregnancy in Nigerians treated with prednisolone. *British Medical Journal* **iv:** 461–466.
Fleming AF, Ghatoura G, Harrison KA et al (1986) The prevention of anaemia in pregnancy in primigravidae in the guinea savanna of Nigeria. *Annals of Tropical Medicine and Parasitology* **80:** 211–233.
Fullerton W & Turner A (1962) Exchange blood transfusion treatment of severe anaemia in pregnancy. *Lancet* **i:** 75–78.
Gilles H, Lawson J, Sibelas M et al (1969) Malaria, anaemia and pregnancy. *Annals of Tropical Medicine and Parasitology* **63:** 245–262.
Greenwood B, Stratton D & Williamson W (1978) A study of the role of immunological factors in the pathogenesis of the anaemia of acute malaria. *Transactions of the Royal Society of Tropical Medicine and Hygiene* **72:** 378–385.
Greenwood B, Bradley A, Greenwood A et al (1987) Mortality and morbidity from malaria among children in a rural area of The Gambia, west Africa. *Transactions of the Royal Society of Tropical Medicine and Hygiene* **81:** 478–486.
Gupta C, Alam A, Mathur P & Dutta G (1982) A new look at nonparasitised red cells of malaria-infected monkeys. *Nature* **299:** 259–261.
Hendrickse R, Hasan A, Olumide L & Akinkunmi A (1971) Malaria in early childhood. *Annals of Tropical Medicine and Parasitology* **65:** 1–20.
Hill A, Allsopp C, Kwiatkowski D et al (1991) Common West African HLA antigens are associated with protection from severe malaria. *Nature* **352:** 595–600.
Howard R & Mitchell G (1979) Accelerated clearance of uninfected red cells from *P. berghei*-infected mice. *Australian Journal of Experimental Medicine and Biological Science* **57:** 455.
Jeje O, Kelton J & Blajchman M (1983) Quantitation of red cell membrane associated immunoglobulin in children with *Plasmodium falciparum* parasitaemia. *British Journal of Haematology* **54:** 567–572.
Jones P, Pickett L, Anderson M & Pasvol G (1990) Human parvovirus infection in children and severe anaemia seen in an area endemic for malaria. *Journal of Tropical Medicine and Hygiene* **93:** 67–70.
Knuttgen H (1963) Das menschliche Knochenmark bei akuten Malaria Infektionen. *Zeitschrift fur Tropenmedizin und Parasitologie* **14:** 423–466.
Knuttgen H (1987) The bone marrow of non-immune Europeans in acute malaria infection: a tropical review. *Annals of Tropical Medicine and Parasitology* **81:** 567–576.
Lee S, Looareesuwan S, Wattanagoon Y et al (1989) Antibody-dependent red cell removal during *P. falciparum* malaria: the clearance of red cells sensitized with an IgG anti-D. *British Journal of Haematology* **73:** 396–402.
Looareesuwan S, Phillips R, White N et al (1985) Quinine and severe falciparum malaria in late pregnancy. *Lancet* **i:** 4–8.
Looareesuwan S, Merry A, Phillips R et al (1987a) Reduced erythrocyte survival following clearance of malarial parasitaemia in Thai patients. *British Journal of Haematology* **67:** 473–478.
Looareesuwan S, Ho M, Wattanagoon Y et al (1987b) Dynamic alteration in splenic function during acute falciparum malaria. *New England Journal of Medicine* **317:** 675–679.
McGregor I, Williams K, Billewicz W & Thomson A (1966) Haemoglobin concentration and anaemia in young West African (Gambian) children. *Transactions of the Royal Society of Tropical Medicine and Hygiene* **60:** 650–667.
McGregor I, Wilson M & Billewicz W (1983) Malaria infection of the placenta in The Gambia, West Africa; its incidence and relationship to stillbirth, birthweight and placental weight. *Transactions of the Royal Society of Tropical Medicine and Hygiene* **77:** 232–244.
Maegraith B (1948) *Pathological Processes in Malaria and Blackwater Fever*. Oxford: Blackwell Scientific.

Merry A & Thompson E (1984) The role of quantitative tests in immunohaematology; determination of the significance of erythrocyte-bound IgG; investigation of some of the parameters affecting the sensitivity of the antiglobulin-test. *Biotest Bulletin* **5:** 130–144.

Merry A, Looareesuwan S, Phillips R et al (1986) Evidence against immune haemolysis in falciparum malaria in Thailand. *British Journal of Haematology* **64:** 187–194.

Molineaux L & Gramiccia G (1980) *The Garki Project*, 311 pp. Geneva: World Health Organization.

Molyneux M, Taylor T, Wirima J & Borgstein A (1989) Clinical features and prognostic indicators in paediatric cerebral malaria: a study of 131 comatose Malawian children. *Quarterly Journal of Medicine* **71:** 441–459.

Oppenheimer S, Gibson F, Macfarlane S et al (1984) Iron supplementation and malaria. *Lancet* **i:** 389–390.

Pasvol G (1986) The anaemia of malaria. *Quarterly Journal of Medicine* **58:** 217–219.

Pasvol G & Jungery M (1983) Glycophorins and red cell invasion by *Plasmodium falciparum. Ciba Foundation Symposium* **94:** 174–195.

Phillips R, Looareesuwan S, Warrell D et al (1986) The importance of anaemia in cerebral and uncomplicated falciparum malaria: role of complications, dyserythropoiesis and iron sequestration. *Quarterly Journal of Medicine* **58:** 305–323.

Rosenberg E, Strickland G, Yang S & Whalen G (1973) IgM antibodies to red cells and autoimmune anemia in patients with malaria. *The American Journal of Tropical Medicine and Hygiene* **22:** 146–152.

Sheagren J, Tobie J, Fox L & Wolff S (1970) Reticuloendothelial system: phagocytic function in naturally acquired human malaria. *Journal of Laboratory and Clinical Medicine* **75:** 481–487.

Smalley M, Abdalla S & Brown J (1980) The distribution of *Plasmodium falciparum* in the peripheral blood and bone marrow of Gambian children. *Transactions of the Royal Society of Tropical Medicine and Hygiene* **75:** 103–105.

Spitz S (1946) The pathology of acute falciparum malaria. *Military Surgery* **99:** 555–572.

Srichaikul T, Wasanasomsithi M, Poshyachinda V et al (1969) Ferrokinetic studies in erythropoiesis in malaria. *Archives of Internal Medicine* **124:** 623–628.

Srichaikul T, Panikbutr N & Jeumtrakul P (1967) Bone marrow changes in human malaria. *Annals of Tropical Medicine and Parasitology* **8:** 40–50.

Taliaferro W & Mulligan H (1937) The histopathology of malaria with special reference to the function and origin of the macrophages in defence. *Journal of Indian Medical Research* **29:** 1–138.

Thorn J (1988) Parvovirus B19: historical and clinical review. *Reviews of Infectious Diseases* **10:** 1005–1011.

Topley E (1968) Common anaemia in rural Gambia: III. A spontaneously remitting anaemia possibly precipitated by malarial parasitaemia. *Transactions of the Royal Society of Tropical Medicine and Hygiene* **62:** 602–606.

Topley E, Knight R & Woodruff AW (1973) The direct antiglobulin test and immunoconglutinin titres in patients with malaria. *Transactions of the Royal Society of Tropical Medicine and Hygiene* **67:** 51–57.

Van der Meulen F, Debruin H, Goosen P et al (1980) Quantitative aspects of the destruction of red cells sensitized with non-complement binding IgG antibodies. *British Journal of Haematology* **46:** 47–56.

Vial H & Phillipott JR (1984) A reevaluation of the status of cholesterol in erythrocytes infected by *Plasmodium knowlesi* and *P. falciparum. Molecular and Biochemical Parasitology* **13:** 53–65.

Villeval J-L, Metcalf D & Lew A (1990) Changes in haemopoietic and regulator levels in mice during fatal or nonfatal malaria infections. I. Erythropoietic populations. *Experimental Parasitology* **71:** 364–374.

Warrell D, Looareesuwan S, Warrell M et al (1982) Dexamethasone proves deleterious in cerebral malaria. A double-blind trial in 100 comatose patients. *New England Journal of Medicine* **306:** 313–319.

Warrell D, Molyneux M & Beales PE (1990) Severe and complicated malaria *Transactions of the Royal Society of Tropical Medicine and Hygiene* **84** supplement 2: 1–65.

Weatherall D, Abdalla S & Pippard M (1983) The anaemia of *Plasmodium falciparum* malaria. *Ciba Foundation Symposium* **94:** 74–97.

Weiss L (1983) Hematopoietic tissue in malaria: facilitation of erythrocytic recycling by bone marrow in *Plasmodium berghei*-infected mice. *Journal of Parasitology* **69:** 307–318.

Wickramasinghe S, Abdalla S & Weatherall D (1982) Cell cycle distribution of erythroblasts in *P. falciparum* malaria. *Scandinavian Journal of Haematology* **29:** 83–88.

Wickramasinghe S, Phillips R, Looareesuwan S et al (1987) The bone marrow in human cerebral malaria: parasite sequestration within sinusoids. *British Journal of Haematology* **66:** 295–306.

Wickramasinghe S, Looareesuwan S, Nagachinta B & White N (1989) Dyserythropoiesis and ineffective erythropoiesis in *Plasmodium vivax* malaria. *British Journal of Haematology* **72:** 91–99.

Zuckerman A (1964) Autoimmunization and other types of indirect damage to host cells as factors in certain protozoan diseases. *Experimental Parasitology* **15:** 138–183.

4

Genetic epidemiology of the β^s gene

RONALD L. NAGEL
ALAN F. FLEMING

It was calculated in 1983 that sickle-cell trait (haemoglobin (Hb) AS) was carried by about 60 million people, of whom 50 million were in sub-Saharan Africa (Figure 1) (World Health Organization Working Group, 1983). The global figure may be as high as 78 million in 1992. There are born each year

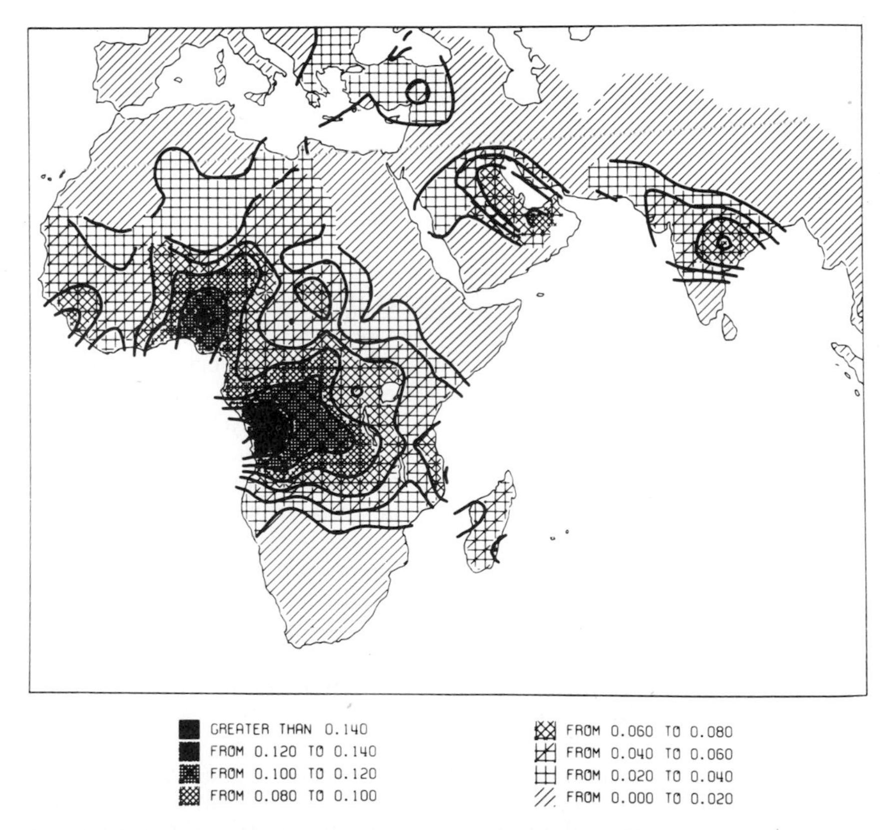

Figure 1. The frequency distribution of the β^s gene in the Old World, according to Bodner and Cavalli-Sforza (1976) with permission of the authors and publishers.

Baillière's Clinical Haematology—
Vol. 5, No. 2, April 1992
ISBN 0–7020–1627–6

about 156 000 infants with sickle-cell disease, of whom 130 000 are in Africa and 33 000 in Nigeria alone: the majority have sickle-cell anaemia (homozygous HbSS), but others have HbSC, especially in Burkina Faso and Ghana, or HbS/β-thalassaemia, especially in Liberia, the Mediterranean area and the Americas (reviewed in Fleming, 1987).

The β^s gene is found in human populations at gene frequencies higher than those explained by mutational pressure alone, that is, higher than 1%. Hence, the sickle mutation is a polymorphic trait. Since homozygous HbSS and the double heterozygous HbSC and HbS/β-thalassaemias have reduced fitness, the high frequency of the heterozygous trait (HbAS) implies that a state of balanced polymorphism exists, in which the advantage of the heterozygous trait partially compensates for the disadvantages of sickle-cell disease (Bodner and Cavalli-Sforza, 1976).

When concerned with the genetic epidemiology of the β^s gene, five basic questions come to mind. (1) What is the distribution of the gene frequency of the β^s gene among the populations of the world today? (2) In how many of the populations (or geographical sites) in which the β^s gene is found today did the mutation arise autochthonously? In other words, is the mutation unicentric (it originated in one population and was distributed around the world by gene flow), or was it multicentric (it originated in several populations independently)? (3) In how many populations was the β^s gene introduced by gene flow from other locations? (4) When did the β^s mutation occur? (5) What is the mechanism underlying the balanced polymorphism of the β^s gene?

β^s GENE FREQUENCY IN THE WORLD TODAY

The β^s gene is found at high frequencies in Africa, especially in the sub-Saharan region but also in north Africa (Belhani et al, 1984; Jain, 1985). It is also found at lower frequencies in several populations to the north and east of the Mediterranean (Portugal, Spain, southern Italy, Sicily, Greece, Turkey and Israel). In addition, the β^s gene has been described at polymorphic frequencies in the Arabian Peninsula, Iraq, Iran, Afghanistan, India and the (formerly Soviet) Republics of Georgia, Azarbijan, Turkomen and Tadhaskistan. In the Old World, the β^s gene is found predominantly in black African populations, but also among a diversity of Caucasian populations (Europeans, Transcaucasians, Central Asians, Arabs and Indians) (Lehmann and Cutbush, 1952; Perrine et al, 1972; Bodner and Cavalli-Sforza, 1976; Haghshenass et al, 1977; Brittenham et al, 1979; Alkasab et al, 1981; Tokarev and Spivak, 1982; Aluoch et al, 1986; Monteiro et al, 1989).

In Africa, the distribution of the frequency of the β^s gene is around three main geographical locations, each one exhibiting a centre of very high frequency: one is around the lower Niger and Benue Rivers in central west Africa (centre = 0.12–0.14; minimum: 0.02); another is centred around the

Congo or Zaire (centre = 0.12–0.14; minimum 0.02); and a third one is around Senegal in Atlantic west Africa (centre = 0.08–0.10; minimum 0.02) (Bodner and Cavalli-Sforza, 1976) (Figure 1).

In the New World, the β^s gene is absent in Amerindian populations, but it is found in many populations that have had an admixture with black African or Mediterranean populations. The presence of the β^s gene is high in the USA, Canada, coastal isolates in Mexico, central America, Caribbean nations (e.g. Cuba and Jamaica) and several south American countries including Colombia, Venezuela, Guyana, Surinam, French Guiana, Brazil and Peru, but it is almost absent in Bolivia, Paraguay, Chile, Uruguay and Argentina (Pons and Oms, 1934; Chediak et al, 1939; Mera, 1943; Tomlinson, 1945; Herrara Cabral, 1950; Barnola et al, 1953; Kalmus, 1957; Fuzman et al, 1964; Zago and Costa, 1985; Granda et al, 1991).

Some of the geographical locations outlined above are inhabited by more than one ethnic group, so a more detailed description is required. For example, in Israel the β^s gene has been found exclusively among Arab Israelis (Roth et al, 1978a). In Turkey, it is found in 13.2–16.8% of the Eti-Turks, an Arabic speaking people living on the Cilician peninsular of the eastern end of the southern coast, between Mersin and Iskenderun (Aluoch et al, 1986); other foci are around Antalya (2.3%) on the Mediterranean coast (Aksoy et al, 1980) and in immigrants from several Balkan countries who settled in eastern Thrace, on the borders with Bulgaria and Greece, after the collapse of the Ottoman Empire (Aksoy, 1985). The Ottoman Empire forcibly recruited African troops, and distributed several African genes within its borders; the other classical example is HbO^{Arab}, first described in Israeli Arabs (Ramot et al, 1960). In Greece, the β^s gene is found at high frequencies, but only in several isolated populations living in Makedhonia (Macedonia), Thessaloniki where prevalence of sickle-cell trait reaches 30% on the Khalkidhiki peninsula and the Peloponnisos (Christakis et al, 1990, 1991). In Europe, the individuals carrying the β^s gene are generally physically indistinguishable from the general population.

In India, the situation is particularly interesting as the β^s gene is almost entirely restricted to the so called 'tribal' groups. The 'tribals' of India correspond to isolated, dispersed and endogamic Caucasian communities (totalling about 50 million individuals) that exist today in central and southern India, and live outside of the mainstream of Indian life and its caste system. Some scholars consider them descendants of early inhabitants of the Indian subcontinent (Bhowmik, 1971). The presence of HbS was first reported by Lehmann and Cutbush (1952) in the tribal populations of the Nilgiris in the southern State of Tamil-Nadu. Since then, high frequencies of the β^s gene (between 0.05 and 0.194) have been reported among about 50 different tribal populations in other areas of India (Shukla and Solanki, 1958; Batabyal and Wilson, 1958; Chatterjea, 1966; Roy and Roy Chaudhuri, 1967; Brittenham et al, 1979; Deka, 1981; Kar et al, 1987).

In the New World, the distribution of the β^s gene follows the extent of an admixture with Africans, and it is found preferentially among minorities of black origin.

POPULATIONS IN WHICH β^s MUTATIONS AROSE AUTOCHTHONOUSLY

Today, the genetic data available allows us to define the following minimum number of independent origins of the β^s gene: it appeared four times in Africa, and once somewhere between the Horn of Oman and southern India.

Africa

The frequency of the β^s gene in Africa has three major high frequency sites surrounded by a descending decline of frequencies (Figure 1) (Bodner and Cavalli-Sforza, 1976). Do these areas correspond to independent origins of the β^s gene, or are all the carriers in Africa related to a single original mutation? Until the advent of molecular biology a couple of decades ago, this was an unanswerable question.

The central strategy to resolve this question has been to define polymorphic sites (DNA sequences that tend to be different in different individuals) around the β^s gene and ask whether these polymorphic sites are the same in all carriers or whether they vary among carriers. The reason why the answer is informative is that polymorphic sites *near* the mutation will have a high probability of inheritance with the mutation (en masse) (Nagel and Ranney, 1990). But if the mutation occurred more than once, it would have had the chance of being associated with a different set of polymorphic sites as 'fellow travellers'; this is the tell-tale sign of multicentricity (Figure 2). The discovery by Kan and Dozy (1978, 1980) that the β^s globin gene was in linkage disequilibrium (that is, not all β^s genes were linked to the same site) with a polymorphic site (located in the 5′ flanking region of the gene identified with the *Hpa*I endonuclease enzyme) posed an intriguing question. The data showed that in African-Americans homozygous for HbS, the abnormal gene was linked to the absence of this polymorphic site in 60% of the population, while in the remaining 40% there was linkage to its presence.

These findings strongly suggested that the β^s globin gene could have arisen in two different mutational events that occurred in two different types of chromosomes 11, distinguishable by their *Hpa*I polymorphism. The other possibility was that a mutation in the *Hpa*I site had followed the sickle mutation on the same chromosome. When Kan and Dozy (1980) extended their studies in Africa, they interpreted their data to mean that the *Hpa*I(+) type was characteristic of East Africans and the *Hpa*(−) type was characteristic of West Africans. These findings were followed by more detailed studies by Mears et al (1981a, 1981b) who found that the *Hpa*I polymorphism was territorially segregated in Africa in three (not two) locations: Atlantic west Africa and Bantu-speaking central Africa had *Hpa*(−) linked β^s genes, while central west Africa had *Hpa*I(+) linked β^s genes. The more extensive investigation by Pagnier et al (1984), that involved 11 polymorphic sites of the β-chain cluster (instead of only one), definitely established that the β^s gene was associated with three distinctly different chromosomes identifiable by their specific array of DNA polymorphic sites or haplotypes, each virtually exclusively present in three separate geographical areas of Africa (Figure 2). These have been designated Benin, Senegal and Bantu (originally called CAR for Central African Republic). This finding entirely

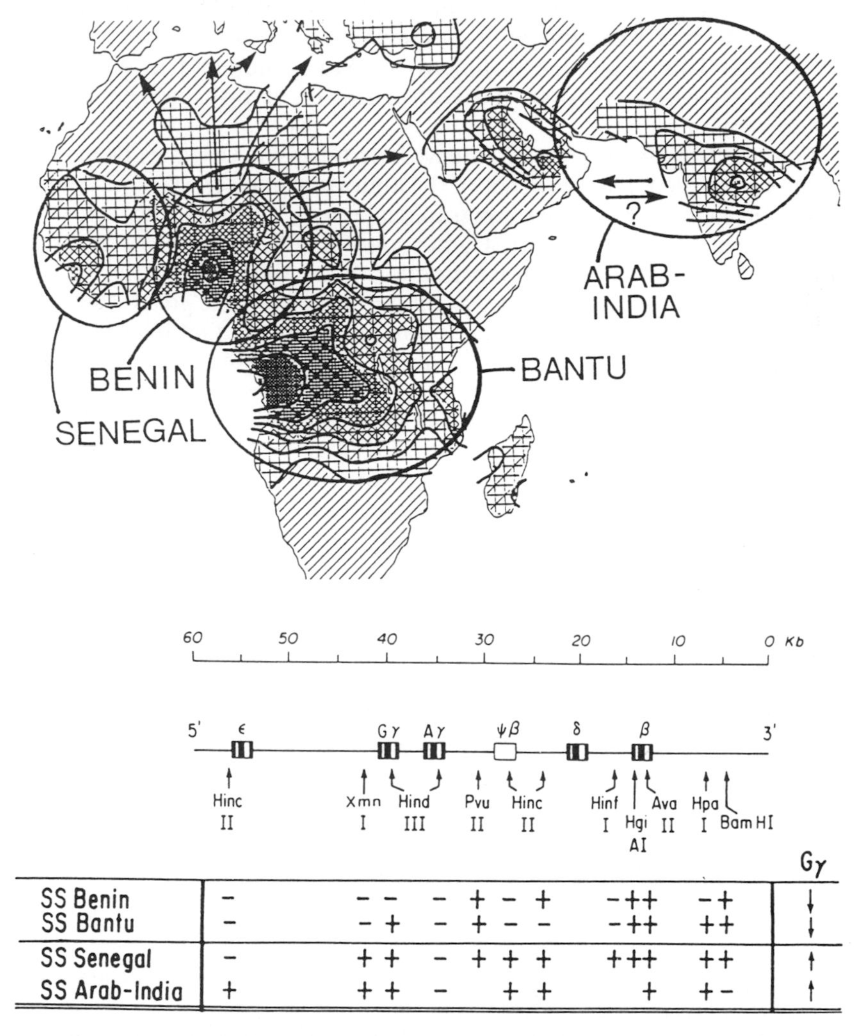

Figure 2. A map illustrating the incidence of HbS in the African continent, the Mediterranean, the Middle East and the Indian subcontinent according to Bodner and Cavalli-Sforza (1976). The approximate boundaries of the four major β^s-linked haplotypes have been superimposed. The arrows depict the possible routes of gene flow of (1) the Benin haplotype to north Africa, Spain, Sicily, Greece, Turkey and western Arabia, and (2) the Arab-India haplotype between the eastern oases of Arabia and the Indian subcontinent. The middle of the figure depicts the β-like gene clusters and indicates by arrows the endonuclease-definable polymorphic sites. From Ragusa et al (1988) and Nagel and Ranney (1990) with permission of the authors and publishers.

eliminated the possibility that the *Hpa*I linkage disequilibrium was subsequent to the β^s mutation.

Recently, a fourth African haplotype, differing from these three in both the 5′ and 3′ regions of the haplotype, has been found in the Eton ethnic group by Lapouméroulie et al (1989). This haplotype, designated Cameroon, had previously been encountered sporadically in the New World, but its association with a specific ethnic group had not been recognized. This haplotype is linked to $A_{\gamma}T$ gene, and is identical to haplotype II which is associated with a subset of β-thalassaemia in the Mediterranean.

Thus, the β^s gene originated at least four times in Africa. Subsequently, major expansion of the frequency of the abnormal gene crossed many ethnic groups in each of the three geographical areas. In addition, a 'private' haplotype of the Eton group (Cameroon), a fourth origin of the sickle mutation in Africa, was also expanded, presumably by malaria, to reach polymorphic frequencies, but it was limited to one ethnic group (the Eton) with some spillover into the Ewondo (an ethnic group that lives in a contiguous geographical area in central Cameroon) (N. Green and R.L. Nagel, unpublished observations).

In the Senegal and the Bantu areas, less than 10% of the chromosomes bearing the β^s gene are atypical; that is they do not correspond to the typical Senegal or Bantu haplotype. A study in the Central African Republic (in which HbS-carrying individuals have the Bantu haplotype) showed that almost all atypicals can be explained by crossing-over events around the 'hot spot' of recombination 5′ to the gene (Srinivas et al, 1988). This crossing-over occurred because the 5′ portion of the haplotype is different from the typical haplotype, but the 3′ portion is identical. In Benin, very few atypical haplotypes have been found. This fact could be the result of the high frequency of the Benin haplotype in the normal population (60%). Hence, many crossing-over events would go undetected.

Several investigators, ourselves included, have noticed a higher frequency of atypicals among African-Americans carrying the β^s gene. Since this population is admixed 20% with Caucasians (on average) (Workman et al, 1963), the β^s chromosomes have the opportunity to pair with chromosomes of Caucasian origin (which are different in frequency), as well as haplotypes of other regions of Africa away from their original geographical origin.

The origin of major haplotypes from recombination events has been postulated (Livingstone, 1989), but this hypothesis can be discarded because recombination would generate at least two different haplotypes associated with β^s in a given geographical area.

Two groups (Wainscoat et al, 1983; Antonarakis et al, 1984) reported on the haplotype linkages to β^s in Jamaica in a black population generated by forced migration to the new continent from Africa during the seventeenth century. While more than 20 haplotypes were found in association with the β^s mutation, the three haplotypes described by Pagnier et al (1984) accounted for more than 95% of the cases. The remainder are thought to represent 'private' haplotype linkages generated by fresh mutations (as the Cameroon haplotype) by gene conversion or, perhaps, by more classical

		HinfI				RsaI				
		-1069	-989	-780	-710	-551	-543 ... -521	-491	Framework	(AT)xTy
Reference		G	C	A	T	T	CAT ATATATATAT AT....TTTT TTTC	A	1	(AT)7T7
β^S	Senegal	G	C	A	G	T	CAT ATATATATAT ATAT.....T TTTT	A	1	(AT)8T4
	Benin	A	G	A	T	T	TAT ATATATATAT ATAT.....T TTTC	C	2	(AT)8T4
	Bantu	G	G	A	T	C	CAT ATATATATAT ....TTTTTT TTTC	A	1	(AT)6T9
	Cameroon	G	C	A	T	T	CAT ATATATATAT ATAT....TT TTTC	A	2	(AT)8T5
	India	G	G	A	T	C	CAT ATATATATAT ATATAT..TT TTTC	A	2	(AT)9T5

Figure 3. The area 5′ to the β gene in which an area of $(AT)_x$ $(T)_y$ repeats is found. (From Trabuchet et al, 1989).

crossing-over events around the putative 'hot spot' 5′ to the β gene (Chakravarti et al, 1984).

Additionally, recent evidence of the separate origin of the three major haplotypes in Africa has been provided by Chebloune et al (1988) and Trabuchet et al (1989) in studies of the area 5′ to the gene in which an area of $(AT)_x(T)_y$ repeats is found. These repeats are unique for each of the four haplotypes (including the Arab-India, see below) (Figure 3). Based on the original data obtained in the Central African Republic and *Hpa*I data from Kan and Dozy (1980), Nagel (1984) postulated that the Bantu haplotype was associated with the β^s gene throughout the Bantu-speaking area of equatorial and southern Africa. Further studies have confirmed this hypothesis. Ojwang et al (1987) (studying populations in western Kenya) and Ramsay and Jenkins (1987) (studying populations in Zimbabwe, Namibia, Zambia and Malawi) found the β^s gene linked to the Bantu haplotype.

Eastern oases of Saudi Arabia and India

A linkage disequilibrium between β^s and a novel haplotype, the Arab-India, was discovered independently by Wainscoat et al (1985), Bakioglu et al (1985) and Miller et al (1987) in HbSS patients from the eastern oases of Saudi Arabia.

The first report of the Arab-India gene haplotype also being associated with the sickle mutation in India was that of Kulozik et al (1986), who studied the tribal population near Calcutta. This haplotype accounts for over 90% of the β^s-associated haplotypes in India, while two other haplotypes are found less frequently; one may have arisen by crossing-over 5′ to the gene. In India, HbSS individuals have an unusually high incidence of (-α/αα) thalassaemia (as does the normal tribal population), and the common haplotype is associated with a high G^γ and HbF expression. Labie et al (1989) have contributed recently to the epidemiology of the β^s in India by asking whether the same haplotype is linked to β^s in tribal populations living in the Indian subcontinent thousands of miles from each other and in total isolation. Three tribal groups, separated by more than 2000 miles (3200 km), were studied: the Irulas, Kurumbes, Paniyas and Badaga scheduled tribes inhabiting the rain forest in the Nilgiris (Blue Mountains) of the western Ghat of the Deccan in southern India; the Ganit and Kokini tribes living in Surat, State of Gujarat, in the western border of central India; the third group were the Domb and Khond tribal groups near Orissa (also studied by the British group) and the Khond of Andhra Pradesh, all of them in the eastern border of central India (near Calcutta). No communication or contact of any kind exists today (nor has it for a long time) between the three populations studied (Figure 4).

The finding of the same haplotype associated with the β^s gene in Orissa, in the southern tribal populations, as well as in western central India, has important epidemiological and anthropological implications. This observation strongly suggests that the mutation had an unicentric origin. Moreover, and quite unexpectedly, it demonstrates that these tribal populations were in close contact with each other at one point (unicentric geographical origin

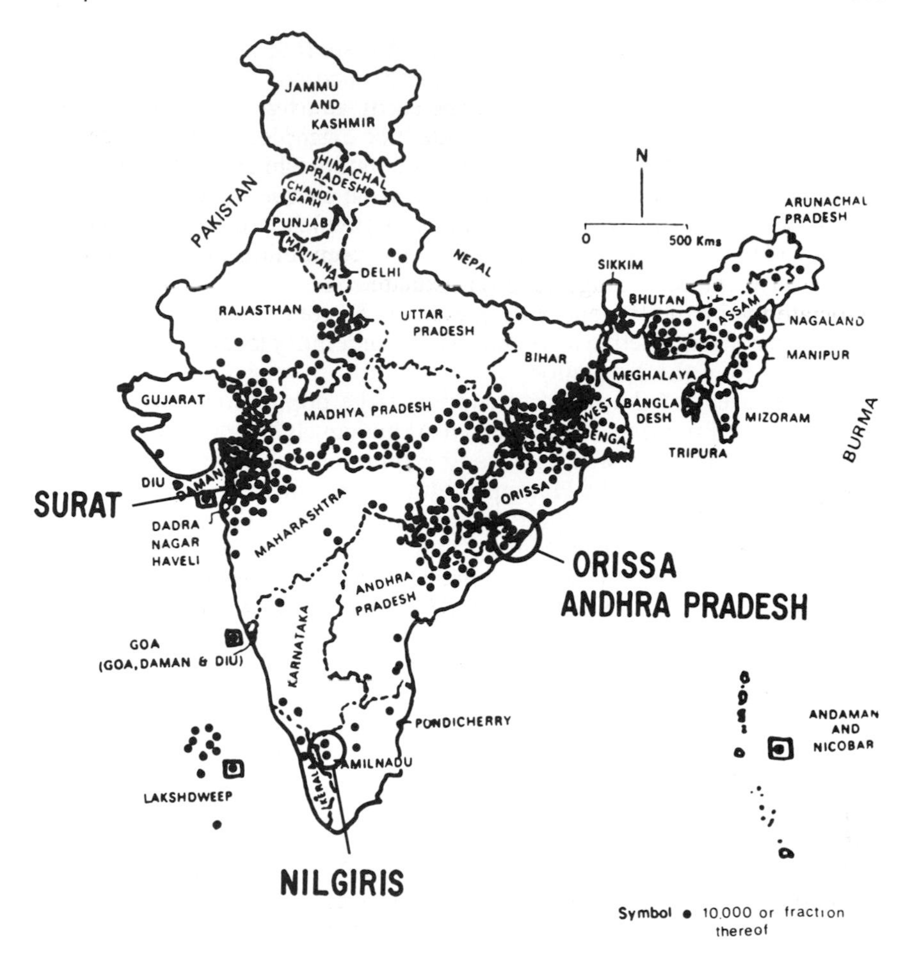

Figure 4. Map of the distribution of the scheduled tribes in India (as of 1971). Each dot corresponds to 100 000 individuals or a fraction thereof. The populations studied for β haplotypes are circled. From Labie et al (1989) with permission of the authors and publishers.

of these populations). Since today these populations live totally isolated by endogamy and cultural traditions, and are surrounded by mainstream Indian populations that do not bear the β^s gene, there must have been an ancestral home for the tribals of India (see below).

WHEN DID THE β^s MUTATION OCCUR?

How old is the β^s mutation? No definitive data exist. The consensus is that the expansion of the mutation occurs in coincidence with malaria becoming endemic in human populations. There are strong reasons to believe that this happens when man progresses from food-gathering to food-producing, because agriculture strongly favours the endemicity of *Plasmodia* (Wiesenfeld, 1967). (1) The water sources created by and for agriculture provide excellent breeding places for mosquitoes. For example, slashing and burning of forest results in open sunlit pools of water, which are the preferred breeding sites of *Anopheles gambiae*. Irrigation channels and dams lead to shaded vegetated water-edges and swamps, which are preferred by *A. funestis*. (2) As food becomes plentiful, the population of man increases vastly and displaces other primates; man becomes the preferred host of parasites of primates, such as *Plasmodia* (Livingstone, 1971, 1976). (3) The people are concentrated in large numbers in sedentary locations close to the breeding sites of the mosquitoes.

The first areas of the world to support large populations through agriculture were all riverine: the Sumerian/Akkadian civilization was based on the Mesopotamian rivers of Tigris and Euphrates; the Egyptian kingdoms developed on the Nile; the Harappa culture flourished on the banks of the Indus and its tributaries in the Punjab; Chinese civilization started on the Hwang Ho (Yellow) and Yangtze Kiang rivers. Of these, the least well-known is the Harappa civilization, which flourished between about 2500 BC and 1600 BC (Piggot, 1950; Wheeler, 1968).

Arab-India β^s mutation

The Indus valley was at that time within the western range of the monsoon rains. It was forested, and experienced flooding with deposition of silt. The Harappa civilization was based on the cultivation of barley, wheat and other crops, and animal husbandry. These supported a centralized administration under priest-kings, in two fortified twin cities, Mohenjo-Daro on the right bank of the Indus (320 km (200 miles) north of Karachi) and Harappa on the left bank of the river Ravi (160 km (100 miles) south-west of Lahore). There were many other small towns and settlements. At its height, the population was possibly five million in what is now Sind and Punjab (McEvedy and Jones, 1978). Skeletal remains showed that there was an ethnically mixed population, with a high proportion of people that, according to some, are related to the Indian tribal groups of today. Based on the *Rigveda*, some authors interpret that around 1600 BC, the Harappa civilization was utterly destroyed by Indo-European invaders coming from the west, the Aryans from whom the majority of the population of northern India today are descended. Nevertheless, continuous flooding and internal strife might have contributed equally, or more, to its disappearance.

Labie and coworkers (1989) have presented the hypothesis that the ancestral home of the Indian tribal groups and the unicentric origin of the Arab-India β^s gene might have been the margins of the Indus river (Figure 5). This is based on the following considerations. (1) The Indus river is geographically close to other populations that carry the same β^s linked-haplotype (Shiite Arabs living in eastern oases near the Horn of Oman). Since the β^s is linked to high HbF expression in the Arab-India haplotype (Labie et al, 1989), and high HbF is reported in subjects with sickle-cell

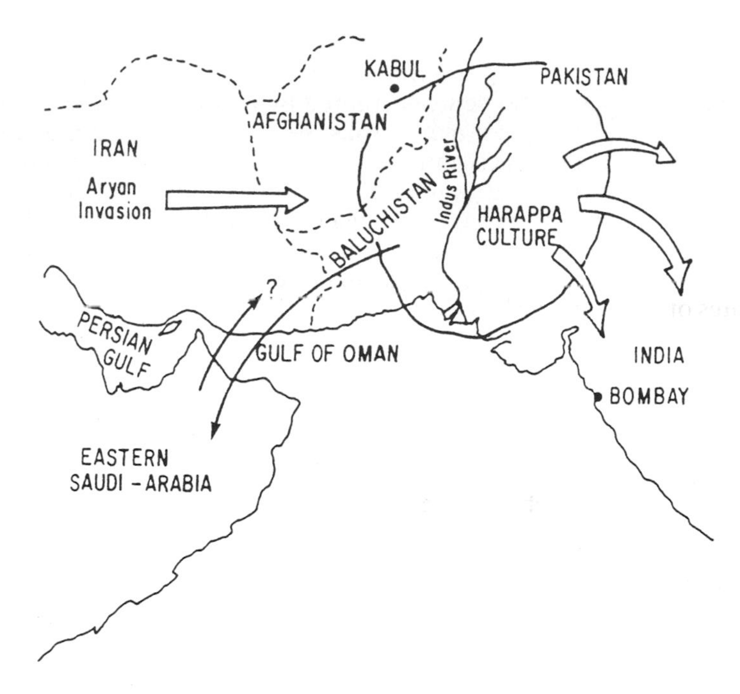

Figure 5. Hypothesis of the geographical area involved in the origin of the β^s gene in India. The open arrows on the right-hand side depict the dispersion of the Harappan culture members after the collapse of their civilization and the Aryan invasion (left-hand side open arrows). Solid arrows depict the potential gene flow of the β^s gene between the Indian subcontinent and the Arabic peninsula. From Labie et al (1989) with permission of the authors and publishers.

anaemia in Iran, possibly Afghanistan, and the Transcaucasian and Central-asians population of the southern republics of the Commonwealth of Independent States (formerly the USSR) (Tokarev and Spivak, 1982), this haplotype might turn out to be predominant in the region. (2) The Indus basin at the time of the Harappa culture was an area capable of sustaining significant malaria endemicity, because of developed agriculture and irrigation methods, a factor indispensable to the selection and expansion for the β^s gene. (3) Skeletal remains of Harappans reveal bone alterations judged characteristic of HbSS disease by Kennedy (1981), although a more conservative estimation is that these findings are compatible with, but not conclusive proof of, the presence of HbSS disease in this population (Labie et al, 1989). Of course, until further archaeological and anthropological data become available, this interpretation has to be considered solely as a working hypothesis.

If the Arab-India mutation did, in effect, occur during the high time of the Harappa culture, the time frame of its appearance might be in the order of 4000 years ago.

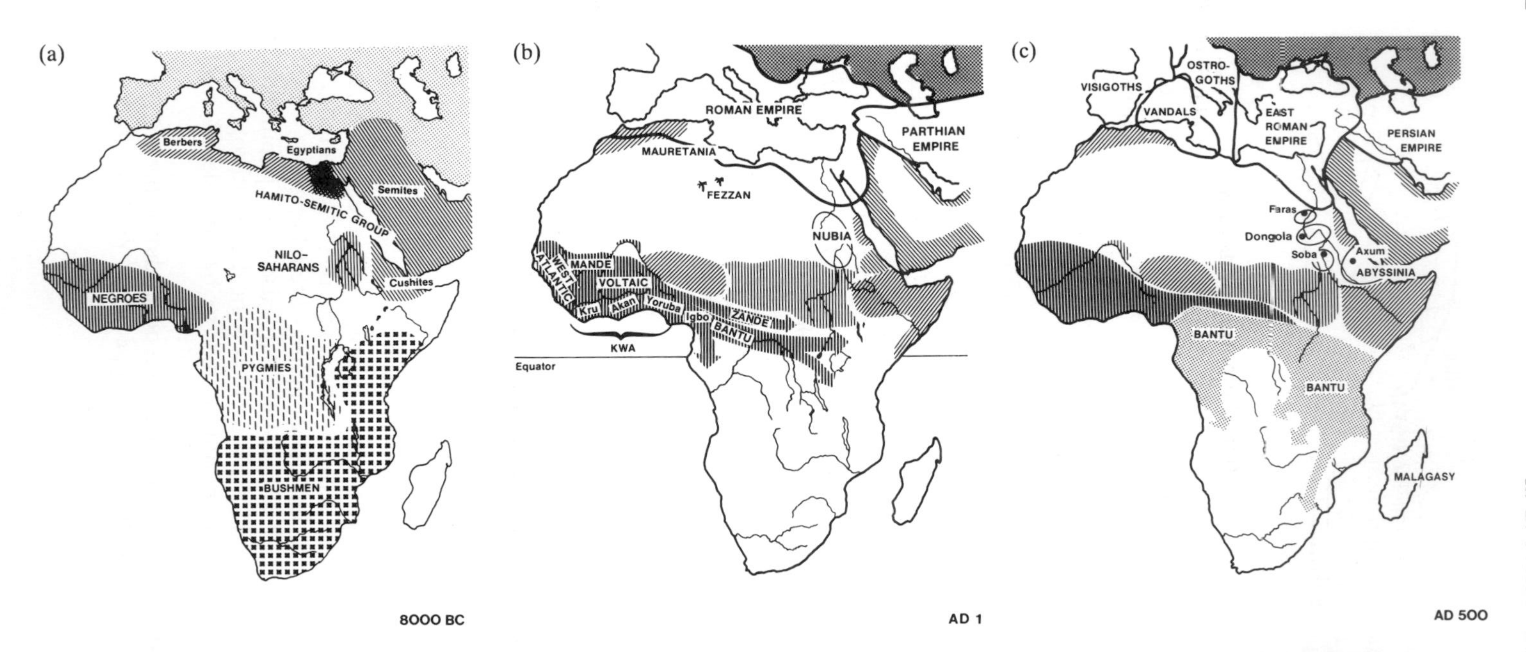

Figure 6. Africa: (a) 8000 BC, (b) AD 1, and (c) AD 500. Originally, black Africans inhabited only west Africa. By the beginning of the Christian era, they can be divided linguistically: the speakers of the west Atlantic languages lived where the Senegal β^s haplotype is found today; the Kwa language speakers lived where the Benin β^s haplotype is found today. The Bantu surge started in the eastern regions of present day Nigeria, expanding and engulfing the territories previously occupied by the Pygmies and the San (previously called Bushmen). The distribution of the Bantu β^s haplotype may be explained if it arose shortly before or shortly after the beginning of the Bantu surge (see text). From McEvedy (1980) with permission of the author and publishers.

Senegal and Benin β^s mutations

During the third millennium BC, neolithic techniques from the upper Nile were carried by Nilo-Saharans and Cushite pastoralists along the Sahel corridor, the strip of steppe immediately south of the Sahara, to west Africa (McEvedy, 1980). The Blacks to the south and west learnt neolithic techniques and cultivated mainly sorghum and millet. The population grew slowly until the acquisition of iron-working techniques about 250 BC was followed by an upsurge of population to around three million in AD 1 (McEvedy and Jones, 1978). Then the populations of west Africa could be divided linguistically: the west Atlantic family of languages (today including Fulani and Woloff) were spoken in the area where the Senegal β^s mutation is now found; the Kwa family (including Kru, Akran, Yoruba and Ibo) were spoken where the Benin β^s mutation is found (Figure 6). It is reasonable to hypothesize a time frame of about 2000–3000 years before the present to the mutations leading to the Senegal and Benin β^s haplotypes.

Bantu and Cameroon β^s mutations

The forest area of southern Nigeria is separated from Cameroon by rivers, marshes and mountains. The Blacks lived to the west and the Pygmies to the east of these barriers, but the technical advances and growing population of Blacks allowed for migration into Cameroon, beginning slowly in the last millennium BC, but gaining momentum at the end of the pre-Christian and early Christian centuries. The surge of population led to the displacement of the Pygmies, who were then confined to the dense forests of the Zaire basin, and of the San (formerly called Bushmen), who were driven into the Kalahari desert, with repopulation of central, eastern and southern Africa by people who were uniformly speakers of Bantu languages (Figure 6) (McEvedy, 1980).

The geographical distribution of the Bantu haplotype provides biological evidence of the common origin of the people presently living in equatorial, eastern and southern Africa, and supports the Bantu expansion hypothesis, previously based exclusively on the linguistic connection of the languages spoken by the different ethnic groups in this area (Greenberg, 1973). This expansion is likely to have occurred by fluvial means as suggested by Greenberg (1973) and could have missed Cameroon entirely and surfaced in present-day Central African Republic and Congo/Zaire. This interpretation is compatible with the almost entire absence of Bantu haplotype and the presence of the Benin haplotype among most of the β^s carriers among the Cameroonians studied up to now, except for the Eton and some Ewondo, who exhibit the Cameroon haplotype (N. Green and R. L. Nagel, unpublished observations).

Therefore, the β^s mutation linked to the Bantu haplotype could have occurred either just before the Bantu expansion about 2000 years ago, or shortly afterwards. If before, it would have occurred east of the Niger and south of the Benue river (present-day Nigeria) and might still be found in that area. If shortly after, it is unlikely to be found at significant frequency in

Nigeria. No data are available on haplotypes studies of populations living around the margins of the Benue and lower Niger rivers. In the southern tip of Africa, the black population of South Africa has a very low frequency of the β^s gene. It is attractive to postulate that the near absence of β^s in the South African black population, who are supposedly descended from the head of the surge, could suggest that the β^s mutation occurred after the Bantu expansion had already begun. Nevertheless, the β^s gene frequency could have declined to its present low level in the South African black population due to the lack of selective advantage of the heterozygote (and the continuous lethal or semilethal character of the homozygote) due to the absence of malaria in that particular habitat.

POPULATIONS IN WHICH THE β^s GENES WERE INTRODUCED BY GENE FLOW

The Mediterranean

The existence of populations with HbS on both shores of the Mediterranean has been recognized for many years. It has long been suspected that the β^s gene in Sicily was introduced by gene flow from Africa. Studies of the β^s gene haplotypes in β^s and β^A-bearing chromosomes in Sicily strongly suggest that the β^s gene in Sicily was introduced from central west Africa, probably via north Africa (Maggio et al, 1986; Ragusa et al, 1988). The β^s-bearing chromosome in Sicilians is the Benin type in all cases studied, a haplotype absent in the normal population of that island (see Figure 3). Furthermore, there is a negative *Taq*I site in the intergenic region of all β^s chromosomes from the Sicilian population, a characteristic also shared by the Benin haplotype in Africa, and not found in Caucasians. Sandler et al (1978) found a high frequency of blood groups characteristic of African populations among Sicilian carriers of the β^s gene.

Other studies have found the β^s gene linked to the Benin haplotype in Morocco and Algeria (Mears et al, 1981a). All the β^s genes found in Egypt have been associated with the Benin haplotype (DiRienzo et al, 1987), which is found also in the majority of patients with sickle-cell anaemia in the western portion of Saudi Arabia. This contrasts with the β^s gene in the eastern oases of Saudi Arabia which is linked to the Arab-India β^s gene (see above). The Benin haplotype also accounts for all of the β^s chromosomes studied in Greece (Kollia et al, 1987) and among the Eti-Turks of Turkey (Aluoch et al, 1986). The low HbF associated with HbSS disease in Arabs from Israel suggest that they too are of the Benin type, although the Bantu haplotype is another possibility. The Arabs of Iraq have not been studied.

In conclusion, the β^s gene found in all of north Africa and the Mediterranean is of the Benin type, and must have originated entirely from central west Africa.

The oldest route from tropical Africa to the Mediterranean was down the Nile (Figure 7), and there is evidence that a few African slaves were supplied by the route in classical Greek and Roman times. Branches of this route

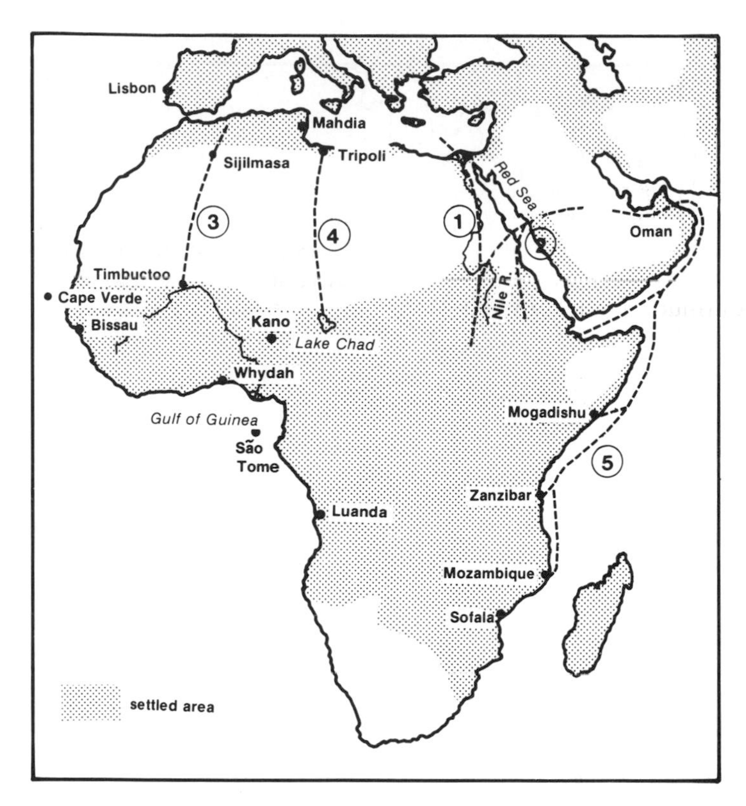

Figure 7. Trans-Saharan Tuareg and Indian Ocean Arab trade routes, and Portuguese slaving stations, operating at different times from the ninth century AD up to the end of the nineteenth century AD (see text). Modified from McEvedy and Jones (1978) with permission of the authors and publishers.

were developed to western Arabia following the rise of Arabic power in the seventh century AD. Further trans-Saharan routes were not opened until the breeding, maintenance and use of camels were mastered in the early eighth century AD. One route ran between the Senegal river/upper Niger and Morocco. This was quickly superseded by two Tuareg camel routes, one between Songhay on the bend of the Niger (Timbuctoo) and the Magreb (Morocco, Algeria and Tunisia), the second between Kanem around Lake Chad and Tripoli in Libya (Figure 7) (Bovill, 1958). The northern markets of these routes were provided by the expansion of the Arab (Umayyad) Empire at the end of the seventh century AD.

North of the Mediterranean, much of the Iberian peninsula was under Arab-Berber rule from AD 711 (Figure 8), and they were not expelled finally until the fall of Granada in AD 1492. Of particular interest is the invasion of Sicily from Tunisia in AD 827. Sicily remained under Arab rule for over 250 years and the Arabs were influential even longer. The Arabs in Sicily developed a system of agriculture based on terracing and syphon irrigation to grow cotton, papyrus, citrus, date palm and sugar cane. It would be

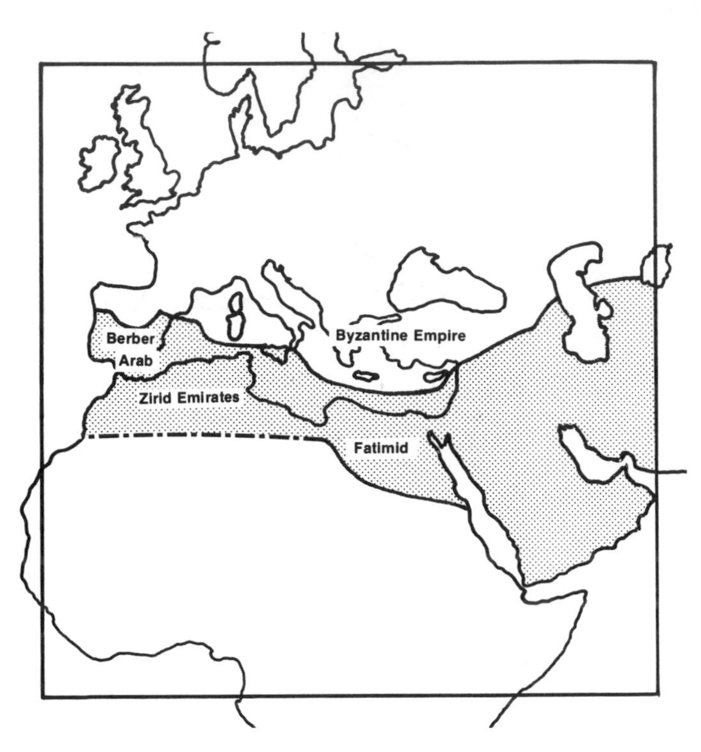

Figure 8. Arab rule in the Mediterranean in the early eleventh century AD. Spain had been almost wholly conquered by Arabs and Berbers in AD 711; the area of Islamic rule was reduced gradually until Granada fell in AD 1492. Sicily was invaded from Tunisia in AD 827 and remained under Arab rule until the invasion by the Normans at the end of the eleventh century AD.

reasonable to hypothesize that the Benin β^s gene was introduced into Sicily, and Spain to a lesser extent, during these centuries. In support of the Arab introduction of the β^s gene in Sicily is the high frequency (0.06) of this gene in the town of Butera, known to have been an Arab fortification during the Arab domination, and inhabited by African troops under Arab command. This strategic site in the valley near the port of Gela dominates one of the traditional invasion routes of Sicily, and General Patton, a history buff, used the same route in the invasion of Sicily during World War II.

The next Islamic power to rule extensively north of the Mediterranean was the Turkish Ottoman Empire, which conquered Constantinople (Istanbul) in 1453 and reached its height in the mid-seventeenth century (Figure 9). The trans-Saharan trade routes carried nearly one million slaves between 1500 and 1810, when the trade was outlawed by the European powers, and about the same number between 1810 and 1880 (McEvedy and Jones, 1978). The most popular slaves were from the Hausa markets of northern Nigeria, such as Kano: the slaves crossed the desert to Tripoli, where the survivors were sold mostly to Turkey and Egypt (Bovill, 1958). As mentioned before, many were posted as soldiers to the Balkans and are the most probable

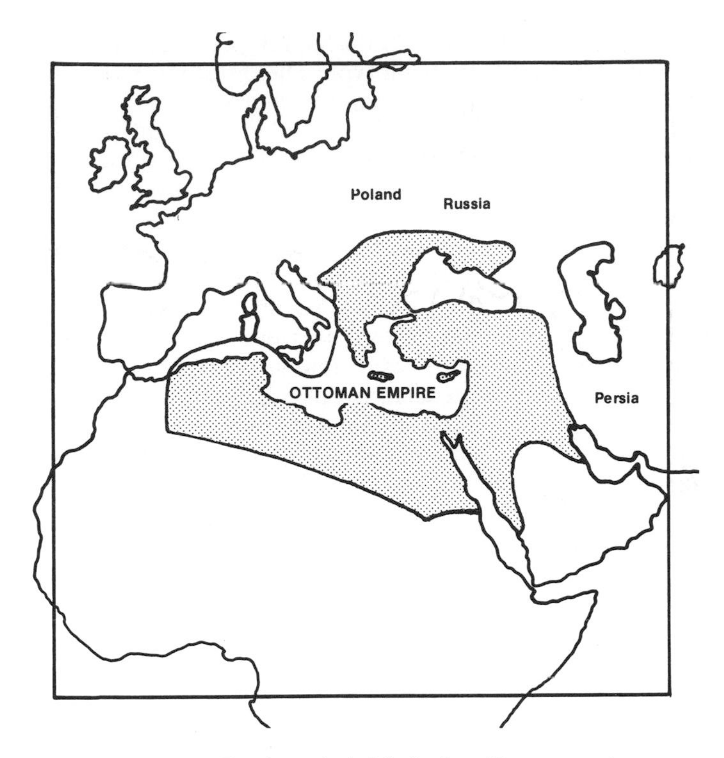

Figure 9. The Ottoman Empire at its height in the mid-seventeenth century AD.

ancestors of sickle-cell gene carriers in Greece, Thracian Turkey and elsewhere in the Balkans.

It is noticeable that the Benin β^s gene is found within the boundaries of the Ottoman Empire, and not in eastern Arabia (Figure 9).

Arabia

In the nineteenth century AD, Arabs from the eastern Arabian coast, especially Oman, opened up sea routes along the east coast of Africa, and developed the Swahili civilization with a chain of port towns as far south as Sofala in Mozambique (see Figure 7). Slave-raiding into the interior of east Africa continued into the second half of the nineteenth century. Probably a total of 800 000 slaves from east Africa reached Oman, and many were re-exported to Iran and India (McEvedy and Jones, 1978). So far the Bantu haplotype has not been identified in eastern Arabia and India, but it may be anticipated that further studies could reveal its presence in a population in which the Arab-India haplotype predominates. In the rest of the Arabian peninsula β^s is linked to the Benin haplotype, which in all probability reflects the Arab and Ottoman slave trades.

Recently, Padmos et al (1991) have compared sickle-cell anaemia (HbSS) in eastern Arabians with the Arab-India haplotype, and in western Arabians with predominantly the Benin haplotype. The differences were remarkable despite the otherwise common genetic background and similar environments of the two groups. Eastern patients had *higher* total haemoglobin and HbF, and *lower* HbA_2, mean cell volume (MCV), reticulocyte counts and platelet counts. Clinical differences include *more* persistent splenomegaly, a *more* normal body build, *greater* subscapular skin-fold thickness, *less* dactylitis and *less* acute chest syndrome in eastern than western Arabic patients. On the other hand, bone pathology (painful crises, osteomyelitis and avascular necrosis of the femoral head) had similar frequencies in the two groups. The disease in the Eastern province was generally milder, with less haemolysis and anaemia, and fewer of some of the infarctive complications such as autosplenectomy, probably the consequences of high HbF associated with the Arab-India haplotype and more frequent α-thalassaemia. In contrast, other complications of sickle-cell disease, especially bone pathology, are under pathophysiological and genetic control not related to HbF levels and α-thalassaemia (Nagel and Fabry, 1985; Billett et al, 1986; Baum et al, 1987).

Portugal

The Portuguese commenced slaving from Senegal right from the beginning of their maritime expansion in the middle of the fifteenth century (Boxer, 1969). Over the next 400 years, they conducted their slave trade from Cape Verde Islands, Bissau, São Tomé in the Bight of Biafra, the Slave Coast (Benin and western Nigeria), Angola and Mozambique (see Figure 7). The presence of all three common African β^s-associated haplotypes, found in a small group of Portuguese people (Monteiro et al, 1989), probably reflects the wide ranging Portuguese naval explorations, and long-standing participation in a slave trade to Europe, although this was a minor concern compared with the Atlantic slave trade (Curtin, 1969). Hence, the appearance of the β^s gene in Portugal is probably much more recent (since the sixteenth century) than in Sicily.

South and East Africa

Although Africa has quite obviously been an exporter of the sickle gene, it should be remembered that Africa has also imported sickle genes from the Indian subcontinent. The Johannesburg Indian community has a sickle-cell trait rate from 1 to 2%, and, of 11 carriers tested, all have been found to have the Arab-India mutation (A. Krause, personal communication). There have been no studies reported on the population of Indian descent in east Africa.

The Americas and the Caribbean

Since the β^s gene is absent in Amerindian populations, the presence of β^s in African-Americans (and occasionally among European-Americans) is the result of gene flow from Africa during the 400 years of the Atlantic slave trade (Curtin, 1969) or, more recently, as part of Mediterranean immigration.

The geographical origins of slaves imported from Africa varied with time, with the European power involved in the trade, and with the port of destination in the New Continent. The Portuguese were the most active in the sixteenth century, the Dutch in the seventeenth century, and the British in the eighteenth century; the rate of exportation rose in each century, from about 1000 per year in 1500, to 5000 per year in 1600, to 30 000 per year in 1700, to a plateau of 75 000 per year between 1750 and 1810. After the European ban on the slave trade in 1810, a further 2.35 million were carried, predominantly by the Portuguese again, until the closure of the slave markets in Brazil and Cuba in 1880. The largest numbers came from west Africa, followed by the west coast of central Africa, with relatively few from the east coast (Table 1) (McEvedy and Jones, 1978). Hence, the mix of β^s haplotypes found in several south and central American countries, Caribbean countries and the USA might vary.

Table 1. Numbers of African slaves (in millions) transported to the Americas, and the distribution of their ports of departure.

Date (AD)	Senegal to Nigeria	Cameroon to Angola	Mozambique
1500–1810	5.75	3.75	0.5
1810–1880	0.7	1.3	0.35
Total	6.45	5.05	0.85

From McEvedy and Jones (1978).

Studies of the haplotypes in Jamaica (Wainscoat et al, 1983; Antonarakis et al, 1984) indicated that the three major African haplotypes were most frequently associated with β^s in populations generated by recent gene flow, the eighteenth-century British Atlantic slave trade. Nagel (1984) used Curtin's classical analysis (1969) of the Atlantic slave trade and found that, remarkably, the numbers calculated from the haplotype data agreed very well with the slave trade projections as to port of origin of the slaves imported to Jamaica.

The haplotype frequencies of African-Americans in different areas of the USA appears to reflect the bias of the South Carolina slave market, in which individuals of Senegalese origin were preferred (Curtin, 1969). South Carolina markets avoided individuals from the Bight of Benin, who would have had the Benin haplotype. Some differences in the frequency of haplotypes linked to β^s in different regions of the USA are observed. Nagel's (1984) calculation of the data of Antonarakis and coworkers (1984) on Baltimore HbSS patients mainly showed a deficiency of Senegal haplotype suggesting that carriers of this haplotype were in part re-exported by the Virginia trade to the South Carolina slave trade. The frequency distribution well reflects the British slave trade. A higher frequency of the Senegal haplotype is expected in the deep South, as opposed to the border states.

UNICENTRIC OR MULTICENTRIC ORIGIN OF THE MUTATION

Based on the early data of Kan and Dozy (1978) on African-Americans, Kurnit (1979) asked how many crossing-overs between the β^s gene and a 7.6 kb site 3′ to it (the *Hpa*I polymorphic site) will need to occur to reach a 13% frequency of the *Hpa*I(−). He concluded that the β^s mutation must have occurred tens of thousands years ago. Unfortunately, the premise on which this analysis was based was wrong. The *Hpa*I polymorphism was not subsequent to the β^s mutation, but preceded it, as both the analysis of multipolymorphic sites and the analysis of African β^A chromosomes have shown. In addition, for the Kurnit analysis to be right, the *Hpa*I(+) and *Hpa*I(−) will have to coexist. This only occurred in America through the vagaries of the slave trade, but not in Africa, where the gene originated. In Africa, no ethnic group has been described in which *Hpa*I(+) coexists with *Hpa*I(−) haplotypes. Bodmer and Solomon (1979) corrected Kurnit on only one point: they pointed out that the mutation could have been 'laying around' and the expansion by malaria and the origin of the mutation need to be separated. The reason that both analyses are incorrect (Kurnit claiming multicentricity) and Bodmer and Solomon (claiming unicentricity) is that these authors did not have the benefit of the data that came afterwards.

Nevertheless, the possibility that dormant (not expanded) β^s mutations could have occurred in Africa and elsewhere before agriculture cannot be discounted. In effect, this possibility is a bit of a red herring: it is unlikely, without positive selection, that a mutation will remain in a population when the homozygote has an extremely low fitness, as sickle-cell anaemia used to have in Africa. But repeated mutations could have arisen and disappeared over a long period of time. What really matters is what mutations were around when malaria became endemic and the number of β^s carriers expanded abruptly. We can exclude that all or several of the major haplotypes coexisted in any significant number in the African locations described, since all of them would have been expanded simultaneously (although not necessarily with the same intensity) and they would coexist today in the same geographical locations. The geographical segregation of the β^s-linked haplotype is a strong argument for the expansion of a single β^s mutation in each geographical area, and suggests that there was, in all probability, a single mutation in a position of being expanded in each of the geographical areas discussed above.

MALARIA AND THE β^s GENE

There are only two possible ways in which the β^s gene can be maintained at high frequency in a population in the face of the genetic unfitness of homozygotes (and doubly heterozygotes); these are (1) a high rate of mutation replacing the loss of genes in each generation, or (2) an advantage for the gene in the heterozygous state. A high rate of mutation can be dismissed as: (1) the mutation has been rare in human evolution, only five such mutations achieving polymorphic frequency (see above); (2) studies of communities have not demonstrated any carriers of HbS who could not be accounted for by inheritance from their parents (legal or biological) (Lambotte-Legrand and Lambotte-Legrand, 1951; Neel, 1956); and (3) the distribution of genotypes in the newborn follows the Hardy–Weinberg law (Fleming et al, 1979), which would not be the case with gene replacement through mutation.

Genetic advantage can either be through survival advantage or through an increase in fertility.

Survival advantage

Higher relative fitness and rates of survival of HbAS compared with HbAA subjects have been demonstrated in several populations in Africa (Allison, 1956; Roberts and Boyo, 1962; Cavalli-Sforza and Bodmer, 1971; Edington and Gilles, 1976). In Garki, northern Nigeria, 24% of newborns had sickle-cell trait (as expected from gene frequency), but this rose to 29% by the age of 5 years, at which level it remained in all older age groups (Table 2) (Fleming et al, 1979). The fitness ratio AS : AA was 1.21 and the differential survival was 1.29, which was similar to the fitness ratio and sufficient to explain it. There was an almost complete elimination of infants born with sickle-cell anaemia by the age of 5 years from this community, which experienced inadequate nutrition, poor hygiene and hyperendemic malaria, and where modern medicine and mosquito avoidance were not practised (Table 2); there was less than 2% of the expected number of HbSS over the age of 5 years (Molineaux et al, 1979).

Table 2. Haemoglobin electrophoretic patterns in the whole population sample in Garki (1970–1972) classified by age, and the newborn during 3 years (1971–1974).

	Age (years)											
	Newborn		<1		1–4		5–9		10–14		>15	
Hb	No.	%	No.	%	No.	%	No.	%	No.	%	No.	%
AA	394	73.8	47	71.2	84	71.0	302	68.9	142	71.4	1178	70.2
AS	126	23.6	16	24.2	73	28.2	133	30.4	56	28.2	486	29.0
SS	11	2.1	2	3.0	1	0.4	0	0	1	0.5	0	0

For the sake of simplicity 22 (0.7%) subjects with HbAC have been omitted. From Fleming et al (1979).

Partial protection against P. falciparum

The evidence that sickle-cell trait affords partial protection against severe *P. falciparum* parasitaemia and its often fatal complications comes from observations based on geographical distribution, population studies, data from patients in hospitals including post-mortem studies, and in vitro experiments, which have also thrown light on possible mechanisms.

Geographical distribution. The β^s gene is found at polymorphic frequency only in populations living in those areas where *P. falciparum* is or was until recently endemic, or in populations with significant descent from the original populations (see Figure 1). Within these areas, close positive correlations between rates of transmission of malaria and β^s gene frequency are seen. However, it seems that the maximum advantage is experienced not where malaria is holoendemic, but where it is hyperendemic (Raper, 1960; Livingstone, 1971). For example, sickle-cell trait has been reported at highest frequency amongst the Kanuri (27.9%) and Bede (32.6%) in Bornu (Roberts et al, 1960), the Hausa (29%) in Garki (Fleming et al, 1979) in the sudan savanna of Nigeria, and the inhabitants of the high grasslands of Cameroon (32%) (Mbantenkhu, 1979) and Nigeria (32%) (Udeozo and Ele, 1975). The probable explanation is that where malaria is holoendemic (transmission continuous, unvaried and high throughout the year), subjects with sickle-cell trait experience advantage for one short period of life, between the decline of maternally-derived protection and the acquisition of high levels of protective immunity by both HbAA and HbAS individuals; where malaria is hyperendemic (transmission continuous, but low during the dry season), the advantage of sickle-cell trait lasts longer or recurs in successive seasons of high transmission.

Population studies. Significantly lower frequencies and densities of *P. falciparum* parasitaemia have been demonstrated in preschool children with sickle-cell trait compared with those with only normal haemoglobin in several African populations (Allison, 1954; Fleming et al, 1979, 1985; Bernstein et al, 1980) and in an Indian population living in Malaya (Joishy et al, 1988). Maternally-derived protection functioned during about the first 6 months of life, and parasitaemias were infrequent and not intense in the newborn in Garki: later with intense parasitaemia, a parasitological advantage for sickle-cell trait carriers started suddenly around the age of 30 weeks (Figure 10) and then slowly diminished to be no longer evident after 3 years of age (Fleming et al, 1979).

Those series which have not shown any significant partial protection against malaria have either (1) not studied the non-immune population, that is in African children aged between about 6 months and 5 years (Michel et al, 1981); (2) have included too few children of the critical age (Carnevale et al, 1981); or (3) been in populations with low *P. falciparum* rates (Vaisse et al, 1981), possibly the result of self-medication.

It is likely that there will be no future studies on communities who do not have access to potent antimalarials and who do not practise mosquito avoidance. The removal or breakdown of mosquito control, or travel from urban areas with low transmission to rural areas with high transmission, can result in the parasitological advantage of sickle-cell trait being apparent in older age groups, even adults, who have relatively low antimalarial immunity (Fleming et al, 1979; Willcox et al, 1983).

Hospital-based studies. Numerous series of ill African children in hospitals or in post-mortem material have shown that subjects with sickle-cell trait are

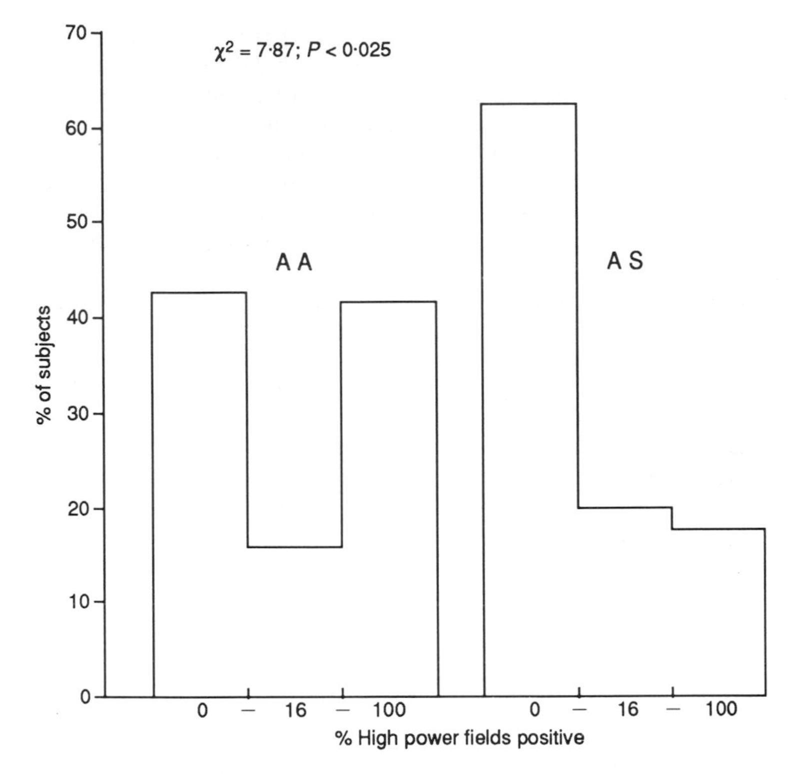

Figure 10. Distribution of HbAA ($n = 119$) and HbAS ($n = 40$) in 35-week-old infants at Garki, northern Nigeria, according to the percentage of microscopy fields positive for *P. falciparum* asexual forms (three classes: zero; 0.1–16.0%; 16.1–100%). From Fleming et al (1979) with permission of the authors and publishers.

under-represented amongst patients with the most intense *P. falciparum* parasitaemias, those with complicated malaria including cerebral malaria, and those who die from severe or complicated malaria (Beet, 1946; Allison, 1957; Edington and Watson-Williams, 1965; Gilles et al, 1967; reviewed by Livingstone, 1971; Allison and Eugui, 1982). A recent study by Hill et al (1991) on children in the Gambia has demonstrated that HbAS is associated with a 92% reduction in the relative risk of severe malaria likely to cause death, defined as cerebral malaria or severe malarial anaemia (Hb <50 g/l). No protection against *P. malariae* or *P. ovale* has been demonstrated (Allison, 1957; Fleming et al, 1979).

Increased fertility

Distinction needs to be made between regions where malaria is stable (i.e. hyperendemic or holoendemic) and levels of immunity in the population are high, and where it is unstable (i.e. mesoendemic, hypoendemic or epidemic) and immunity is low or absent in adults. With stable malaria, acquired immunity to *P. falciparum* is diminished during pregnancy, especially first pregnancies, and there is an increase of parasite frequency and density up to a plateau in mid-pregnancy (reviewed by Fleming, 1989a). Sickle-cell trait was associated with a partial protection against intense parasitaemia in northern Nigerian primigravidae (Fleming et al, 1984): however, this parasitological advantage was not translated into a better haematological state, except that HbAS has been shown to protect against severe anaemia (haematocrit <0.23) associated with gross splenomegaly (>10 cm below the costal margin) in pregnancy in Ibadan (Fleming et al, 1968). Where *P. falciparum* is stable, increased fertility of women with sickle-cell trait is unlikely to contribute significantly to genetic fitness (reviewed Allison, 1956; Cavalli-Sforza and Bodmer, 1971). Fertility of HbAA and HbAS women did not differ significantly in Garki (Fleming et al, 1979) or in malarial endemic Costa Rica (Madrigal, 1989).

Where malaria is unstable, women of all parities are liable to develop severe and complicated malaria during pregnancy (reviewed by Fleming, 1989a). In this situation, sickle-cell trait can be associated with better health during pregnancy and increased fertility sufficient to make a major contribution to greater genetic fitness, for example amongst the Black Caribs (Firschein, 1961: reviewed by Cavalli-Sforza and Bodmer, 1971).

Sickle-cell trait and immunity

Plasma immunoglobins (Ig) and titres of specific antimalarial antibodies rise with age. Subjects with sickle-cell trait had significantly lower mean Ig, especially IgM, and lower titres of antibodies against *P. falciparum* compared with subjects with normal adult haemoglobin only, and the difference between the two genotypes increased with age (Figure 11) (Cornille-Brøgger et al, 1979). It is unlikely that HbAS subjects had a limited ability to produce antibody or a more rapid catabolism of Ig, but the more probable explanation is that they had less malarial antigenic stimulus, and that this remained true in older children and adults, long after any parasitological advantage of HbAS could be demonstrated.

Reduced malarial antigenic load may explain the almost complete protection offered by sickle-cell trait against development of hyper-reactive malarial splenomegaly (previously called the tropical splenomegaly syndrome) (Fleming et al, 1968; Hamilton et al, 1969; Bryceson et al, 1976), a condition seen in patients with acquired antimalarial immunity and characterized by lymphocytic proliferation and overproduction of IgM and antibodies against *P. falciparum*.

Lower frequency of splenomegaly in non-immune children exposed to malaria has been reported (Beet, 1947; Monekosso and Ibiama, 1966), but differences did not achieve significance (Bowman, 1968), although it has been claimed that the average spleen size is smaller (Boyo, 1972).

Malaria is itself immunosuppressive, and it may be hypothesized that protection against malaria should be followed by improved immune responses to other infections or immunizations. Greenwood et al (1980) demonstrated that the antibody responses of Nigerian children with sickle-

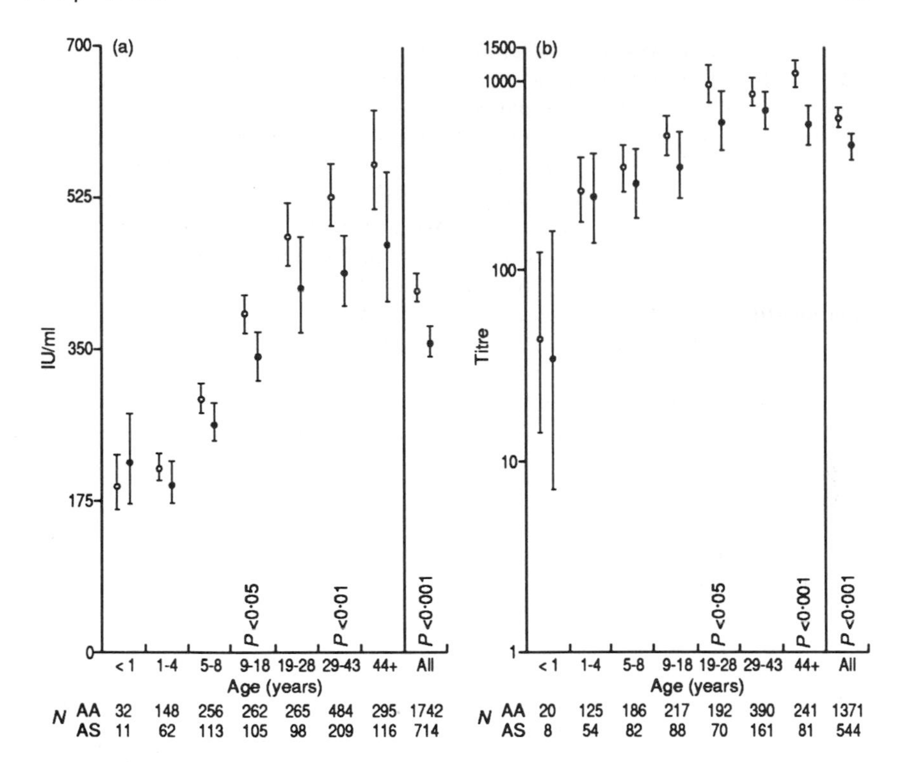

Figure 11. (a) Immunoglobulin M. (b) Indirect haemagglutination test against *P. falciparum*. The geometric mean and its 95% confidence limits in haemoglobin AA (○) and haemoglobin AS (●), in the population of Garki, northern Nigeria. From Cornille-Brøgger et al (1979) with permission of the authors and publishers.

cell trait to group C meningococcal polysaccharide vaccine were, on average, better than in children with HbAA. In an environment of many endemic infections, the advantages of sickle-cell trait may reach beyond the immediate effects of the limitation of *P. falciparum* parasitaemia.

Mechanism of the balanced polymorphism of the β^s gene

The first mechanistic explanation for the restriction of *P. falciparum* in β^s carriers came from Luzzatto and collaborators (1970), who reported in 1970 that the rate of sickling of the parasitized HbAS red cells was 2–8 times greater than the non-parasitized cells in the same blood. This finding suggested that the parasite had unwittingly increased the chances of sickling, and hence, the probability of being detected by the spleen and removed from the circulation. In other words, the parasite had undertaken a suicidal infection.

Roth et al (1978b) provided further evidence of the soundness of this hypothesis by measuring sickling curves on parasitized red cells in culture, and also at physiological levels of nitrogen-induced deoxygenation (conditions similar to venous haemoglobin, i.e. oxygen saturations of about 50%). Differences in sickling were detectable between parasitized and non-parasitized sickle-trait red cells.

The mechanism by which the parasitized HbAS cells sickle is most probably the reduction of the intracellular pH. Bookchin et al (1976) demonstrated that a decreased intracellular pH induces the appearance of morphological sickling in unparasitized red cells. *P. falciparum* is known to increase glycolysis significantly in the red cell cytoplasm, with the corresponding production of lactic and glutamic acid (Friedman, 1979a). Nevertheless, the invasion of HbAS red cells and their subsequent sickling and removal by the spleen is not the only mechanism involved. Friedman (1978) demonstrated that HbAS cells at 17% oxygen normally sustained the growth of *P. falciparum*, but the reduction of oxygen to 3% (after 2 days of normal growth in 17% oxygen), was accompanied by a failure of the parasite to thrive and its ultimate death in 48 hours. This finding strongly suggested that the parasites which survive the suicidal invasion of HbAS cells during their ring form stage have another hurdle to jump during the deep vascular schizogony, the period in which the parasitized red cells, during the early trophozoite stage, grow knobs in the red cell surface (Raventos-Suarez et al, 1985) and adhere to the endothelium surfaces of venules (Rock et al, 1988). The venules, bedecked with adherent parasitized HbAS cells, become partially or totally obstructed, a situation that leads to hypoxia and low pH, conditions that favour sickling of the HbAS cells, and in which the parasite does not thrive.

The mechanism of death of parasites in sickled HbAS cells is not definitively established but there are two possible mechanisms, not mutually exclusive. (1) Sickling of HbAS is accompanied by the loss of water concomitant with the loss of K^+, progressively increasing mean corpuscular haemoglobin concentration and, hence, further increasing HbS polymerization (this reaction is affected by the twentieth power of the initial HbS concentration) (Friedman, 1979a). The main proof for the role of K^+ or loss of cell water was the decrease in sickling observed when HbAS cells were suspended in high extracellular K^+, an observation confirmed by Olson and Nagel (1986). It would be of interest to establish if the K^+ efflux is through Ca^{2+}-dependent K^+ channels activated by the intracellular increases in Ca^{2+} that accompanies sickling, or by a parasitized-cell specific mechanism. Early suggestions of an intrinsic effect of low intracellular K^+ secondary to K^+ efflux detrimental to parasite growth was based on the K^+ requirements for *P. lophurie* culture (Friedman et al, 1979). Nevertheless, Ginsberg et al (1986) and Tanabe et al (1986) have shown that ouabain-treated red cells, enriched in intracellular Na^+, sustain the growth of the parasite normally. (2) The second mechanism operating in the ultimate death of the *P. falciparum* parasite in the HbAS red cells could be that the polymer is an inappropriate substrate for the proteases of the parasite, as suggested by Eaton and Hofrichter (1987), or that the polymer interferes intrinsically with some critical function of the parasite.

Pasvol confirmed the inhibition of parasite growth in deoxygenated HbAS cells, but in addition reported a significant decrease in invasion rate (Pasvol et al, 1978; Pasvol, 1980). Olson and Nagel's (1986) data in synchronized cultures, a method that can detect invasion quite sensitively, are not compatible with this last claim.

In summary, the carriers of HbAS cells have innate partial resistance to dying from *P. falciparum* malaria by at least two mechanisms: (1) the dramatic increase in sickling rates of parasitized HbAS cells (compared with the almost never sickled non-parasitized HbAS cells) makes them particularly prone to be removed from the circulation by the spleen; (2) the parasites that have escaped the first line of defence find themselves incapable of prospering during the deep vascular schizogony.

These two mechanisms are compatible with the epidemiological data that suggests that the AS carriers are not immune to contracting the disease, but are less likely to die from it. This mechanism renders the carriers fitter than individuals with normal haemoglobin and increases their chance to reproduce. Their advantage is balanced with the decreased fitness of the homozygote for HbS eventually reaching an equilibrium in the β^s gene frequency.

Sickle-cell disease and malaria

Whatever the intracellular mechanisms by which *P. falciparum* growth is limited in HbAS red cells are, the same apply in HbSS red cells. In vitro development of late forms of the parasite was inhibited in HbSS cells at low oxygen tension (Friedman, 1978; Pasvol et al, 1978; Pasvol, 1980); in fact, and as might be expected, the decline of growth was faster in HbSS than in HbAS cells, with death and lysis of most or all intracellular parasites within 24 hours of incubation with low oxygen, as compared to 48 hours in HbAS cells (Friedman, 1978). Electron microscopy suggested that parasites in HbSS cells were being impaled by needle-like deoxyhaemoglobin S aggregates (Friedman, 1979b), but it remains uncertain whether this appearance has any in vivo equivalent. When HbAA, AS and SS red cells were infected with *P. falciparum* and incubated with monocytes from the same donors, phagocytosis of parasitized red cells was greater in both HbAS and HbSS cells compared to HbAA (Luzzatto and Pinching, 1990); the *enhancement* of erythrophagocytosis of parasitized HbAS cells was twice that of HbSS cells, but the initial rate of erythrophagocytosis of unparasitized HbSS cells was high, and the parasites seemed to be in about equally suicidal positions in both types of HbS-containing cells.

In the only published field study of malaria in subjects with sickle-cell anaemia in a community, as opposed to hospital-based studies, HbSS subjects at Garki did not have significantly less than expected *P. falciparum* frequency (unlike HbAS), but did have lower than median *P. falciparum* densities while below the age of 5 years (like HbAS); over 1 year of age they tended to have below average titres of antibodies against *P. falciparum* antigens (like HbAS), compatible with there being less antigenic stimulus (Molineaux et al, 1979). HbSS children had significantly less than expected *P. malariae* parasitaemias and antibodies against *P. malariae*, suggesting that HbS in the proportions found in the red cells of homozygotes inhibits this parasite as well.

However, in the clinical setting, these observations are almost meaningless, as malarial parasitaemia, even if mild, precipitates haemolytic and infarctive crises in patients with sickle-cell disease. In otherwise unselected hospital patients, those with HbSS were reported to be more likely than HbAA (10 versus 2%) to have obvious parasitaemias (defined as at least one parasite in every other ×450 field on a thin blood film) (Luzzatto, 1974; Luzzatto and Pinching, 1990); however, it should be noted that parasite densities were considerably lower in the HbSS than the HbAA patients, suggesting that *P. falciparum* may be both inhibited in growth and a common cause of clinical disease in patients with sickle-cell disease. *P. falciparum* frequently causes severe haemolytic crises and profound anaemia in patients with sickle-cell disease (Rey et al, 1966; Adeloye et al, 1971; Fleming and Werblińska, 1982; Akinyanju and Johnson, 1987), and this used to be the most commonly observed cause of death (Trowell et al, 1957; Rey et al, 1966; Kagwa-Nyanzi, 1970; reviewed by Fleming, 1989b). The role of deficient spleens and autosplenectomy (the latter almost invariably found after 10 to 15 years of age) might also reduce innate resistance.

Malaria is also the factor most often identified as precipitating infarctive crises, especially bone-pain crises (Edington, 1953; Konotey-Ahulu, 1971, 1974; Maharajan et al, 1983; reviewed by Fleming, 1989b). Prompt antimalarial therapy for patients in crisis and continuous antimalarial prophylaxis for patients in the steady state are cornerstones in the management of sickle-cell disease, and have contributed to the well-being of Africans with sickle-cell disease more than any other intervention over the past four decades (Oyejide et al, 1982, 1985; Fleming, 1989b).

SUMMARY

The β^s gene arose at least four times in Africa, with three of these mutations expanding through diverse ethnic groups, but limited to definite geographical areas: Atlantic west Africa for the Senegal haplotype linked β^s; central west Africa for the Benin haplotype; and equatorial, eastern and southern Africa for the Bantu haplotype. The fourth mutation (linked to the Cameroon haplotype) is restricted to a single ethnic group, the Eton of central Cameroon. The Benin haplotype linked β^s gene was spread by gene flow to the Mediterranean (north, south and east) and to the western portions of Saudi Arabia. An independent mutation linked to a fifth haplotype, Arab-India, is found among the tribals of India (independent from their geographical origin) and in the eastern oases of Saudi Arabia. It is also suspected of being associated with the β^s gene found in Afghanistan, Iran, Transcaucasia and central Asia.

The selective force involved in the expansion of the gene was most likely *P. falciparum* malaria, and the time of the gene frequency increase was likely to have been during the expansion of agriculture about 4000 or more years ago in India and about 3000 years ago in Africa.

The partial protection against severe and life-threatening malaria is through the limitation of *P. falciparum* parasitaemia. This is a complex process which involves at least two mechanisms: early intraerythrocyte parasite forms are in a suicidal position through increasing the tendency of HbAS cell to sickle and then be destroyed by the spleen; intraerythrocyte growth is inhibited during deep vascular schizogony.

Although there is evidence that *P. falciparum* (and *P. malariae*) parasitaemias are limited in HbSS red cells, malaria is a major trigger to haemolytic and infarctive crises in sickle-cell disease, and a common cause of morbidity and mortality.

Acknowledgements

We wish to thank Ms Gayle Spring, Ms Linda Thompson-Biggs, Ms Felicity English and Dr Ivan Dukes for their skilled and careful help in the preparation of this manuscript, and Mr E D Swanepoel (Department of Illustration, SAIMR) for the preparation of figures. The work summarized here has been made possible by grants from the National Institutes of Health (nos HL21016 and HL38655) and by grant G3/181/70 from the World Health Organization.

REFERENCES

Adeloye A, Luzzatto L & Edington GM (1971) Severe malarial infection in a patient with sickle-cell anaemia. *British Medical Journal* **ii:** 445–446.

Akinyanju O & Johnson AO (1987) Acute illness in Nigerian children with sickle cell anaemia. *Annals of Tropical Paediatrics* **7:** 181–186.

Aksoy M (1985) Hemoglobinopathies in Turkey. *Hemoglobin* **9:** 209–216.

Aksoy M, Dinçol G & Erdem S (1980) Survey of haemoglobin variants, β-thalassaemia, glucose-6-phosphate-dehydrogenase deficiency and haptoglobin types in Turkish people living in Manavgat, Serik and Boztepe (Anatalya). *Human Heredity* **30:** 3–6.

Alkasab FM, Al-Alusi FA, Adnani MS et al (1981) The prevalence of sickle cell disease in Abu-Al-Khasib district of southern Iraq. *Journal of Tropical Medicine and Hygiene* **84:** 77–80.

Allison AC (1954) Protection afforded by sickle cell trait against subterrain malarial infection. *British Medical Journal* **i:** 290–294.

Allison AC (1956) The sickle-cell and haemoglobin C genes in some African populations. *Annals of Human Genetics* **21:** 67–89.

Allison AC (1957) Malaria in carriers of the sickle-cell trait and in newborn children. *Experimental Parasitology* **6:** 418–447.

Allison AC & Eugui EM (1982) A radical interpretation of immunity to malaria parasites. *Lancet* **ii:** 1431–1433.

Aluoch JR, Kilinc Y, Aksoy M et al (1986) Sickle cell anaemia among Eti-Turks: haematological, clinical and genetic observations. *British Journal of Haematology* **64:** 44–55.

Antonarakis SE, Boehm CD, Serjeant GR et al (1984) Origin of the β^s-globin gene in Blacks: the contribution of recurrent mutation or gene conversion or both. *Proceedings of the National Academy of Sciences of the USA* **81:** 853–856.

Bakioglu I, Hattori Y, Kutlar A et al (1985) Five adults with mild sickle cell anemia share a $beta^s$ chromosome with the same haplotype. *American Journal of Hematology* **20:** 297–300.

Barnola J, Tovar-Escobar G & Potenza L (1953) Enfermedad por celulas falciformes. *Archivos Venezolanos de Peuricultura y Pediatria* **16:** 293–376.

Batabyal JN & Wilson JMG (1958) Sickle cell anemia in Assam. *Journal of the Indian Medical Association* **30:** 8–16.

Baum KF, Dunn DT, Maude GH & Serjeant GR (1987) The painful crisis of homozygous sickle-cell disease. A study of risk factors. *Archives of Internal Medicine* **147:** 1231–1234.

Beet EA (1946) Sickle cell disease in Balovale District of Northern Rhodesia. *East African Medical Journal* **23:** 75–86.

Beet EA (1947) Sickle cell disease in Northern Rhodesia. *East African Medical Journal* **24:** 212–222.
Belhani M, Morle L, Godet J et al (1984) Sickle cell β-thalassaemia compared with sickle cell anaemia in Algeria. *Scandinavian Journal of Haematology* **32:** 346–350.
Bernstein SC, Bowman JE & Kaptue Noche L (1980) Population studies in Cameroon. Hemoglobin S, glucose-6-phosphate-dehydrogenase deficiency and falciparum malaria. *Human Heredity* **30:** 251–258.
Bhowmik KL (1971) *Tribal India: A Profile in Indian Ethnology*. Calcutta: World Press.
Billett HH, Kim K, Fabry ME & Nagel RL (1986) The percentage of dense red cells does not predict incidence of sickle cell painful crisis. *Blood* **68:** 301–303.
Bodmer E & Solomon WF (1979) Evolution of sickle variant gene. *Lancet* **i:** 923.
Bodner J & Cavalli-Sforza LL (1976) *Genetics, Evolution and Man*. San Francisco: WH Freeman.
Bookchin RM, Balazs T & Landau LC (1976) Determinants of red cell sickling: effects of varying pH and of increasing intracellular hemoglobin concentration by osmotic shrinkage. *Journal of Laboratory and Clinical Medicine* **87:** 597–616.
Bovill EW (1958) *The Golden Trade of the Moors*. London: Oxford University Press.
Bowman JE (1968) Splenomegaly and the sickle-cell trait. *Lancet* **i:** 1200.
Boxer CR (1969) *The Portuguese Seaborne Empire 1415–1825*. London: Hutchinson.
Boyo AE (1972) Malariometric indices and hemoglobin type. *American Journal of Tropical Medicine and Hygiene* **21:** 863–867.
Brittenham G, Lozoff B, Harris JW et al (1979) Sickle cell anemia and trait in southern India: further studies. *American Journal of Hematology* **6:** 107–123.
Bryceson ADM, Fleming AF & Edington GM (1976) Splenomegaly in northern Nigeria. *Acta Tropica* **33:** 185–214.
Carnevale P, Bosseno MF, Lallemant M et al (1981) Le paludisme à *Plasmodium falciparum* et le gène de la drépanocytose en République populaire du Congo. I. Relation entre la parasitémie et le trait drépanocytaire à Djoumouna (région de Brazzaville). *Annales de Génetique* **24:** 100–104.
Cavalli-Sforza LL & Bodmer WF (1971) *The Genetics of Human Populations*, pp 148–154. San Francisco: WH Freeman.
Chakravarti A, Buetow KH, Antonarakis SE et al (1984) Nonuniform recombination within the human β-globin gene cluster. *American Journal of Human Genetics* **36:** 1239–1258.
Chatterjea JB (1966) Haemoglobinopathies, glucose-6-phosphate-dehydrogenase deficiency and allied problems in the Indian subcontinent. *Bulletin of the World Health Organization* **35:** 29–48.
Chebloune Y, Pagnier J, Trabuchet G et al (1988) Structural analysis of the 5′ flanking region of the β-globin gene in African sickle cell anemia patients: further evidence for three origins of the sickle mutation in Africa. *Proceedings of the National Academy of Sciences of the USA* **85:** 4431–4435.
Chediak M, Calderon JC & Vargas GP (1939) Anemia a hematies falciformes. Contribucion a su estudio en Cuba. *Archivos de Medicina Interna* **5:** 313–370.
Christakis J, Vavatsi N, Hassapopoulou H et al (1990) Comparison of homozygous sickle cell disease in northern Greece and Jamaica. *Lancet* **335:** 637–640.
Christakis J, Vavatsi N, Hassapopoulou H et al (1991) A comparison of sickle cell syndromes in northern Greece. *British Journal of Haematology* **77:** 386–391.
Cornille-Brøgger R, Fleming AF, Kagan I et al (1979) Abnormal haemoglobins in the sudan savanna of Nigeria. II. Immunological response to malaria in normals and subjects with sickle cell trait. *Annals of Tropical Medicine and Parasitology* **73:** 173–183.
Curtin PD (1969) *The Atlantic Slave Trade. A Census*. Milwaukee: University of Wisconsin Press.
Deka R (1981) Fertility and haemoglobin genotypes: a population study in Upper Assam (India). *Human Genetics* **59:** 172–174.
DiRienzo A, Felicetti J, Terrenato L et al (1987) RFLP's in β^{thal} and β^{s} chromosomes in Egypt. *Second International Symposium on Thalassaemia in Crete*.
Eaton WA & Hofrichter J (1987) Hemoglobin S gelation and sickle cell disease. *Blood* **70:** 1245–1266.
Edington GM (1953) Sickle-cell anaemia in the Accra district of the Gold Coast. *British Medical Journal* **ii:** 957–961.

Edington GM & Gilles HM (1976) *Pathology in the Tropics* 2nd edn, p. 466. London: Edward Arnold.
Edington GM & Watson-Williams EJ (1965) Sickling, haemoglobin C, glucose-6-phosphate-dehydrogenase deficiency and malaria in Western Nigeria. In Jonix JHP (ed.) *Abnormal Haemoglobins in Africa,* pp 393–401. Oxford: Blackwell Scientific.
Firschein IL (1961) Population dynamics of the sickle-cell trait in the Black Caribs of British Honduras, Central America. *American Journal of Human Genetics* **13:** 233–248.
Fleming AF (1987) Anaemia as a world health problem. In Weatherall DJ, Ledingham JGG & Warrell DA (eds) *Oxford Textbook of Medicine* 2nd edn, pp 19.72–19.79. Oxford University Press.
Fleming AF (1989a) Tropical obstetrics and gynaecology. 1. Anaemia in pregnancy in tropical Africa. *Transactions of the Royal Society of Tropical Medicine and Hygiene* **83:** 441–448.
Fleming AF (1989b) The presentation, management and prevention of crisis in sickle cell disease in Africa. *Blood Reviews* **3:** 18–28.
Fleming AF & Werblińska B (1982) Anaemia in childhood in the guinea savanna of Nigeria. *Annals of Tropical Paediatrics* **2:** 161–173.
Fleming AF, Allan NC & Stenhouse NS (1968) Splenomegaly and sickle-cell trait. *Lancet* **ii:** 574.
Fleming AF, Storey J, Molineaux L et al (1979) Abnormal haemoglobins in the sudan savanna of Nigeria. I. Prevalence of haemoglobins and relationships between sickle-cell trait, malaria and survival. *Annals of Tropical Medicine and Parasitology* **73:** 161–172.
Fleming AF, Harrison KA, Briggs ND et al (1984) Anaemia in young primigravidae in the guinea savanna of Nigeria; sickle-cell trait gives partial protection against malaria. *Annals of Tropical Medicine and Parasitology* **78:** 395–404.
Fleming AF, Akintunde A, Attai EDE et al (1985) Malaria and haemoglobin genotype in young northern Nigerian children. *Annals of Tropical Medicine and Parasitology* **79:** 1–5.
Friedman MJ (1978) Erythrocytic mechanism of sickle cell resistance to malaria. *Proceedings of the National Academy of Sciences of the USA* **75:** 1994–1997.
Friedman MJ (1979a) Oxidant damage mediates variant red cell resistance to malaria. *Nature* **280:** 245–247.
Friedman MJ (1979b) Ultrastructural damage to the malaria parasite in the sickled cell. *Journal of Protozoology* **26:** 195–199.
Friedman MJ, Roth EF, Nagel RL & Trager W (1979) *Plasmodium falciparum:* physiological interactions with the human sickle cell. *Experimental Parasitology* **47:** 73–80.
Fuzman LC, Etcheverry BR, Muranda RM et al (1964) Hemoglobinas anormales y hemoglobinopatias en Chile. Drepanocitosis. *Proceedings of the 9th Congress of the International Society of Hematology 1962, Mexico* **3:** 71–80.
Gilles HM, Fletcher KA, Hendrickse RG et al (1967) Glucose-6-phosphate-dehydrogenase deficiency, sickling, and malaria in African children in south western Nigeria. *Lancet* **i:** 138–140.
Ginsburg H, Handeli S, Friedman S et al (1986) Effects of red blood cell potassium and hypertonicity on the growth of *Plasmodium falciparum* in culture. *Zeitschift für Parasitenkunde* **72:** 185–192.
Granda H, Gispert S, Dorticos A et al (1991) Cuban programme for prevention of sickle cell disease. *Lancet* **337:** 152–153.
Greenberg JH (1973) African languages. In Skinner EP (ed.) *Peoples and Cultures of Africa* p 84. New York: Doubleday/National History Press.
Greenwood BM, Bradley AK, Blakebrough IS et al (1980) The immune response to a meningococcal polysaccharide vaccine in an African village. *Transactions of the Royal Society of Tropical Medicine and Hygiene* **74:** 340–346.
Haghshenass M, Ismail-Beigi F, Clegg JB & Weatherall DJ (1977) Mild-sickle cell anaemia in Iran associated with high levels of fetal haemoglobin. *Journal of Medical Genetics* **14:** 168–171.
Hamilton PJS, Morrow RH, Ziegler JL et al (1969) Absence of sickle cell trait in patients with tropical splenomegaly syndrome. *Lancet* **ii:** 109.
Herrera Cabral JM (1950) *Revista Medica Dominicana* **5:** 265. Quoted in WA Collier and DA de la Parra (1952) Sickle-cell trait in Surinam Creoles. *Tropical and Geographical Medicine* **6:** 517–521.

Hill AVS, Allsopp CEM, Kwiatkowski D et al (1991) Common West African HLA antigens are associated with protection from severe malaria. *Nature* **352:** 595–600.

Jain RC (1985) Sickle cell and thalassaemic genes in Libya. *Transactions of the Royal Society of Tropical Medicine and Hygiene* **79:** 132–133.

Joishy SK, Hassan K, Lopes M & Lie-Injo LE (1988) Clinical, genetic and fertility studies of Indians with β^s-globin gene and the influence of HbS on *Plasmodium falciparum* malaria infection. *Transactions of the Royal Society of Tropical Medicine and Hygiene* **82:** 515–519.

Kagwa-Nyanzi JA (1970) Causes of death amongst sickle cell anaemia patients in Mulago Hospital, Kampala, Uganda. *East African Medical Journal* **47:** 337–343.

Kalmus H (1957) Defective colour vision, PTC tasting and drepanocytosis in samples from fifteen Brazilian populations. *Annals of Human Genetics* **21:** 313–317.

Kan YW & Dozy AM (1978) Polymorphism of DNA sequence adjacent to the human β-globin structural gene: relationship to sickle mutation. *Proceedings of the National Academy of Sciences of the USA* **75:** 5631–5635.

Kan YW & Dozy AM (1980) Evolution of the hemoglobin S and C genes in world populations. *Science* **209:** 388–391.

Kar BC, Devi S, Dash KC & Das M (1987) The sickle cell gene is widespread in India. *Transactions of the Royal Society of Tropical Medicine and Hygiene* **81:** 273–275.

Kennedy KAR (1981) Skeletal biology: when bones tell tales. *Archeology* **34:** 17–24.

Kollia P, Karababa PH, Sinopoulou K et al (1987) Distribution of the beta-gene cluster haplotypes in Greece. Feasibility of prenatal diagnosis of thalassaemia. *Second International Symposium of Thalassaemia in Crete.*

Konotey-Ahulu FID (1971) Malaria and sickle cell disease. *British Medical Journal* **ii:** 710–711.

Konotey-Ahulu FID (1974) The sickle cell diseases. *Archives of Internal Medicine* **133:** 611–619.

Kulozik AE, Wainscoat JS, Serjeant GR et al (1986) Geographical survey of β^s-globin gene haplotypes: evidence for an independent Asian origin of the sickle-cell mutation. *American Journal of Human Genetics* **39:** 239–244.

Kurnit DM (1979) Evolution of sickle variant gene. *Lancet* **i:** 104.

Labie D, Srinivas R, Dunda O et al (1989) Haplotypes in tribal Indians bearing the sickle gene: evidence for the unicentric origin of the β^s mutation and the unicentric origin of tribal populations of India. *Human Biology* **61:** 479–491.

Lambotte-Legrand J & Lambotte-Legrand C (1951) L'anémie a hematies falciformes chez l'enfant indigene du Bas-Congo. *Annales de le Société Belge de Médecine Tropicale* **31:** 207–234.

Lapouméroulie D, Dunda O, Trabuchet G et al (1989) A novel sickle gene of yet another origin in Africa: the Cameroon type. *Blood* **74** (supplement 1): 63a.

Lehmann H & Cutbush M (1952) Sickle cell-trait in southern India. *British Medical Journal* **i:** 289–290.

Livingstone FB (1971) Malaria and human polymorphisms. *Annual Review of Genetics* **5:** 33–64.

Livingstone FB (1976) Hemoglobin history in west Africa. *Human Biology* **48:** 487–500.

Livingstone FB (1989) Who gave whom hemoglobin S: the use of restriction site haplotype variation for the interpretation of the evolution of the β^σ-globin gene. *American Journal of Human Biology* **1:** 289–302.

Luzzatto L (1974) Genetic factors in malaria. *Bulletin of the World Health Organization* **50:** 195–202.

Luzzatto L & Pinching AJ (1990) Innate resistance to malaria: the intraerythrocytic cycle. Commentary. *Blood Cells* **16:** 340–347.

Luzzatto L, Nwachuku-Jarrett ES & Reddy S (1970) Increased sickling of parasitised erythrocytes as mechanism of resistance against malaria in the sickle-cell trait. *Lancet* **i:** 319–322.

McEvedy C (1980) *The Penguin Atlas of African History*. Harmondsworth: Penguin.

McEvedy C & Jones R (1978) *Atlas of World Population History*, pp 204–218. Harmondsworth: Penguin.

Madrigal L (1989) Hemoglobin genotype, fertility, and the malaria hypothesis. *Human Biology* **61:** 311–325.

Maggio A, Acuto S, LoGioco P et al (1986) β^A and β^{thal} DNA haplotypes in Sicily. *Human Genetics* **72:** 229–230.

Maharajan R, Fleming AF & Egler LJ (1983) Pattern of infections among patients with sickle-cell anaemia requiring hospital admission. *Nigerian Journal of Paediatrics* **10:** 13–17.
Mbantenkhu FJ (1979) Rôle de la polygamie dans la distribution du gène drépanocytaire. *Seminaire Provincial de la Santé Publique de l'Ouest Cameroun.*
Mears JG, Lachman HM, Cabannes R et al (1981a) The sickle gene: its origin and diffusion from West Africa. *Journal of Clinical Investigation* **68:** 606–610.
Mears JG, Beldjord C, Benabadji M et al (1981b) The sickle gene polymorphism in north Africa. *Blood* **58:** 599–601.
Mera B (1943) Preliminares del estudio de la meniscocitemia en Colombia. *Boletin de la Oficina Sanitaria Pan-Americana* **22:** 680–682.
Michel R, Carnevale P, Bosseno MF et al (1981) La paludisme à *Plasmodium falciparum* et le gène de la drépanocytose en République populaire du Congo. I. Prévalence du paludisme et du trait drépanocytaire en milieu scolaire dans la région Brazzavilloise. *Médecine Tropicale* **41:** 403–412.
Miller BA, Olivieri N, Salameh M et al (1987) Molecular analysis of the high-hemoglobin F phenotype in Saudi Arabian sickle cell anemia. *New England Journal of Medicine* **316:** 224–250.
Molineaux L, Fleming AF, Cornille-Brøgger R et al (1979) Abnormal haemoglobins in the sudan savanna of Nigeria. III. Malaria, immunoglobulins and antimalarial antibodies in sickle-cell disease. *Annals of Tropical Medicine and Parasitology* **73:** 301–310.
Monekosso GL & Ibiama AA (1966) Splenomegaly and sickle-cell trait in a malaria-endemic village. *Lancet* **i:** 1347–1348.
Monteiro C, Rueff J, Falcao AB et al (1989) The frequencies and origin of the sickle mutation in the district of Corciche/Portugal. *Human Genetics* **82:** 255–258.
Nagel RL (1984) The origin of hemoglobin S gene. Clinical, genetic and anthropological consequences. *Einstein Quarterly Journal of Biology and Medicine* **2:** 53–62.
Nagel RL & Fabry ME (1985) The many pathophysiologies of sickle cell anemia. *American Journal of Hematology* **20:** 195–199.
Nagel RL & Ranney HM (1990) Genetic epidemiology of structural mutations of the β-globin gene. *Seminars in Hematology* **27:** 342–359.
Neel JV (1956) The genetics of human haemoglobin differences: problems and perspectives. *Annals of Human Genetics* **21:** 1–30.
Ojwang PJ, Ogada T, Beris P et al (1987) Haplotypes and α globin gene analyses in sickle cell anaemia patients from Kenya. *British Journal of Haematology* **65:** 211–215.
Olson JA & Nagel RL (1986) Synchronized cultures of *P. falciparum* in abnormal red cells: the mechanism of the inhibition of growth in HbCC cells. *Blood* **67:** 977–1001.
Oyejide OC, Adeyokunnu AA, Kraus JF & Fanti C (1982) A comparative study of the morbidity associated with sickle cell anemia among patients in Ibadan (Nigeria) and Oakland (USA). *Tropical and Geographical Medicine* **34:** 341–345.
Oyejide OC, Abilgaard C & Fanti C (1985) A comparative study of hematocrit values of sickle cell patients in Ibadan (Nigeria) and Oakland (CA, USA). *Journal of Tropical Pediatrics* **31:** 328–331.
Padmos MA, Roberts GT, Sackey K et al (1991). Two different forms of homozygous sickle cell disease occur in Saudi Arabia. *British Journal of Haematology* **79:** 93–98.
Pagnier J, Mears JG, Dunda-Belkhodja O et al (1984) Evidence for the multicentric origin of the sickle cell hemoglobin gene in Africa. *Proceedings of the National Academy of Sciences of the USA* **81:** 1771–1773.
Pasvol G (1980) The interaction between sickle haemoglobin and the malarial parasite *Plasmodium falciparum. Transactions of the Royal Society of Tropical Medicine and Hygiene* **74:** 701–705.
Pasvol G, Weatherall DJ & Wilson RJM (1978) Cellular mechanism for the protective effect of haemoglobin S against *P. falciparum* malaria. *Nature* **274:** 701–703.
Perrine RP, Brown MJ, Clegg JB et al (1972) Benign sickle-cell anaemia. *Lancet* **ii:** 1163–1167.
Piggott S (1950) *Prehistoric India*, pp 132–289. Harmondsworth: Penguin.
Pons JA & Oms M (1934) Incidencia del rasgo meniscocitico (eritrocitos semilunares) en Puerto Rico. *Boletin de la Asociacion Medica de Puerto Rico* **41:** 1132–1144.
Ragusa A, Lombardo M, Sortino G et al (1988) β^s gene in Sicily is in linkage disequilibrium with the Benin haplotype: implications for gene flow. *American Journal of Hematology* **27:** 139–141.

Ramot B, Fisher S, Remex D et al (1960) Haemoglobin O in an Arab family. *British Medical Journal* **ii:** 1262–1264.
Ramsay M & Jenkins T (1987) Globin gene-associated restriction-fragment-length polymorphisms in southern African peoples. *American Journal of Human Genetics* **41:** 1132–1144.
Raper AB (1960) Sickling and malaria. *Transactions of the Royal Society of Tropical Medicine and Hygiene* **54:** 503–504.
Raventos-Suarez C, Kaul DK, Macaluso F & Nagel RL (1985) Membrane knobs are required for the microcirculatory obstruction induced by *Plasmodium falciparum*-infected erythrocytes. *Proceedings of the National Academy of Sciences of the USA* **82:** 3829–3833.
Rey M, Quenum C & Guerin M (1966) Paludisme pernicieux mortel chez un drépanocytaire. *Bulletin de la Société Médicale d'Afrique Noire de Langue Française* **11:** 802–807.
Roberts DF & Boyo AE (1962) Abnormal haemoglobins in childhood among the Yoruba. *Human Biology* **34:** 20–37.
Roberts DF, Lehmann H & Boyo AE (1960) Abnormal hemoglobins in Bornu. *American Journal of Physical Anthropology* **18:** 5–11.
Rock EP, Roth EF Jr, Rojas-Corona RR et al (1988) Thrombospondin mediates the cytoadherence of *Plasmodium falciparum*-infected red cells to vascular endothelium in shear flow conditions. *Blood* **71:** 71–75.
Roth EF Jr, Rachmilewitz E, Schifter A & Nagel RL (1978a) Benign sickle cell anemia in Israeli-Arabs with high red cell 2,3-diphosphoglycerate. *Acta Haematologica* **59:** 237–245.
Roth EF Jr, Friedman M, Ueda Y et al (1978b) Sickling rates of human AS red cells infected in vitro with *Plasmodium falciparum* malaria. *Science* **202:** 650–652.
Roy DN & Roy Chaudhuri SK (1967) Sickle cell trait in the tribal population in Madhya Pradesh and Orissa (India). *Journal of the Indian Medical Association* **48:** 150–152.
Sandler GS, Schilirò G, Russo A et al (1978) Blood group phenotypes and the origin of sickle cell hemoglobin in Sicilians. *Acta Haematologica* **60:** 350–357.
Shukla RN & Solanki BR (1958) Sickle cell trait in central India. *Lancet* **i:** 297–298.
Srinivas R, Dunda O, Krishnamoorthy R et al (1988) Atypical haplotypes linked to the β^s gene in Africa are likely to be the product of recombination. *American Journal of Hematology* **29:** 60–62.
Tanabe K, Izumo A & Kageyama K (1986) Growth of *Plasmodium falciparum* in sodium-enriched human erythrocytes. *American Journal of Tropical Medicine and Hygiene* **35:** 476–478.
Tokarev YN & Spivak VA (1982) Heterogeneity and distribution of hemoglobinopathies in some parts of the USSR. *Hemoglobin* **6:** 653–660.
Tomlinson WJ (1945) The incidence of sicklemia and sickle cell anemia in 3000 Canal Zone examinations upon natives of Central America. *American Journal of Medical Sciences* **209:** 181–186.
Trabuchet G, Elion J, Baudot G et al (1989) Origin and spread of β-globin gene mutations in India, Africa and Mediterranean: analysis of the 5′ flanking and intragenic sequences of β^s and β^c genes. *Human Biology* **63:** 241–252.
Trowell HC, Raper AB & Welbourn HF (1957) The natural history of homozygous sickle cell anaemia in central Africa. *Quarterly Journal of Medicine* **26:** 401–422.
Udeozo IOK & Ele E (1975) Distribution of haemoglobin electrophoretic patterns among Igbo patients attending the University of Nigeria teaching hospital, Enugu. *Abstracts of the Joint Annual Conference of the Nigerian Society for Immunology, Nigerian Society of Haematology and Blood Transfusion and the Association of Pathologists of Nigeria*, p. 69.
Vaisse D, Michel R, Carnevale P et al (1981) Le paludisme à *Plasmodium falciparum* et le gène de la drépanocytose in République populaire du Congo. II. Manifestations cliniques du paludisme selon la parasitémie et le génotype hémoglobinique. *Médecine Tropicale* **41:** 413–423.
Wainscoat JS, Bell JI, Thein SL et al (1983) Multiple origins of the sickle mutation: evidence from β^s globin gene cluster polymorphisms. *Molecular Biological Medicine* **1:** 191–197.
Wainscoat JS, Thein SL, Higgs DR et al (1985) A genetic marker for elevated levels of haemoglobin F in homozygous sickle cell disease? *British Journal of Haematology* **60:** 261–268.
Wheeler M (1968) *The Indus Civilization* 3rd edn. Cambridge: Cambridge University Press.
Wiesenfeld SL (1967) Sickle-cell trait in human biological and cultural evolution. *Science* **157:** 1134–1140.

Willcox M, Björkman A, Brohult J et al (1983) A case-control study in Liberia of *Plasmodium falciparum* malaria in haemoglobin S and β-thalassaemia traits. *Annals of Tropical Medicine and Parasitology* **77:** 239–246.
Workman PL, Blumberg BS & Cooper AJ (1963) Selection, gene migration and polymorphic stability in a US White and Negro population. *American Journal of Human Genetics* **36:** 495–465.
World Health Organization Working Group (1983) Community control of hereditary anaemias: memorandum from a WHO meeting. *Bulletin of the World Health Organization* **61:** 63–80.
Zago MA & Costa FF (1985) Hereditary haemoglobin disorders in Brazil. *Transactions of the Royal Society of Tropical Medicine and Hygiene* **79:** 385–388.

5

Glucose-6-phosphate dehydrogenase deficiency

O. SODEINDE

Deficiency of glucose-6-phosphate dehydrogenase (G6PD). (EC 1.1.1.49) is the most common enzymopathy in human populations. It combines this with the unique phenomenon of X-chromosome inactivation, because of the siting of its gene locus on that chromosome (Xq28). The relative ease with which blood can be obtained for testing makes the study of the red cell enzyme a subject of keen interest. Thus, about 400 variants have been described since the early reports of this disorder appeared less than 40 years ago (Beutler, 1959; 1991).

G6PD catalyses the first and rate-limiting step of the hexose monophosphate (pentose phosphate) pathway. This pathway generates reduced nicotinamide adenine dinucleotide phosphate (NADPH), which is essential for many biosynthetic reactions and for the protection of biological molecules in membranes and elsewhere against oxidant damage. This function is vital for the erythrocyte, which has no alternative source of NADPH. In other cells, with less extreme degrees of differentiation, other enzymes like hexokinase can produce some NADPH in the presence of low G6PD activity.

The second function of the hexose monophosphate shunt is to generate ribose, without which the production of nucleotide coenzymes, the replication of nucleic acids, and therefore cell division, cannot occur. For this reason, it is not surprising that G6PD has been detected in virtually every cell type of every contemporary organism so far tested. Thus, G6PD is a typical 'household' or 'housekeeping' enzyme. Total absence of G6PD enzyme activity is probably incompatible with life, at least in multicellular organisms.

Apart from the clinical importance of G6PD deficiency, which affects large segments of the human population, this enzyme is of interest from a purely biological viewpoint. Analyses of variants present at cellular level in heterozygotes have been used to demonstrate the clonal origin of human tumours (Fialkow, 1979), as well as certain embryonal cells (Sobis et al, 1991).

Classification of variants

The over 300 alleleic variants of G6PD are classified as shown in Table 1. Less than one-third of them are common, i.e. polymorphic, this being

Baillière's Clinical Haematology—
Vol. 5, No. 2, April 1992
ISBN 0-7020-1627-6

Table 1. Classification of G6PD variants.

Class*	No. polymorphic	Electrophoretic mobility			% with electrophoretic change	Total
		Fast	Normal	Slow		
I	1 (1)	20	30	32	63	82
II	49 (45)	29	39	41	64	109
III	22 (30)	25	13	36	82	74
IV	14 (32)	15	2	26	95	43
V	0	2	0	0	100	2
Total	86 (28)	91	84	135	73	310

Values in parentheses are percentages.
*Class I, associated with chronic non-spherocytic haemolytic anaemia (CNSHA); class II, severely deficient less than 10% residual activity; class III, moderately deficient: 10–60% residual activity; class IV, normal activity: 60–150%; class V, increased enzyme activity.
From Betke et al (1967), Yoshida et al (1971) and Beutler (1983).

defined arbitrarily as a frequency of >1% of the males in that particular population. The majority of polymorphic variants belong to classes II and III, and it is these which constitute public health problems in communities where they occur.

Some 10 years ago, G6PD deficiency was reviewed in this series (Bienzle, 1981; Panich, 1981). Since then, several excellent reviews have appeared (Luzzatto and Battistuzzi, 1985; WHO Working Group, 1989a; Beutler, 1991). However, the focus in this review is on the epidemiology of this disorder.

EPIDEMIOLOGY

World distribution

The world distribution of polymorphic G6PD deficient variants is summarized graphically in Figure 1. The actual population frequency figures for various regions is summarized also in Table 2, although the range is from 62% in Kurdish Jews (Szeinberg, 1973) to 0.1% in Japan and northern Europe (WHO Working Group, 1989b). Detailed figures for individual countries can be found in the unpublished WHO document (WHO/HDP/WG/G6PD/85.9), which is obtainable from the Hereditary Diseases Programme, Division of Noncommunicable Diseases, WHO, Geneva. However, the limitations in the applicability of these figures must be stressed. In a number of countries no published figures are available and the data in the tables have been derived from what is known for neighbouring countries. In some countries, especially in tropical Africa, only a handful of epidemiological surveys conducted at a few centres are available. Yet, micromapping in other places (e.g. Sardinia) has shown that otherwise genetically relatively homogeneous communities in geographical proximity may have significantly different gene frequencies for G6PD deficiency (Siniscalco et al, 1966; Terrenato, 1976). For the foregoing reasons, the figures in Table 2 and

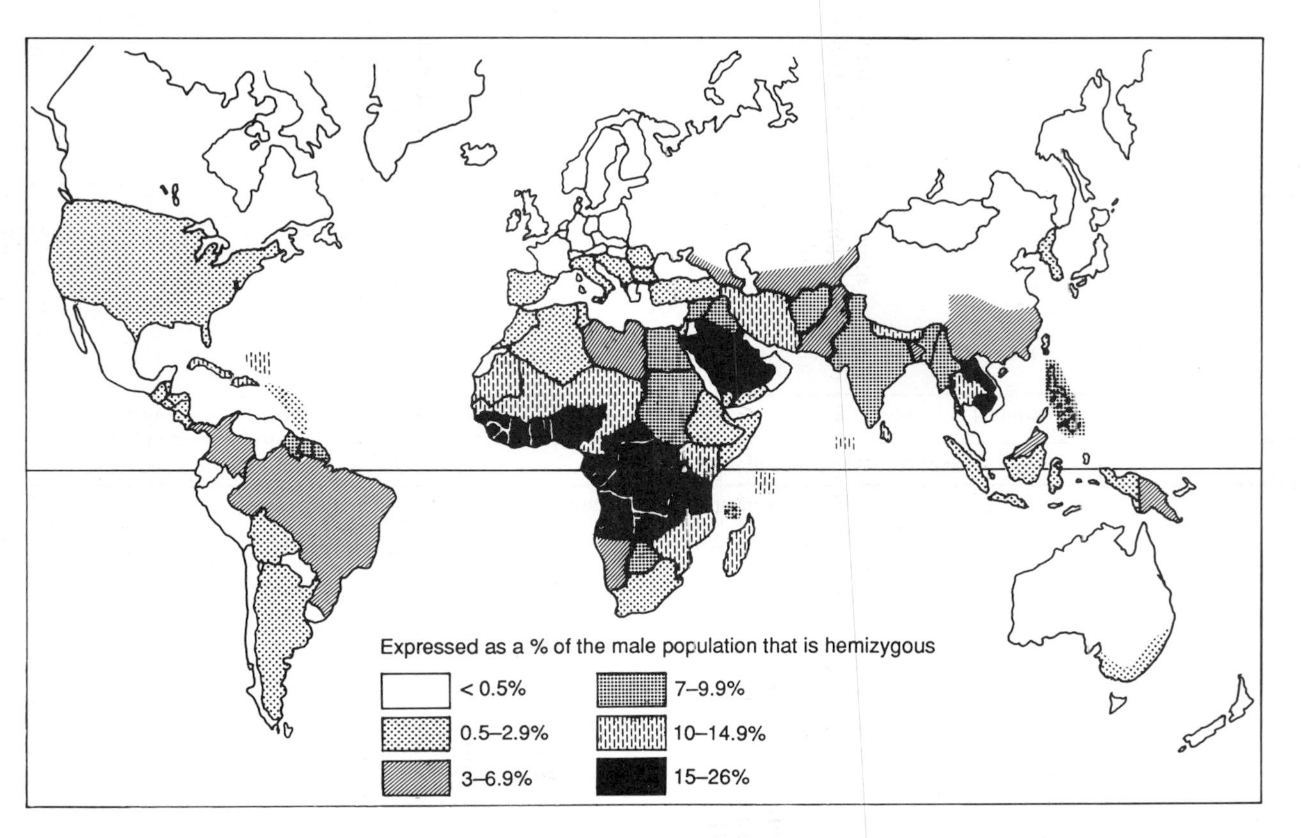

Figure 1. World distribution of G6PD deficiency. (From WHO Working Group, 1989a).

Table 2. Summary of estimated incidence of G6PD deficiency in the regions of the world.

	Population (millions)	Annual births (thousands)	Males hemizygous (%)	Annual births (thousands) of			♀ Homozygous (%) of all deficient
				♂ Hemizygous	♀ Homozygous	♀ Heterozygous	
Africa							
North	116.1	4951	3.8	142.8	20.2	264.8	12.4
East (north)	37.9	1869	1.0	9.4	0.1	18.7	1.0
East (south)	81.7	3910	13.2	258.4	34.6	447.2	11.8
South	33.9	1299	0.9	15.7	0.6	30.4	4.0
Islands	11.2	469	13.2	31.0	4.3	52.8	12.2
Sub-saharan	212.0	10161	17.1	870.7	161.7	1148.2	15.1
Total	492.8	22650	11.7	1327.9	221.5	2232.1	14.3
Americas							
North	257	4183	1.8	36.8	3.2	74.2	8
Central	97	3394	0.5	8.8	0.2	15.8	2.2
South	252	8243	3.4	145.5	7.2	274.4	4.8
Caribbean	31.2	833	9.6	40.0	4.2	70.9	9.5
Total	637.2	16653	2.7	231.1	18.8	435.3	6.1

Asia							
North-west	161.5	6 649	7.2	239.5	52.1	424.4	17.9
South	923.5	33 397	6.3	1 046.1	77.9	1 951.0	6.9
East (north)	791.0	16 246	0.1	8.9	—	20.8	—
East (south)	803.0	21 992	5.24	576.5	38.4	970.5	6.2
Total	2 663.1	78 112	4.8	1 872.1	168.4	3 368.9	8.4
Europe							
West	236.5	2 954	0.3	4.2	—	8.4	—
East	79.2	1 311	0.1	—	—	—	—
South	171.7	2 403	1.3	16.0	0.8	30.4	4.5
CIS (USSR)	267.0	5 130	0.8	18.6	1.5	35.8	6.8
Total	754.4	11 798	0.7	38.8	2.3	74.6	5.1
Oceana total	23.2	475	1.9	4.7	0.3	9.0	6.3
Global total	4 570	130 000	5.25	3 475	411	6 120	10.6
% of total annual births				2.7	0.3	4.7	
					7.7		

—, No data available

the relevant publications should be regarded as stimuli for more epidemiological studies (including micromapping) on G6PD deficiency. Meanwhile, the available data can be summarized to the effect that lower frequencies of G6PD deficiency are associated with higher altitudes, especially above 1000 m. Thus, within tropical (sub-Saharan) Africa, deficiency gene frequencies are 0.26, 0.20 and 0.197 in low altitude Côte d'Ivoire, Nigeria and Zaire respectively. These contrast with 0.12, 0.112 and 0.126 for higher altitude Kenya, Uganda and Zimbabwe respectively. This summary, of course, excludes populations in which inbreeding (consanguinity) is prominent. Examples include many Jewish populations (Szeinberg, 1973; Milbauer et al, 1973) as well as the Kel Kummer Tuaregs in west Africa (Junien et al, 1982). Also excluded would be populations in which genetic drift is obviously the dominant factor, as exemplified by the Negro populations of the West Indies, north and south America.

Epidemiological tools

Standard methods for G6PD testing stipulate the use of fresh blood in suitable anticoagulant (Betke et al, 1967; Beutler et al, 1979). Although dried blood collected on filter paper is more convenient and has been used for large scale screening of newborns in Europe (Solem et al, 1985), this was considered unsuitable for the hot humid tropics. However, recent evidence shows that, in such climates as well, specimens collected in this way are indeed suitable for the fluorescent spot (screening) test as well as G6PD electrophoresis (O. Sodeinde et al, unpublished observations).

POLYMORPHISM AND MALARIA

The early observations on the close correlation between the prevalence of G6PD deficiency and falciparum malaria, past or current, led to the 'malaria hypothesis' (Motulsky and Campbell-Kraut, 1961; Allison, 1964). Since then, a plethora of evidence has accumulated. This has been competently reviewed elsewhere (Bienzle, 1981; Panich, 1981; Luzzatto and Battistuzzi, 1985). In epidemiological studies of G6PD alleles random inactivation of the X-chromosome requires that male subjects should be analysed separately from female ones. Considering those studies in which this has been done, the data on balance provide evidence, in many cases quite compelling, in support of the view that falciparum malaria is the environmental agent of natural selection that enabled an otherwise deleterious gene (i.e. G6PD deficiency) to attain polymorphic frequencies, and that this operates through an advantage (protection) enjoyed by heterozygotes, who are females of necessity in this particular system.

In vitro, the data also support this conclusion (Luzzatto et al, 1983; Usanga and Luzzatto, 1985; Ling and Wilson, 1988; Kurdi-Haidar and Luzzatto, 1990). However, it must be noted that a few gaps still exist in the published reports, the filling of which should render the evidence incontrovertible. The main gap concerns the lack of published reports on G6PD alleles in cerebral malaria, the most severe form of falciparum malaria. For instance, for the haemoglobin S gene, heterozygote advantage against cerebral malaria has been demonstrated in post-mortem studies (Edington, 1967). Hitherto, no similar reports exist for G6PD heterozygotes, but in a recent series in Ibadan, Nigeria, significant under-representation of G6PD deficiency heterozygotes has been observed among patients with cerebral malaria, and the rarity of haemoglobin S gene heterozygotes was confirmed (O. Sodeinde et al, unpublished observations).

Altitude

The higher gene frequencies for G6PD deficiency in west and central Africa as contrasted with east Africa was mentioned earlier. The average altitudes in these two regions are <100 m and 1400 m respectively. In parts of the latter region, lower levels of malaria endemicity with occasional epidemics are known to occur (Bruce-Chwatt, 1985). Thus, higher altitudes (>1000 m), which are known to be associated with lower levels of malaria endemicity, are also associated with lower gene frequencies for G6PD deficiency, not only with respect to the Mediterranean variant (Siniscalco et al, 1966; Terrenato, 1976), but to the A− variant as well.

G6PD polymorphism and non-falciparum human malaria

The malaria–G6PD hypothesis, as initially put forward, concerned *Plasmodium falciparum*. The question as to whether these ideas apply to other human plasmodia is difficult to tackle. This is because the world-wide preponderance of *P. falciparum* means that there are fewer patients with pure non-falciparum malaria available for study. However, quartan malaria nephropathy, a major cause of nephrotic syndrome in the tropics (Hendrickse, 1976), provides an opportunity for the indirect study of the interaction between G6PD polymorphism and *P. malariae*, the parasite associated with this condition. Malaria is still holoendemic in Nigeria (Salako et al, 1990), but the relative rarity of this condition after the eradication of malaria in Guyana (Giglioli, 1962) makes this study desirable. In an on-going study in Ibadan, Nigeria, the first 33 girls cumulated suggest a reduction in the G6PD A−/B heterozygotes (Table 3). If this is borne out at the end of the

Table 3. G6PD types in 33 girls who had childhood nephrotic syndrome.

	Gene frequencies					
G6PD genotype	B/B	B/A−	B/A	A/A−	A/A	A−/A−
Current study ($n=33$)	0.606 (20)	0.03 (1)	0.212 (7)	0.03 (1)	0.091 (3)	0.03 (1)
Control* ($n=100\,000$)	0.3136	0.2461	0.246	0.097	0.048	0.048

Values in parentheses are actual numbers.
* Predicted from the Hardy–Weinberg equilibrium for blood bank donors.

study, it would indicate that the protective effect of G6PD heterozygosity probably covers *P. malariae* too.

Malaria, G6PD deficiency and haemoglobin S

In the population. It is logical to expect that since both variant genes are associated with partial protection against malaria, the population distributions of G6PD deficiency and haemoglobin S would be similar. This expectation holds true if haemoglobinopathies are taken as a group, i.e. including thalassaemias, in those populations where this latter condition is common. There are two notable 'exceptions' to this generalization. One is the indigenous (Amerindian) American population who, despite malaria endemicity, have neither G6PD deficiency nor haemoglobinopathies (Luzzatto and Battistuzzi, 1985). The second is the fact that in Africa south of the Zambezi, G6PD deficiency evidently occurs alone without any sickle-cell disorders (Hitzeroth and Bender, 1980). Much of this region lies within the temperate zone: therefore it is tempting to speculate that the lower environmental temperatures bring about a lower level of malaria endemicity, and that consequently, a smaller biological (survival) advantage against malaria is conferred on heterozygotes. This advantage could still be enough to balance the conceivably lower genetic burden of G6PD deficiency but not that of sickle-cell disease (SCD). In fact, the colder environmental temperatures would tend to increase oxygen demand by the tissues and so increase the genetic burden (clinical illness) of SCD beyond what obtains within the tropics. But direct evidence for this idea is entirely lacking. In any case, neither of these 'exceptions' constitutes an effective argument against the malaria hypothesis with respect to G6PD deficiency.

In individual patients/subjects. It is also logical to wonder whether the simultaneous presence of heterozygosity for haemoglobin S and G6PD deficiency would enhance biological fitness even more than either factor alone. The best group in which to test this idea would be patients with cerebral malaria, but the rarity of haemoglobins A + S among such patients makes such a test difficult. However, it is clear that the advantage conferred by such 'double heterozygosity' is not absolute, since in a series of 122 paediatric patients with cerebral malaria, one girl was shown to have haemoglobin A + S as well as a G6PD genotype A−/B (O. Sodeinde et al, unpublished observations).

Among sickle-cell disease (SCD) patients. Since malaria is a major contributor to morbidity and mortality in SCD patients, a logical extension of the foregoing is to ask whether G6PD deficiency ameliorates or aggravates SCD, especially sickle-cell anaemia (SCA), the clinically most severe form. If either of these happens, then one would expect the frequencies of G6PD deficiency among male SCD patients to be significantly higher or lower, respectively. Among female SCD patients, the frequencies of the genotype A−/B would be higher or lower, respectively. There are no relevant published data on female SCD patients, but in the two large male series from

Nigeria and the USA, the frequency of G6PD (−) was not different from that of the general population (Bienzle et al, 1975; Steinberg et al, 1988). However, the recent report of increased prevalence of G6PD (−) among patients with gallstones (Meloni et al, 1991) suggests that G6PD (−) may still be of significance in the clinical course of the individual SCD patient.

ADVERSE CLINICAL EFFECTS

The main adverse clinical effects of G6PD deficiency are neonatal jaundice and acute haemolytic anaemia induced by food (favism), drugs, certain other chemicals and infections. Certain rare variants are associated with a chronic haemolytic anaemia (see Table 1).

Neonatal jaundice

This has been reviewed extensively in the past (Luzzatto and Testa, 1978; Bienzle, 1981; Panich, 1981; WHO Working Group, 1989a; Beutler, 1991) and elsewhere in these two volumes; however, a few points of epidemiological importance probably bear repetition.

Aflatoxin. This ubiquitous mycotoxin has been found at high concentrations in cord blood and breast milk of patients in tropical Africa (Lamplugh et al, 1988). Since aflatoxin has a serious effect on liver cells, it may play a major role in neonatal jaundice by worsening the 'immaturity' of the neonatal liver.

Menthol-containing balms. Olowe and Ransome-Kuti (1980) pointed to 'mentholated' dusting powders as an important source of exposure to oxidants. Of similar importance are a wide range of menthol-containing balms which are applied as dressings to the umbilical cord, rubbed on the chest to 'prevent or treat colds' or into the nostrils for a similar reason. Unlike the dusting powders, which are usually present in homes in which there are newborns or older infants, these balms are present in virtually every home in many communities in tropical areas.

Neonatal transfusions. It is obvious that blood for exchange transfusion and transfusion for favism and other forms of acute haemolytic anaemia should have normal G6PD activity (WHO Working Party, 1989a), but it is not often remembered that this requirement should apply to all neonatal transfusions. This includes the correction of iatrogenic anaemia, often associated with the need for blood tests in the care of critically ill neonates, especially those of low birth weight. Otherwise, in certain communities like Nigeria, there would be roughly a 20% chance at each transfusion of converting a neonate with normal enzyme activity into a haematological mosaic, with 25% enzyme-deficient red cells. This would enhance the risk of subsequent jaundice should sepsis occur.

Food-induced haemolysis

The most important here is favism. It is difficult to predict which G6PD-deficient patient will develop haemolysis after eating fava beans, a Mediterranean staple. Only about 25% of them do so, although it is more common among children under 5 years old. Divisine and isouramil are thought to be the haemolytic agents. Haemolysis is not related to the quantities of beans consumed (Hedayat et al, 1981; Battistuzzi et al, 1982; Arese and De Flora, 1990). This interpatient variation may be due to other genetic factors, but there are also intrapatient variations. It appears that the genetics of the *Vicia*

Table 4. Drugs to be avoided in G6PD deficiency.

Antimalarials	*Analgesics*
Primaquine [people with the African A− variant may take it at reduced dosage, 15 mg daily or 45 mg twice weekly under surveillance]	Acetylsalicylic acid (aspirin): moderate doses can be used.
Pamaquine	Acetophenitidin (phenacetin)
Chloroquine (may be used under surveillance when required for prophylaxis or treatment of malaria)	Safe alternative: paracetamol
Sulphonamides and sulphones	*Anthelmintics*
Sulphanilamide	**β-Naphthol**
Sulphapyridine	**Bilbophan**
Sulphadimidine	**Niridazole**
Sulphacetamide (Albucid)	
Sulphafurazole (Gantrisin)	
Salicylazosulphapyridine (Salazopyrin)	
Dapsone*	
Sulphoxone*	
Glucosulphone sodium (Promin)	
Co-trimoxazole	
Other antibacterial compounds	*Miscellaneous*
Nitrofurans: Nitrofurantoin	**Vitamin K analogues** (1 mg of menaphthone can be given to babies)
Furazolidone	**Naphthalene*** (moth balls)
Nitrofurazone	**Probenecid**
[Nalidixic acid]	**Diamercaprol (BAL)**
Chloramphenicol	**Methylene blue**
p-Aminosalicylic acid	**Arsine***
	Phenythydrazine*
	Acetylphenylhydrazine*
	Toluidine blue
	Mepacrine

- Drugs given in **bold** print should be avoided by people with all forms of G6PD deficiency.
- Drugs in normal print should be avoided, in addition, by G6PD-deficient persons of Mediterranean, Middle Eastern, and Asian origin.
- Items in normal print and within square brackets apply only to people with the African A− variant.

* These drugs may cause haemolysis in normal individuals if given in large doses. Many other drugs may produce haemolysis in particular individuals.
(From WHO Working Group, 1989a).

faba plant may provide a useful complementary approach to the control of favism, if plant varieties could be bred (and propagated) which are not associated with the precipitation of favism.

Favism has been associated with G6PD Mediterranean but not with G6PD A−. However, with respect to the latter, one report of food-induced haemolysis has been made from Nigeria. The agent appears to be a food-colouring dye sometimes used in preparing barbecued meat (Williams et al, 1988). It is of little epidemiological importance since only a small minority of vendors use this dye.

Drug-induced haemolysis

Historically, the discovery of G6PD deficiency occurred while investigating primaquine-induced haemolytic anaemia. Table 4 lists the drugs to be avoided by G6PD-deficient individuals. Small differences exist between mildly deficient variants (e.g. A−) and more severely deficient ones (e.g. Mediterranean, Mahidol and Canton). It has been argued that the continued presence of aspirin on the list is unjustified (Beutler, 1991), but in this particular case there is another reason for avoiding the drug in all newborns, not just in the G6PD deficient. This is because aspirin has a high binding ratio to plasma albumin, to which unconjugated bilirubin also binds. Aspirin would tend therefore to displace bilirubin from those albumin binding sites into the intracellular compartment, with a greater risk of irreversible brain damage (kernicterus). In older children, the association with the Reye syndrome is a reason to avoid aspirin. The risk here is probably epidemiologically small but real. Meanwhile, no entirely satisfactory in vitro test to predict haemolysis is yet available (Gaetani et al, 1976; Horton and Calabiese, 1986; Bashan et al, 1988).

Infection-induced haemolysis

Quantitatively, this is more important than the other precipitants of haemolysis (Burka et al, 1966; Effiong and Laditan, 1976; Beutler, 1991). Although neonatal jaundice is the most common clinical problem in most populations, infection is present in a large proportion of those neonates. In addition, in older children and adults, bacterial (e.g. typhoid and pneumococcal pneumonia) as well as viral (e.g. hepatitis A and B) infections are known to precipitate jaundice (Choremis et al, 1966; Morrow et al, 1968; Owusu et al, 1972; Williams et al, 1976; Oluboyede et al, 1979). Jaundice is known to occur in malaria, probably the most common human protozoal infection worldwide, but there is no clear association of malarial haemolysis with G6PD deficiency, except perhaps in the case of blackwater fever (WHO Division of Control of Tropical Diseases, 1990). The haemolysis which occurs in the foregoing conditions is dose dependent in the case of drugs and probably severity dependent in the case of infections. It is also self-limiting. However, when massive, the haemolysis can become life threatening (Wong, 1972, 1977; Luzzatto, 1975; Luzzatto and Testa, 1978; Bienzle, 1981; Panich, 1981; Beutler, 1983).

Chloroquine-induced pruritus

A peculiar pattern of pruritus has for some time been known to follow the use of certain antimalarials (Ekpechi and Okoro, 1964; Sowunmi et al, 1989). This self-limiting but distressing side-effect of chloroquine is seen virtually exclusively in negroid races, in which G6PD A− is also mainly found. This codistribution raises the question of an epidemiological association between these two factors. No published data on this matter could be found, but the preliminary results of an ongoing study in Ibadan, Nigeria are summarized in Table 5. Among male patients, G6PD A− occurred more frequently in the group of those who developed pruritus after taking chloroquine than in the group who did not.

Table 5. G6PD alleles in 125 chloroquine-treated male patients.

	Chloroquine-induced pruritus		
G6PD allele	Yes	No	Subtotal
B	40	50	90
A	5	10	15
A−	12(21.1)*	8(11.8)*	20
Total	57	68	125

* G6PD deficiency (%) in parenthesis. Prevalence of G6PD deficiency (i.e. G6PD A−) was significantly higher among patients who developed chloroquine-induced pruritus than among those who did not ($P < 0.05$).

G6PD deficiency and environmental pollution

In recent times, there has been a growing world-wide concern about the implications of environmental pollution, not only for human and animal health, but also for the overall ecology of the Earth. The vulnerability of a given organism to many of these pollutants may depend on its ability to generate reductive molecules such as NADPH for which G6PD is important. Thus, the increasing interest in how G6PD-deficient individuals handle certain environmental pollutants should yield valuable data for the formulation of public health policies in occupational health. This is particularly true for pollutants which have been recognized for a long time as public health problems, for example lead (Cocco et al, 1991).

MOLECULAR GENETICS OF G6PD: EPIDEMIOLOGICAL ASPECTS

The growing understanding of the molecular genetics of G6PD variants has been reviewed recently (Beutler, 1991; Beutler et al, 1991). The mutations associated with chronic haemolytic anaemia (i.e. class I variants) are clustered towards the carboxy end of the molecule (between amino acid residues 362 and 446), while those producing milder clinical effects are near the amino terminal. 'Silent' mutations have been identified (D'Urso et al, 1988), including population markers at DNA level (Fey et al, 1990). Also G6PD Mediterranean, which was thought to be quite heterogeneous, now seems to be far less so, although the mutants in India and Europe probably have different origins (Beutler and Kohl, 1990; Vives-Corrons et al, 1990; Beutler et al, 1991). On the other hand, G6PD A− has been shown to comprise at least three different mutants (Beutler et al, 1989).

Of more clinical interest, however, is whether the relative frequencies of the various mutants within a given 'biochemical phenotype' explain the variations in clinical expression earlier observed. For example, in G6PD A− patients, is the distribution of the three mutants among those who develop jaundice different from the distribution among those who do not? There is good reason to expect that data of this type will grow rapidly, since the polymerase chain reaction requires very little blood (<1 ml), and this is likely to come increasingly within the reach of laboratories in tropical developing countries (Zuo et al, 1990; Stoker, 1990).

SUMMARY

Glucose-6-phosphate dehydrogenase (G6PD) deficiency is the most common human enzymopathy. Because its gene locus is on the X-chromosome it is more common in males than females in all populations. Prevalence rates vary from 62% among Kurdish Jews to the very low rates (0.1% or less in Japan, for example), which are compatible with sporadic cases arising from spontaneous mutations. However, there is at least one population in which G6PD deficiency has not been found, namely the indigenous (Amerindian) population of America. Approximately 400 variants have been described. Despite the clinical burden imposed by this enzymopathy, polymorphic frequencies have been reached in many populations. There is abundant epidemiological evidence that this has happened because of a biological advantage conferred on heterozygotes in falciparum malaria endemic areas. This advantage may apply to quartan malaria as well. Clinical severity varies, from the rare chronic non-spherocytic haemolytic anaemia to progressively milder forms like the Mediterranean and A− types. The other clinical syndromes, i.e. neonatal jaundice and haemolysis caused by infections, foods, drugs and chemicals, are not always predictable. This is because only a fraction of such enzymopathic persons develop these syndromes after exposure to the relevant stimulus. Modern techniques of molecular biology may elucidate why this is so. There is some emerging evidence that the genetic burden or survival value associated with G6PD deficiency may be relevant not only in tropical and infectious diseases, but also in their chemotherapy (e.g. malaria) as well as in the control of a long-recognized environmental pollutant such as lead.

Acknowledgements

The financial assistance of the World Health Organization is gratefully acknowledged.

REFERENCES

Allison AC (1964) Polymorphisms and natural selection in human populations. *Cold Spring Harbor Symposia on Quantitative Biology* **29:** 137–149.
Arese P & De Flora A (1990) Pathophysiology of hemolysis in glucose-6-phosphate dehydrogenase deficiency. *Seminars in Hematology* **27:** 1–40.
Bashan N, Peleg N & Moses SW (1988) Attempts to predict the haemolytic potential of drugs in glucose-6-phosphate dehydrogenase deficiency of the Mediterranean type by an in-vitro test. *Israeli Journal of Medical Sciences* **24:** 61–64.
Battistuzzi G, Morellini M, Meloni T, Gandini E & Luzzatto L (1982) Genetic factors in favism. In Weatherall DJ, Fiorelli G & Gorini S (eds) *Advances in Red Cell Biology*, pp 339–346. New York: Raven.
Betke K, Brewer GJ, Kirkman HN et al (1967) *Standardization of procedures for the study of glucose-6-phosphate dehydrogenase*. Report of a WHO scientific group. Technical Report Series No. 366. Geneva: World Health Organization.
Beutler E (1959) The hemolytic effect of primaquine and related compounds: a review, *Blood* **14:** 103–139.
Beutler E (1983) Glucose-6-phosphate dehydrogenase deficiency. In Stanbury JB, Wyngaarden JB, Fredrikson DS, Goldstein JL & Brown MS (eds) *The Metabolic Basis of Inherited Disease* 5th edn, pp 1629–1653. New York: McGraw-Hill.
Beutler E (1991) Glucose-6-phosphate dehydrogenase deficiency. *New England Journal of Medicine* **324:** 169–174.
Beutler E & Kuhl W (1990) The N1 1311 polymorphism of G6PD: G6PD Mediterranean may have originated independently in Europe and Asia. *American Journal of Human Genetics* **47:** 1008–1012.
Beutler E, Kuhl W, Vives-Corrons J-L & Prchal JT (1989) Molecular heterogeneity of glucose-6-phosphate dehydrogenase A−. *Blood* **74:** 2550–2555.
Beutler E, Kuhl W, Gelbert T & Foreman L (1991) DNA sequence abnormalities of human G6PD variants. *Journal of Biological Chemistry* **266:** 4145–4150.
Bienzle U (1981) Glucose-6-phosphate dehydrogenase deficiency part 1: Tropical Africa. *Clinics in Haematology* **10:** 785–799.
Bienzle U, Sodeinde O, Effiong CE & Luzzatto L (1975) G6PD deficiency and sickle cell anemia: frequency and features of the association in an African community. *Blood* **46:** 591–597.
Bruce-Chwatt LJ (1985) *Essential Malariology*, p 207. London: Heinemann.
Burka ER, Weaver ZIII & Marks PA (1966) Clinical spectrum of hemolytic anemia associated with glucose-6-phosphate dehydrogenase deficiency. *Annals of Internal Medicine* **64:** 817–825.
Choremis C, Kettamis CA, Kyriazakou M & Gavrilidou E (1966) Viral hepatitis in G6PD deficiency. *Lancet* **i:** 269.
Cocco PL, Cocco E, Anni MS et al (1991) Occupational exposure to lead and blood cholesterol in G6PD deficient and normal subjects. *Research Communications in Chemical Pathology and Pharmacology* **72:** 81–96.
D'Urso M, Luzzatto L, Perroni L et al (1988) An extensive search for restriction fragment length polymorphism in the human glucose-6-phosphate dehydrogenase locus has revealed a silent mutation in the coding sequence. *American Journal of Human Genetics* **42:** 735–741.
Edington GM (1967) Pathology of malaria in West Africa. *British Medicial Journal* **1:** 715–718.
Effiong CE & Laditan AAO (1976) Neonatal jaundice in Ibadan: a study of cases seen in the out-patients clinic. *Nigerian Journal of Paediatrics* **3:** 1–8.
Ekpechi OL & Okoro ANA (1964) A pattern of pruritus to chloroquine. *Archives of Dermatology* **89:** 631–632.
Fey MF, Wainscoat JS, Mukwala EC et al (1990) A Pvu III restriction fragment length polymorphism of the glucose-6-phosphate dehydrogenase gene is an African-specific marker. *Human Genetics* **84:** 471–472.
Fialkow PJ (1979) Clonal origin of human tumours. *Annual Review of Medicine* **30:** 135–143.
Gaetani GD, Mareni C, Ravazzolo R & Salvidio E (1976) Haemolytic effect of two sulphonamides evaluated by a new method. *British Journal of Haematology* **32:** 183–191.

Giglioli G (1962) Malaria and renal disease with special reference to British Guiana. II. The effect of malaria eradication on renal disease in British Guiana. *Annals of Tropical Medicine and Parasitology* **56:** 225–241.

Hedayat Sh, Farhud DD, Montazami K & Ghadiran P (1981) The pattern of bean consumption: laboratory findings in patients with favism, G6PD deficient and a control group. *Journal of Tropical Paediatrics* **27:** 110–113.

Hendrickse RG (1976) The quartan malarial nephrotic syndrome. In Hanebuger J, Crosuier J & Maxwell MH (eds) *Advances in Nephrology*, Volume 6, pp 229–247. Chicago: Year Book Medical Publishers Inc.

Hitzeroth HW & Bender K (1980) Erythrocyte G6PD and 6PGD genetic polymorphisms in South African negroes, with a note on G6PD and the malaria hypothesis. *Human Heredity* **54:** 233–242.

Horton HM & Calabiese EJ (1986) Prediction models for human glucose-6-phosphate dehydrogenase deficiency. *Drug Metabolism Review* **17:** 261–281.

Junien C, Chaventre A, Fofana Y et al (1982) Glucose-6-phosphate dehydrogenase and haemoglobin variants in Kel Kummer Tuareg and related groups. *Human Heredity* **32:** 318–328.

Kurdi-Haidar B & Luzzatto L (1990) Expression and characterization of glucose-6-phosphate dehydrogenase of *Plasmodium falciparum*. *Molecular and Biochemical Parasitology* **41:** 83–92.

Lamplugh SM, Hendrikse RG, Apeagyei F & Mwanmut DD (1988) Aflatoxins in breastmilk, neonatal cord blood and serum of pregnant women. *British Medical Journal* **296:** 968.

Ling IT & Wilson RJM (1988) Glucose-6-phosphate dehydrogenase activity of the malaria parasite *P. falciparum*. *Molecular and Biochemical Parasitology* **31:** 47–56.

Luzzatto L (1975) Inherited haemolytic states: Glucose-6-phosphate dehydrogenase deficiency. *Clinics in Haematology* **4:** 83–108.

Luzzatto L & Testa U (1978) Human erythrocyte glucose-6-phosphate dehydrogenase: Structure and function in normal and mutant subjects. *Current Topics in Haematology* **1:** 1–70.

Luzzatto L & Battistuzzi G (1985) Glucose-6-phosphate dehydrogenase. In Harris H & Hirschorn K (eds) *Advances in Human Genetics* **11:** 217–329.

Luzzatto L, Sodeinde O & Martini G (1983) Genetic variation in the host and adaptive phenomena in *Plasmodium falciparum* infection. *Ciba Foundation Symposium* **94:** 159–173.

Meloni T, Forteloni G, Noja G et al (1991) Increased prevalence of G6PD deficiency of patients with cholelithiasis. *Acta Haematologica* **85:** 76–78.

Milbauer B, Peled N & Svirsky S (1973) Neonatal hyperbilirubinaemia and glucose-6-phosphate dehydrogenase deficiency. *Israel Journal of Medical Sciences* **9:** 1547–1552.

Morrow MH, Smetana HF, Sai FT & Edgecomb JH (1968) Unusual features of viral hepatitis in Accra, Ghana. *Annals of Internal Medicine* **68:** 1250–1257.

Motulsky AG & Campbell-Kraut JM (1961) Population genetics of glucose-6-phosphate dehydrogenase deficiency of the red cell. In Blumberg BS (ed.) *Proceedings of the Conference on Genetic polymorphisms and Geographic Variation in Disease*, pp 9–180. New York: Grune & Stratton.

Olowe SA & Ransome-Kuti O (1980) The risk of jaundice in glucose-6-phosphate dehydrogenase deficient babies exposed to menthol. *Acta Paediatrica Scandinavica* **69:** 341–345.

Oluboyede AO, Esan GJF, Francis TI & Luzzatto L (1979) Genetically determined deficiency of glucose-6-phosphate dehydrogenase (type A−) is expressed in the liver. *Journal of Laboratory and Clinical Medicine* **2:** 87–100.

Owusu SK, Foli AK, Konotey-Ahulu FID & Janosi M (1972) Frequency of glucose-6-phosphate dehydrogenase deficiency in typhoid fever in Ghana. *Lancet* **i:** 320.

Panich V (1981) Glucose-6-phosphate dehydrogenase deficiency. Part 2: Tropical Asia. *Clinics in Haematology* **10:** 800–814.

Salako LA, Ajayi FO, Sowunmi A & Walker O (1990) Malaria in Nigeria: a revisit. *Annals of Tropical Medicine and Parasitology* **84:** 2–11.

Siniscalco M, Bernini L, Fillipi G et al (1966) Population genetics of haemoglobin variants, thalassaemia and glucose-6-phosphate dehydrogenase deficiency, with particular reference to the malaria hypothesis. *Bulletin of the World Health Organization* **34:** 379–393.

Sobis H, Verstuyf A & Vandeputte M (1991) Histochemical differences in expression of X-linked glucose-6-phosphate dehydrogenase between ectoderm-derived and endoderm-derived embryonic and extra-embryonic tissues. *Journal of Histochemistry and Cytochemistry* **39:** 569–574.

Solem E, Pirzer C, Siege M et al (1985) Mass screening for glucose-6-phosphate dehydrogenase deficiency: improved fluorescent spot test. *Clinica Chimica Acta* **152:** 135–142.

Sowunmi A, Walker O & Salako LA (1989) Pruritus and antimalarial drugs in Africans. *Lancet* **ii:** 213.

Steinberg MH, West MS, Gallagher D, Mentze W and the Cooperative Study of Sickle Cell Anemia (1988) Effects of glucose-6-phosphate dehydrogenase deficiency upon sickle cell anemia. *Blood* **71:** 748–752.

Stoker NG (1990) The polymerase chain reaction and infectious diseases: hopes and realities. *Transactions of the Royal Society of Tropical Medicine and Hygiene* **84:** 755–758.

Szeinberg A (1973) Investigation of genetic polymorphic traits in Jews: a contribution to the study of population genetics. *Israeli Journal of Medical Sciences* **9:** 1174–1180.

Terrenato L (1976) Variabilita genetica in Sardegna. In *Genetica di Popolazioni*, vol. 14, pp 187–214. Rome: Atti Convegni Lincei.

Usanga EA & Luzzatto L (1985) Adaptation of *Plasmodium falciparum* to glucose-6-phosphate dehydrogenase deficient host red cells by production of parasite-encoded enzymes. *Nature* **313:** 793–795.

Vives-Corrons JL, Kuhl W, Pujades MA & Beutler E (1990) Molecular genetics of G6PD Mediterranean variant and description of a new G6PD mutant G6PD Andalus^{1361A}. *American Journal of Human Genetics* **47:** 575–579.

WHO Working Group (1989a) Glucose-6-phosphate dehydrogenase deficiency. *Bulletin of the World Health Organization* **67:** 601–611.

WHO Working Group (1989b) *Glucose-6-phosphate dehydrogenase deficiency*. Report of a WHO Working Group (unpublished) WHO/HDP/WG/G6PD/85.9. Geneva: World Health Organization.

WHO Division of Control of Tropical Diseases (1990) Severe and complicated malaria, 2nd edn. *Transactions of the Royal Society of Tropical Medicine and Hygiene* **84** (supplement 2)**:** 1–65.

Williams AO, Tugwell P & Edington GM (1976) Glucose-6-phosphate dehydrogenase deficiency and lobar pneumonia. *Archives of Pathology and Laboratory Medicine* **100:** 25–31.

Williams CKO, Osotimehin BO, Ogunmola GB & Awotedu AA (1988) Haemolytic anaemia associated with Nigerian barbecued meat (Red Suya). *African Journal of Medicine and Medical Sciences* **17:** 71–75.

Wong HB (1972) Favism in Singapore. *Journal of the Singapore Paediatric Society* **14:** 17–25.

Wong HB (1977) Acute haemolysis in Southeast Asia. *Medical Progress* **4:** 12–14.

Yoshida A, Beutler E & Motulsky AG (1971) Human glucose-6-phosphate dehydrogenase variants. *Bulletin of the World Health Organization* **45:** 243–253.

Zuo L, Chen E, Du CS, Chang CN & Chiu DTY (1990) Genetic study of Chinese G6PD variants by direct PCR sequencing. *Blood* **76** (supplement): 51A (abstract).

6

Epidemiology of coagulation disorders

A. C. NATHWANI
E. G. D. TUDDENHAM

Haemostasis is the arrest of haemorrhage at sites of vascular injury by various means, including clot formation and platelet aggregation, with subsequent restoration of perfusion by fibrinolysis. It is a remarkable achievement of evolution which reconciles two conflicting requirements, namely that blood should clot extremely rapidly in order to prevent exsanguination and yet preserve liquidity in the circulation. Haemostasis is highly complex, involving an intricate balance between vascular endothelium, platelets, the coagulation cascade, natural anticoagulants and fibrinolysis (Figure 1). When a blood vessel is injured an immediate response is achieved by reflex vasoconstriction and formation of a platelet plug (primary haemostasis). This allows time for the coagulation cascade to form a tough fibrin meshwork (thrombus) that seals off the defect (secondary haemostasis) and provides a scaffold for angiogenic repair of the vascular wall. The manifestations of haemostasis are confined to the area of vascular damage by secretions elaborated by the intact vascular endothelium acting in concert with the circulating natural anticoagulants. Acquired or congenital failure of the system may lead either to bleeding disorders, most of which are now well understood, or to thrombotic disorders which are less well understood and yet represent the most common cause of death in developed countries. There are large differences in the incidence of these disorders (as reported in the literature) between nations and regions. Some of this variation is probably due to under-reporting from the developing countries (especially for haemophilia) but highly significant and interesting differences in mortality from thrombosis worldwide have been identified. We review here the clinical, laboratory and epidemiological aspects of the more common coagulation disorders.

CONGENITAL BLEEDING DISORDERS

The existence of congenital bleeding disorders has been known for a least two millennia amongst communities which practise ritual circumcision. Accounts of these disorders are vividly documented in the early medical

Baillière's Clinical Haematology—
Vol. 5, No. 2, April 1992
ISBN 0–7020–1627–6

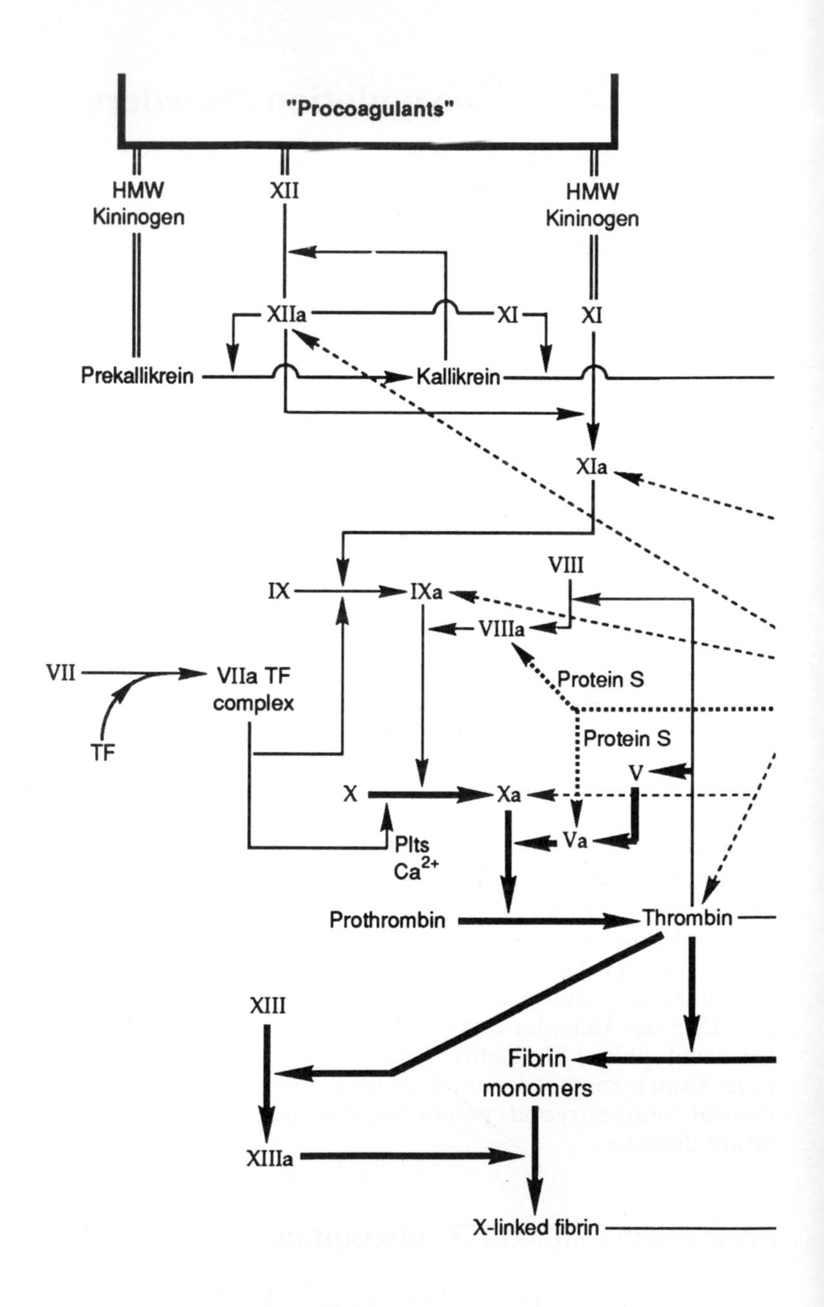

Figure 1. The coagulation and fibrinolytic system.

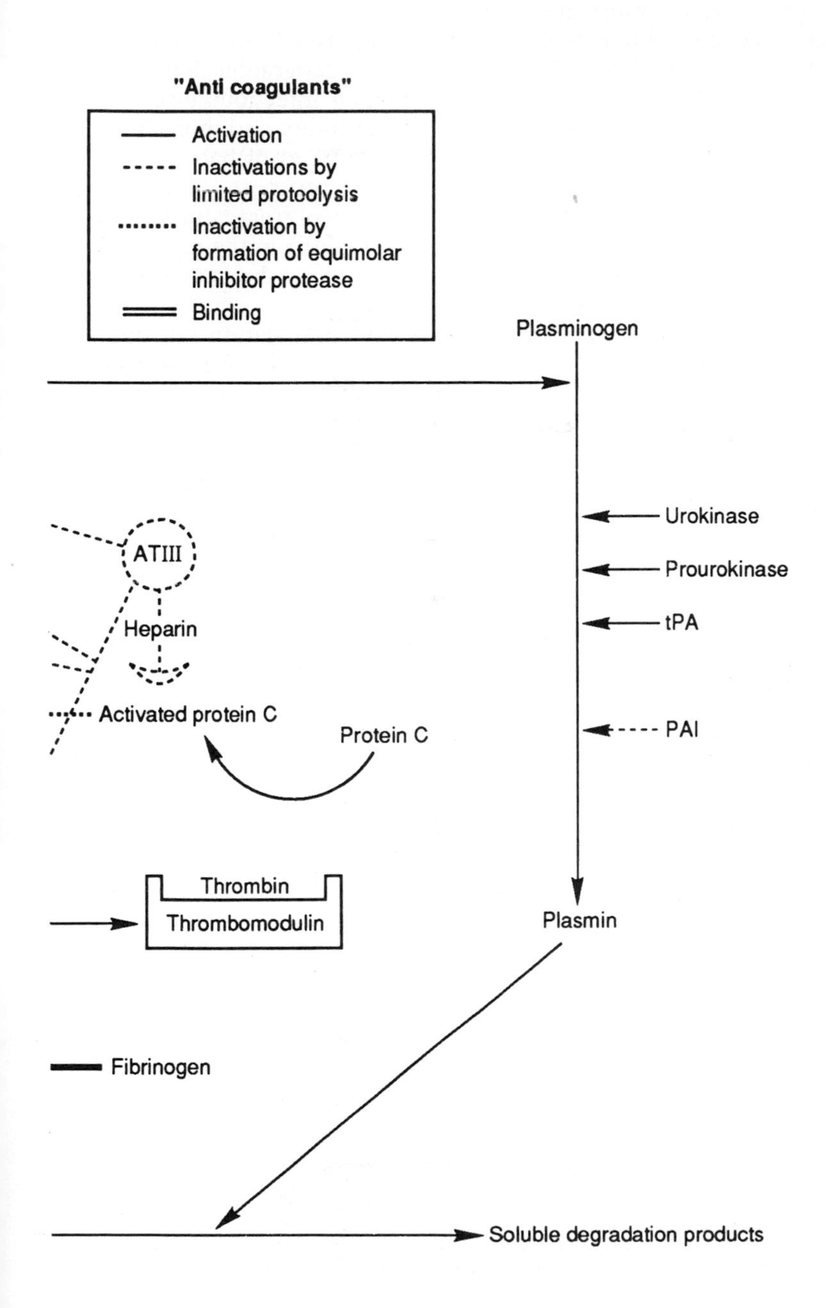
"Anti coagulants"
Activation
Inactivations by limited protoolysis
Inactivation by formation of equimolar inhibitor protease
Binding
Plasminogen
Urokinase
Prourokinase
tPA
PAI
ATIII
Heparin
Activated protein C
Protein C
Thrombin
Thrombomodulin
Plasmin
Fibrinogen
Soluble degradation products

literature because of the lasting impression left by exsanguinating blood loss occurring after trivial injury in sufferers.

It is now recognized that congenital bleeding disorders (broadly termed haemophilias) affect all racial groups without geographical limitations. Although haemophilia is far less prevalent than infectious diseases it is nevertheless a significant cause of crippling morbidity and mortality at an early age. With recent scientific advances most types of haemophilia are eminently treatable and there are now modest prospects of prevention through genetic counselling. Whilst the availability of treatment has revolutionized the life of patients afflicted with haemophilia in the more affluent societies, the rest of the world is only now beginning to direct any resources towards these unfortunate people.

Nearly all the hereditary disorders of blood coagulation are due to a deficiency or abnormality of a single clotting factor, although a few instances of multiple clotting factor deficiency have been described. There are of course as many inherited disorders of coagulation as there are clotting factors, with diverse modes of inheritance (Table 1). They result from either a mutation that diminishes the synthesis of a clotting factor or mutations that produce structurally dysfunctional or unstable clotting proteins. Inheritance of a single defective autosomal gene coding for a clotting factor seldom leads to a serious bleeding problem because the paired normal allele maintains factor levels at about half normal. The uncommon occurrence of homozy-

Table 1. Congenital bleeding disorders.

Disorders (synonyms)	Mode of inheritance*	Identified genetic lesions causing the condition	Approx. incidence per 10^6 population†
Haemophilia A (Classical haemophilia)	XLR	Deletion, missense, nonsense, insertion, splicing error	100
von Willebrand's disease	AD	Substitution	100 or more‡
	AR	Deletion	1
Haemophilia B (Christmas disease)	XLR	Deletion, missense, nonsense, splicing error	20
Haemophilia C (PTA deficiency)	AD		5% in Ashkenazi Jews; others rare
Factor X deficiency	AR	Deletion substitution	1
Factor V deficiency	AR	?	1
Factor VII deficiency	AR	Substitution	1
Factor II deficiency	AR	Missense	1
Afibrinogenaemia	AR	Deletion	1
Dysfibrinogenaemia	AD	Missense	1
Factor XIII deficiency	AR	Missense	1
Hyperplasminaemia: α_2 antiplasmin deficiency	AR	Deletion, insertion, missense	Very rare

* XLR, X-linked recessive; AD, autosomal dominant; AR, autosomal recessive; PTA, plasma thromboplastin antecedent.

† Figures applicable to developed countries.

‡ Recent population survey indicates a much higher incidence of mild von Willebrand's disease.

gosity (e.g. due to consanguineous marriage) is required for clinical expression. An exception to this is found in some types of von Willebrand's disease where an abnormal allele can interfere with the expression of the normal allele, causing dominant autosomal inheritance. Alternatively, if the coding gene is located on the X chromosome, a male inheriting the unpaired defective gene will suffer with a lifelong haemorrhagic disorder. The clinical phenotype, however, is determined not only by the mode of inheritance and the degree of deficiency, but also by the relative importance of the coagulation protein in the clotting cascade.

As most of the congenital bleeding disorders present with a similar bleeding diathesis, distinction between them requires laboratory tests. Some of these laboratory tests are simple (Table 2) and widely available, whilst others can only be performed in specialist centres with trained personnel. Using the simple tests it would be possible to confirm a diagnosis of X-linked haemophilia, but not to differentiate between haemophilia A and B. Mild haemophilia and mild von Willebrand's disease would be indistinguishable. A common pathway defect could be identified but not the distinction between factor V, X or II deficiencies. So called correction tests using adsorbed plasma and serum are cheap and simple to perform but not very reliable. Thus epidemiological data from developing countries based on screening assays are necessarily very limited in regard to specific diagnosis. This fact must be borne in mind when considering the small amount of

Table 2. Laboratory diagnosis of inherited coagulation disorders.

Disorder	Widely available tests				Specific assay (units/dl) (rarely available in developing countries)
	PT	PTTK	TCT	BT	
Haemophilia A	N	↑	N	N	Factor VIII <30 vWF: Ag N Ricof N
von Willebrand's disease	N	↑ or N	N	↑ or N	Factor VIII <50 vWF: Ag <50 or N Ricof <50 or N
Haemophilia B	N	↑	N	N	Factor IX <30
Factor XI deficiency	N	↑	N	N	Factor XI <35
Factor X deficiency	↑	↑	N	N	Factor X <30
Factor V deficiency	↑	↑	N	N or ↑	Factor V <30
Factor VII deficiency	↑	N	N	N	Factor VII <30
Factor II deficiency	↑	↑	N	N	Factor II <30
Afibrinogenaemia	↑	↑	↑	↑	Fibrinogen undetectable
Dysfibrinogenaemia	↑	↑	↑	N	Fibrinogen N or ↓
Factor XIII deficiency	N	N	N	N	Fibrinogen N or ↓ Fibrin solubility ↑
Hyperplasminaemia	N	N	N	N	Euglobulin clot lysis time short α Antiplasmin absent

PT, prothrombin time; PTTK, activated partial thromboplastin time; TCT, thrombin clotting time; BT, bleeding time.
Factor VIII (formerly VIII: c); vWF: Ag, von Willebrand factor antigen (formerly VIIIR: Ag); Ricof, Ristocetin cofactor.
↑, increased; ↓, decreased; N, normal.

data that has been published from these areas of the world, that now contain the majority of the human population and therefore, by inference, the majority of cases of coagulation disorders.

According to the data collected by haemophilia centres the most prevalent of these congenital bleeding disorders appear to be the X-linked haemophilias A and B (see Table 1). However, it is now appreciated that the combined frequency of all the variants of von Willebrand's disorders approaches or surpasses that of haemophilia A. We shall therefore concentrate on these three disorders in our subsequent discussion.

History

Although the existence of a hereditary condition causing death after circumcision at 8 days was recognized in the Talmudic writings of 1700 years ago (Rosner, 1969) and whilst the inheritance of the disease was described in 1800 (Otto, 1803), the first description of the role of antihaemophilic factor (factor VIII) in coagulation was not published until 1937 (Patek and Taylor, 1937). The resolution of sex linked haemophilia into two distinct disorders, haemophilia A (factor VIII deficiency) and haemophilia B (factor IX deficiency) did not occur until 1952 (Biggs et al, 1952). The relationship between hereditary factor VIII deficiency and von Willebrand's disease (first described in 1926) was unclear for most of this century because a deficiency of von Willebrand factor is autosomally inherited and is associated with some degree of factor VIII deficiency. It is now recognized that von Willebrand factor is a product of a gene located on chromosome 12, which is both a protective carrier of factor VIII and a promoter of platelet adhesion. Thus defects in the von Willebrand factor gene result in a decrease in the levels of factor VIII in the plasma and in a prolonged bleeding time. Since 1984 it has been clear that factor VIII, although complexed with von Willebrand factor in plasma, is the product of an X-linked gene, defects of which cause haemophilia A (Vehar et al, 1984).

Clinical features

Haemophilia A or classical haemophilia is caused by a defect in the synthesis of functional procoagulant factor VIII and accounts for about 85% of X-linked haemophilia. The balance of such cases result from deficient production of functional factor IX (haemophilia B). As factor IX is also located on the X chromosome and since factor VIII acts as a cofactor to factor IX in activating factor X (Figure 1), it is clear why haemophilia A and B are clinically indistinguishable. The clinical syndrome of factor VIII or IX deficiency is characterized by repeated painful acute episodes of bleeding into joints or soft tissue, which in severe cases occurs apparently spontaneously. This is the chief burden of haemophilia and in the absence of adequate treatment leads to crippling at an early age. Minor trauma or surgery can result in large haematomas which can be fatal, especially if the bleeding is intracranial or in the respiratory tract. Haematuria, epistaxis, gastrointestinal and retroperitoneal bleeding are other frequent manifestations. The severity and frequency of bleeding are inversely correlated with the residual coagulation factor level. Table 3 summarizes this relationship and gives the relative frequency of categories for haemophilia A based on the UK national data.

Table 3. Haemophilia A: clinical severity*.

Factor VIII (units/dl)	Bleeding tendency†	Relative incidence (% cases)
<2	Severe: frequent spontaneous bleeding into joints, muscles and internal organs	50
2–10	Moderately severe: some 'spontaneous bleeds'; bleeding after minor trauma	30
>10	Mild: bleeding only after significant trauma/surgery	20

* This table is also applicable to factor IX, X, VII and II deficiencies but not to factor XI, V, XIII or von Willebrand factor deficiencies.
† The bleeding severity is quite stable in an individual patient and generally correlates well with the residual plasma level of coagulation factor. Thus a clinical report of a severe bleeding tendency is a reliable indicator of a very low factor level.

Von Willebrand's disease is classically an autosomal dominant condition. The more severely affected patients present with bruising, epistaxis, prolonged bleeding from minor cuts, menorrhagia and excessive but not often life-threatening bleeding after trauma or surgery. On the other hand mild cases may go undetected. Much less common is autosomal recessive von Willebrand disease, where von Willebrand factor is undetectable and factor VIII levels are below 2% of normal. These patients have a bleeding tendency that clinically resembles severe haemophilia A, with haemarthroses, muscle bleeds and life-threatening haemorrhage after trauma as well as the disposition to small vessel bleeding that is characteristic of von Willebrand's disease.

Epidemiological problems

Distorting tendencies with opposite effects will affect the apparent prevalence rates in developing countries. Firstly, only the more severely affected patients are likely to come to diagnosis. Secondly, due to the clinical complication of their disease they are more likely to die and be lost from the data. Conversely, the mildly affected cases will seldom come to diagnosis. Hence the overall effect on the statistics will be to produce much lower rates for all classes of the haemophilias in the developing countries.

The epidemiology of congenital bleeding disorders in the western world is distinctly different from the rest of the world. This is primarily because the West has been at the forefront of recent scientific advances which have resulted in coagulation factor replacement therapy being widely available. Together with a more co-ordinated approach to the management of congenital bleeding disorders, patients in the West are now able to lead near normal lives. Financial restraints, the overwhelming importance of infectious diseases and lack of expertise has meant that congenital bleeding disorders have been neglected in many regions of the world. Consequently the prospects for patients afflicted with these disorders are grim in these regions. In the subsequent discussion we shall highlight the epidemiological consequences of the disparity in the care of these patients, using haemophilia as our model.

Haemophilia in the West

Prevalence

The prevalence of a disease, defined as the number of living patients at a specific time, is a function of the incidence, detection rate, longevity and emigration/immigration. The incidence of haemophilia A was stated to be around 0.5–1 case per 10 000 newborn male infants (World Health Organization, 1972). However, data from countries with advanced health care suggest that the true incidence is nearer 1 per 5000 male infants (see below). Recent advances in medical treatment have resulted in improved reproductive fitness, with the consequent disruption of the equilibrium between mutation and selection. The effect of therapy, however, has been more profound on the life expectancy of the haemophiliac. Patients with severe haemophilia usually did not live beyond early adulthood, while even in mild haemophilia the life expectancy was reduced to about two-thirds of normal life span (Sjoln, 1960; Ramgren, 1962; Ikkala et al, 1982; Larsson, 1985). There is currently a steady increase in life expectancy of haemophiliacs in western countries (Figure 2). Improving reproductive fitness, together with an increasing life expectancy, has resulted in an expansion of the haemophiliac population in the West. The main beneficiaries of the medical advances in haemophilia has been the more severely affected haemophiliacs. Simultaneously their median life expectancy has increased by

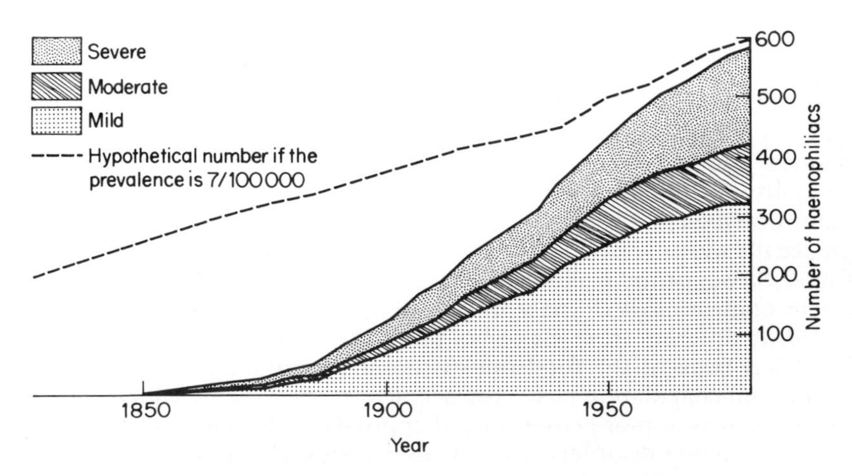

Figure 2. Number of known haemophiliacs in Sweden, allocated into severities, 1831–1980. From Larsson (1985), with permission.

sixfold, from 11.4 years at the beginning of the century (Larsson, 1985) to 69.1 years in 1983 (Rizza and Spooner, 1983; Larsson, 1985) (Figure 3a). Moderately severe haemophiliacs have also experienced more than a doubling of their median life expectancy from 27.5 years to 71.5 years during the same period (Figure 3b). On the other hand the life expectancy of mild haemophiliacs is similar to that of the normal male (Figure 3c).

In spite of these impressive advances, the true prevalence of haemophilia in the West remains controversial. This is partly because of the paucity of national surveys as well as the difficulty in detecting mild and otherwise symptom-free haemophiliacs. Table 4 is a summary of some of the more comprehensive surveys. This shows some notable differences in the prevalence rate, ranging from 3.3 per 100 000 population in Spain to 9.1 per 100 000 population in the UK. Similar variations have also been detected in the prevalence of severe haemophilia, even allowing for the variations in the laboratory definition of severe haemophilia. One of the reasons for this may be that the severe haemophiliacs are more likely to seek treatment because of their more pernicious bleeding complications. Another explanation for this variation may be that many of the reports are not from true national surveys but are either compilations of case reports or reports from individual treatment centres.

In the UK there is a national register which comprises one of the largest and most intensively studied cohorts of haemophiliacs. By the end of 1989 there were 5226 patients with haemophilia A, 1031 patients with haemophilia B and 2510 with von Willebrand's disease recorded in this register (Rizza and Spooner, 1992). Of these, 40% of haemophilia A, 33% of haemophilia B and 45% of patients with von Willebrand's disease were severely affected. The ratio of haemophilia A to haemophilia B was 84 to 16 and this ratio has been relatively constant throughout the western world. An explanation for this consistency may simply be that it reflects the ratio of the

Table 4. Prevalence of haemophilia in different western countries.

Country	Haemophiliacs per 100 000 population	Haemophilia A: Haemophilia B	Proportion of severe cases (%)
UK	9.1	83:11	43*
Switzerland	7.0		
Australia	6.7†		
The Netherlands	8	86:14	45‡
Canada (Alberta)	6.6	84:16	53‡
Norway	6.5	78:22	40‡
Denmark	6.4	80:20	50
USA (Pennsylvania)	5.4	85:15	30‡
France	5.3†	80:20	71
Greece	4.6	87:13	77
Japan	3.6	84:16	56‡
Spain	3.3	87:16	
Sweden	7.0	81:19	30‡

* Factor VIII level <2% of normal.
† Estimated prevalence.
‡ Factor VIII level <1% of normal.
Adapted from Biggs and Rizza (1984), with permission.

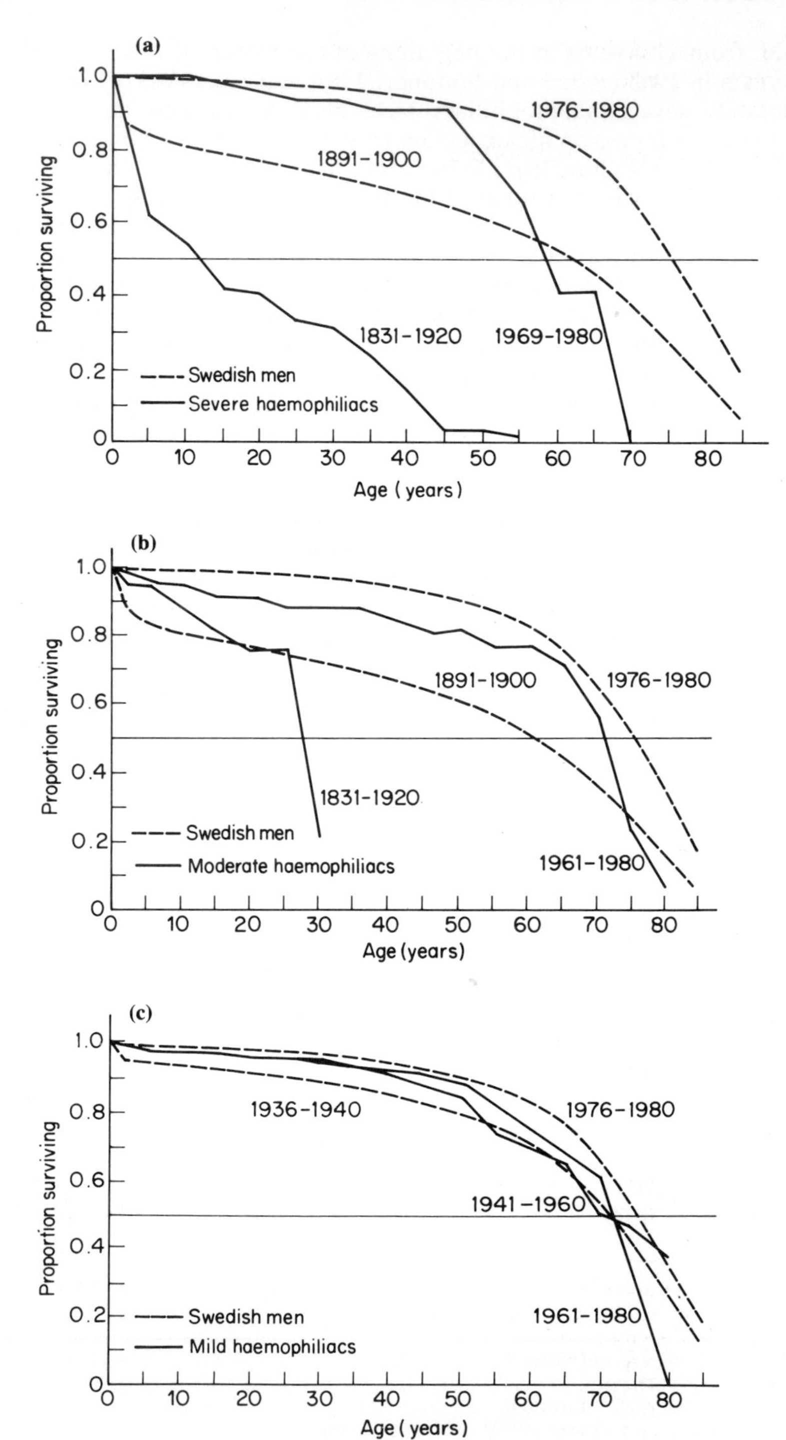
(a)
1.0
0.8
0.6
0.4
0.2
0
Proportion surviving
1976-1980
1891-1900
1831-1920
1969-1980
Swedish men
Severe haemophiliacs
0
10
20
30
40
50
60
70
80
Age (years)
(b)
1.0
0.8
0.6
0.4
0.2
0
Proportion surviving
1891-1900
1976-1980
1831-1920
Swedish men
Moderate haemophiliacs
1961-1980
0
10
20
30
40
50
60
70
80
Age (years)
(c)
1.0
0.8
0.6
0.4
0.2
0
Proportion surviving
1936-1940
1976-1980
1941-1960
Swedish men
Mild haemophiliacs
1961-1980
0
10
20
30
40
50
60
70
80
Age (years)

size of the respective genes (185:35) and therefore of the 'target' for mutations to 'strike'.

Age distribution of haemophiliacs

Not surprisingly, with increasing life expectancy the average age of western haemophiliacs has increased to a mean of around 23 years and a median of around 25 years (Rizza and Spooner, 1992). This has meant that in the UK and elsewhere more haemophiliacs are living to be middle-aged and older (Figure 4). There are fewer patients with severe haemophilia over the age of 50 years, reflecting the previous excess mortality in this age group. At the same time the relative paucity of patients with mild haemophilia below the age of 10 years must be due to the low detection rate in this group in their first decade.

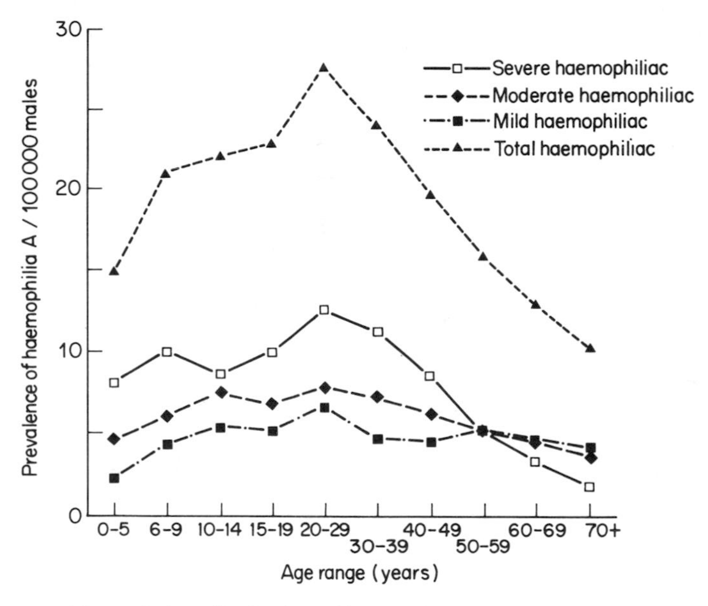

Figure 4. Age distribution of haemophilia A in Britain in 1986.

Treatment

The blood coagulation defects may be corrected temporarily by giving transfusions of materials rich in the appropriate clotting factors. Ideally all

---

Figure 3. **(a)** The proportion of surviving severe haemophiliacs in the periods 1831–1920 and 1969–1980. Corresponding curves for Swedish males, 1891–1900 and 1976–1980, are given for comparison. **(b)** The proportion of surviving moderate haemophiliacs in the periods 1831–1920 and 1961–1980. Corresponding curves for Swedish males, 1891–1900 and 1976–1980, are given for comparison. **(c)** The proportion of surviving mild haemophiliacs for the periods 1941–1960 and 1961–1980. Corresponding curves for Swedish males, 1936–1940 and 1976–1980 are given for comparison. From Larsson (1985), with permission.

severely affected patients would be maintained on long-term prophylaxis with daily or alternate day infusions to keep spontaneous haemorrhage to a minimum. This is seldom possible, except for haemophilia B, due to limitations of supply and finance. In practice most patients are treated on demand, optimally receiving therapy within a few minutes to 1 h of onset of a bleeding episode. This prevents significant leakage of blood into the joints or other tissues, thus allowing normal activity to be resumed almost immediately. In the 1960s it was realized that such prompt treatment could only be achieved if the patient or relative could initiate treatment at the first sign of a bleed. Therefore, home therapy programmes were instituted. In the UK home treatment programmes have been introduced by all the haemophilia centres such that, in 1989, 54% of all haemophiliacs and 71% of the severely affected haemophiliacs were receiving home treatment (Rizza and Spooner, 1992). This has resulted in a dramatic fall in time lost from school or work and a marked reduction in the onset of new and the progression of old joint damage. At the present time most factor VIII and all factor IX used is blood derived (Table 5). More aggressive treatment in conjunction with increasing prevalence has caused the requirements for coagulation factors to escalate. Over the last 12 years there has been a dramatic change in the usage of various blood products, in the UK and the West, for the treatment of haemophiliacs. Whole blood and plasma are now very rarely used for coagulation factor replacement. Cryoprecipitate was the most popular choice in the 1960s and early 1970s, however its use has been superseded in many countries by the more potent and relatively stable coagulation factor concentrates. The latter are more suited to home therapy and consequently home therapy accounts for just under half the total factor VIII consumed in the UK (Rizza and Spooner, 1983).

Unfortunately, the concentrates used for replacement therapy (particularly unpasteurized concentrates and concentrates prepared from paid blood donation) has introduced hazards that are just as dangerous to health as the conditions for which they were prescribed, namely hepatitis and acquired immune deficiency syndrome (AIDS).

Epidemiology of blood product transmitted infections

Hepatitis. The majority of patients who are intensively treated with pooled plasma products develop abnormal liver function tests (Levine et al, 1976). However, the incidence of clinical jaundice amongst haemophiliacs who have received factor concentrates is about 20% (Schulman and Wiechel, 1984). Clinical jaundice appears to be more common amongst patients with haemophilia B compared to those with haemophilia A (Hasiba et al, 1977; Schulman and Wiechel, 1984), suggesting that factor IX concentrates are associated with a higher incidence of hepatitis. Paradoxically, a higher incidence of clinical hepatitis has been reported amongst haemophiliacs with fewer transfusions compared with those requiring multiple transfusions (30 versus 0–2.1%) (Kasper and Kipnis, 1972). The reason for this is not clear, although passively transferred antibody to hepatitis B surface antigen (HBsAb) in multiply transfused patients may be a factor. Over 90% of

Table 5. Therapeutic materials for treatment of haemophilia A and von Willebrand's disease.

Material	Factor VIII (units/ml)	vWF (units/ml)	Donors per unit‡	Advantages	Disadvantages
Fresh frozen plasma (FFP)	1	1	1	1. Low infection hazard 2. Available in many developing countries 3. Very simple to prepare	1. Storage at −20°C 2. High volume/low potency 3. Allergic reactions
Cryoprecipitate	5–10	5–10	1	1. Low infection hazard (unless many units used) 2. Available in some developing countries 3. Simple technology needed for preparation	1. Storage at −20°C 2. Allergic reactions 3. Not heat treated in UK 4. Potency not assayed
Heat/solvent/detergent treated factor VIII concentrate	20–50	Low*	3000–15 000	1. Assayed high potency 2. Low or absent HIV and hepatitis infectivity 3. Storage at 4.0°C 4. Few allergic reactions	1. High cost 2. Heavy load of non-factor VIII protein including iso anti A, anti B, $\beta_2$microglobulin, fibrinogen, etc.
DDAVP	—	—	0	1. No infection risk 2. Totally synthetic 3. Cheap	1. Only effective in mild cases
Porcine factor VIII†	20–50	Low	—	1. No infection risk 2. High purity	1. Animal protein allergic reactions 2. Resistance to treatment
Recombinant factor VII†	—	0	0	1. No infection risk	1. Thrombosis if sepsis present
Monoclonally purified and recombinant factor VIII	5000 units/mg	0	3000–15 000 0	1. No infection risk 2. Totally pure 3. Stable	1. Very high cost

DDAVP, deamino-D-arginine vasopressin.

* Although high concentrations of vWF antigen are present, the size distribution is altered with loss of highly polymerized forms and consequently little effect on the bleeding time in von Willebrand's diseases.

† Reserved for treatment of inhibitor cases.

‡ No. of individuals whose blood donation contributes to a single unit of treatment.

multiply transfused haemophiliacs have antibody to hepatitis B virus surface antigen (HBsAg), suggesting recovery from a previous infection with the virus (Lander et al, 1975). Only a small number of patients (1–5%) have evidence of persistent infection with hepatitis B virus and this is associated with persistent biochemical liver abnormalities. However the large majority of haemophiliacs who have biochemical evidence of persistent hepatitis do not have serological evidence of active hepatitis A or B infections. This fact supports the view that such hepatitis is associated with parental transmission of one or more non-A non-B hepatitis virus (NANB) (Fletcher et al, 1983). Until recently, NANB hepatitis was a diagnosis of exclusion. Now the genome for a NANB hepatitis agent (hepatitis C virus (HCV)) has been cloned (Choo et al, 1989) and anti-HCV antibody was detected in 76% of haemophiliacs with chronic or intermittently elevated liver enzymes. This supports an aetiological role for HCV in the development of chronic liver disease in haemophiliacs (Mannucci et al, 1989). Initially the frequent occurrence of NANB hepatitis did not give rise to major concern because clinically this complication appeared to be mild and self-limiting as compared with the problems associated with haemophilia, which were usually more immediate and pressing. However, histological studies of these patients gave cause for concern. Whilst chronic persistent hepatitis was the most common lesion, a significant proportion of patients showed chronic aggressive hepatitis or even established cirrhosis (Preston et al, 1978; Schimpf, 1986). Serial liver biopsies have shown that chronic persistent hepatitis appears to be much more aggressive in haemophiliacs as progression to chronic active hepatitis and even cirrhosis has been recorded within the relatively short time of 5 years (Hay et al, 1985).

HIV-1 infection. The life-long requirement for blood derived coagulation concentrates has meant that haemophiliacs, as a group, have the highest relative risk of acquiring the human immunodeficiency virus-1 (HIV-1). Retrospective studies show that HIV-1 infection first emerged in the USA in 1978 (Evatt et al, 1985). Amongst haemophiliacs seroconversion had began to occur by 1982 and then rapidly increased in 1983. By 1984 most severe haemophiliacs had been infected by this virus (Machin et al, 1985). The pattern in Europe has lagged behind the USA epidemic by approximately 2 years, with the first UK cases being detected during 1980–1981. In the USA the overall prevalence of HIV-1 is approximately 70% for haemophilia A and 35% for haemophilia B (Centers for Disease Control, 1987). In the UK the overall prevalence in haemophiliacs is 35.5%, with a 40.9% prevalence in haemophilia A and 6.8% in haemophilia B (AIDS Group of the UK, 1986). The lower prevalence of HIV-1 in haemophilia B suggests either that the method of factor IX production destroyed the virus or that the source plasma was less infectious. As all factor IX concentrate used in the UK was of local origin, this probably further lowered the infection rate in haemophilia B in this country. The risk of HIV-1 infection is related to the type, the amount and the source of factor concentrates used. Whilst HIV-1 infection has been reported with all blood products used to treat haemophiliac bleeding, the relative risk of acquiring this infection was much greater with the untreated commercial concentrates which were prepared from plasma pools derived from up to 25 000 paid donors (Table 6).

As far as clinical features of HIV-1 infection are concerned, they are similar in haemophiliacs to those observed in other risk groups, with three exceptions. Firstly, the rate of progression to full blown AIDS is much lower in haemophiliacs as compared with other risk groups: 12% in 3 years in haemophilia versus 30% in homosexuals in the same period (Goedert et al, 1986). The reason for the slower progression to AIDS in haemophiliacs is not clear. Secondly, the incidence of neurological abnormalities associated with the well-recognized infectious mononucleosis-like illness associated with primary HIV infection seems to be greater in haemophiliacs (Tucker et al, 1985). This may be related to the direct inoculation of virus into the bloodstream. Thirdly, the incidence of Kaposi's sarcoma is much lower in haemophiliacs compared with the other risk groups (3 versus 50%). This remarkable difference strongly suggests that an additional agent may be involved in the aetiology of Kaposi's sarcoma, but the nature and ecology of such an agent remains speculative. In spite of the slow rate of progression to AIDS in haemophilia, in the UK in 1988 about 10% of haemophiliacs with HIV-1 infection had AIDS. AIDS is now the main cause of mortality amongst haemophiliacs in the UK, accounting for just under half of all the reported deaths (Rizza and Spooner, 1992).

Table 6. Number of seroconversions to HIV-1 positive in UK haemophiliacs according to type and source of concentrate.

Type/source of concentrate	No. of patients treated	No. HIV-1 antibody positive
Cryoprecipitate	166	2 (1.2)
NHS factor VIII	198	10 (10.1)
Commercial factor VIII	97	44 (45.4)
More than 1 type of factor preparation	1564	830 (53)
Factor IX	324	20 (6.2)
Total treated	2349	916 (38.9)

Values in parentheses are percentages.
From Madhok and Forbes (1990) with permission.

Mortality and causes of death

In spite of remarkable advances in the care of haemophilia over the last 20 years, the mortality is twice as high in haemophiliacs as in the general population, with a relative mortality ratio (the ratio of observed over expected mortality) of 2.1 (Johnson et al, 1985; Rosendaal et al, 1989). The relative mortality ratio is 2.9 in severe haemophilia, as compared with 1.6 in milder cases. Patients with factor inhibitors have a 5.3 times higher risk of dying than patients without. Thus, correcting for this, the relative mortality rate does not differ much by severity of haemophilia. It is also becoming clear that comparatively fewer deaths occur in patients on prophylactic replacement therapy and home therapy as the relative mortality ratio is 1.9

in these patients, compared with 2.5 in patients not on prophylactic therapy (Rizza and Spooner, 1983). However, intensive therapy also carries the risk of serious blood borne viral infections. In the early 1980s cerebral haemorrhage was the main cause of death (Table 7). Over the last 3 years AIDS has become the leading cause of death in haemophiliacs in the UK, with at least 43% of fatalities attributable to this disease. Most of these deaths have occurred amongst the severely affected individuals (80%). Many studies antedating the HIV epidemic observed an excess of cancer deaths (Rizza and Spooner, 1983; Rosendaal et al, 1989). Most of these deaths were due to carcinoma of the lung (Rosendaal et al, 1989). In sharp contrast the number of deaths from ischaemic heart disease is much lower than the national average (Rizza and Spooner, 1983; Rosendaal et al, 1989), suggesting a protective effect of haemophilia against thrombosis. This apart, Table 7 tells a depressing story, since actual mortality per annum has increased in every category (note that the left half covers 3 years and the right 5 years). Ageing of the cohort plus viral infections are the obvious causes.

Table 7. Causes of death in patients with haemophilia (1976–1980 compared with 1987–1989).

	1987–1989			1976–1980
Causes	Severe	Non-severe	Total	Total
AIDS	80 (8)	18 (1)	98 (9)	0
Cerebral haemorrhage	20 (6)	13	33 (6)	26 (5)
Other types of bleeding	6 (2)	1	7 (2)	11 (6)
Postoperative complications	3 (1)	1	4 (1)	6 (2)
Suicide	1	4 (2)	5 (2)	5
Neoplasm	11	10	21	7
Pulmonary embolism	1	1	2	2
Pneumonia	6 (2)	6	12 (2)	4
Hepatitis	9 (2)	1	10 (2)	1 (1)
Myocardial infarction	4	4	8	1
Accident	3	2	5	4
Not known	4	4	8	11 (1)
Miscellaneous non-haemorrhagic conditions	5	7	12	11 (5)
Total	153 (21)	72 (3)	225 (24)	89 (20)

Numbers of patients with antibodies to FVIII given in parentheses.
Data from 1987–1989 compiled from UK Haemophilia Centre Director's returns (by kind permission of the UKHCD committee).
Data from 1976–1980 extracted from Rizza and Spooner (1983).

Haemophilia in the rest of the world

Although effective coagulation factor replacement therapy is the cornerstone of management of bleeding disorders, unfortunately 65% of the world's haemophiliacs do not have the simplest blood products available to them (Brading, 1990). Most of these haemophiliacs dwell in regions of the world where limited resources have meant that haemophilia care has no priority. Most of the available funds for health care are devoted to combating highly prevalent communicable diseases and malnutrition. Health care in these regions is often at a very rudimentary stage, with lack of expertise, equipment and facilities for diagnosing or managing bleeding disorders, with the predictable consequences for life expectancy in haemophiliacs.

For a long time it was felt that inherited bleeding disorders were rare in places such as Africa (Trowell, 1941; Griffiths and Lipschitz, 1949; Gelfand, 1957) and China (Wintrobe et al, 1974). This misunderstanding occurred because of the lack of clinical awareness and social acceptability on a background of overwhelming morbidity and mortality from infectious diseases. Also, in many regions belief in supernatural forces, sorcery, witchcraft and spirits still prevails (Good and Kimani, 1980). Consequently the services of a traditional healer are sought before turning to scientific medicine. As a result many of the cases that were diagnosed represented those who had not died of haemorrhage following trauma or tribal rituals (Kitonyi and Kasili, 1981).

Although the true incidence of bleeding disorders in developing countries remains obscure, as more reports emerge from these societies it is now becoming clear that haemophilia and other bleeding disorders are not as uncommon as originally thought, and indeed may be prevalent on the western world scale. A compilation of some of the more recent data is shown in Tables 8–10. The gross variation in the prevalence rate and distribution of classical haemophilia is quite impressive. Whilst it would be tempting to ascribe these differences to the small population samples and lack of discriminatory laboratory tests, this would not explain the difference amongst the more authoritative studies (Kitonyi and Kasili, 1981; Karabus, 1984; Rojas, 1984; Rueda, 1984). In fact a number of the studies also report a tribal difference in the prevalence rate (Omer and Zadia, 1973; Kitonyi and Kasili, 1981). There are no obvious explanations for this, although in some circumstances social customs may play a part. For example, in the Middle East and many parts of India, a high degree of consanguinity has resulted in a higher incidence of autosomal recessive conditions such as Glanzmann's thrombasthenia (Khanduri et al, 1981; Awidi, 1984). Similarly, in-breeding is one reason for a higher incidence of factor XI deficiency amongst Ashkenazi Jews. But the founder effect cannot be the only reason in that case since at least four different mutations have been found, implying a selective heterozygote advantage that may have operated in the past, similar to Tay–Sachs disease which is prevalent in the same group (O'Brien, 1991).

Studies in which the severity of haemophilia has been graded also show a heterogeneous distribution. In many parts of Africa (Kasili, 1983) the mild and moderately severe forms of the disease predominate over the severe form. This is probably a result of inadequate replacement therapy and thus the moderately severe and mild forms represent those patients who have survived haemostatic challenges. On the other hand, in regions of South Africa (Cohn et al, 1990) and Korea (Kim et al, 1988) the more severe form of the disease is more prevalent. In comparison to the West the majority of the patients are below the age of 20 years and very few patients exceed the age of 40 years (Figure 5). The life expectancy has increased only marginally in the last 20 years, from 15.6 to 22.4 years, as compared with the average life expectancy of a normal male of 58.8 years (Cruz-Coke and Rivera, 1980).

Table 8. Prevalence and treatment options of inherited bleeding disorders in Africa.

	Prevalence of inherited bleeding disorders						Treatment options				
	Number of patients registered at haemophilia centres										
Country	HA	HB	vWD	Others	HA:HB	Prevalence/ 100 000 males	Blood products widely used*	24 h emergency service†	Self treatment	Number severely affected (%)	Reference
Egypt	675 (67.5)	133 (13.3)	77 (7.7)	(11.5)	5:1	2.51	2, 3, 4	3	limited extent	—	El Shinnawi (1984)
Ivory Coast	NK (83.2)	NK (16.8)	—	—	5:1	‡	5	—	No	—	Essien (1981)
Kenya	66 (63)	22 (21)	10 (9.5)	7 (6.5)	3.0:1	8.62	3	1	No	21	Kitonyi and Kasili (1981)
Nigeria	NK (69.4)	NK (14.3)	—	—	4.9:1	‡	2, 3	2	No	41.2	Essien (1981)
South Africa	647 (66)	127 (13)	140 (14.4)	58 (6)	5.0:1	6.02	2, 3, 4	3	Approx. 15%	—	Karabus (1984)
Sudan	18 (50.0)	4 (11.0)	10.8 (28)	3.96 (11)	4.5:1	‡	—	—	—	—	Omer and Zadia (1973)
Tanzania	(100)	—	—	—	—	‡	1.2	—	No	—	Williams (1976)
Tunisia	64 (55)	21 (18)	20 (17)	97 (10)	3.0:1	2.25	2, 3	—	No	—	Mohsen (1984)
Uganda	8 (87)	1 (12.5)	—	—	7:1	‡	—	—	No	—	Lothe (1968)
Zambia	12 (100)	—	—	—	—	‡	—	—	No	—	Chintu (1976)
Zimbabwe	108 (90)	12 (10)	—	—	9:1	4.21	2, 3	1	No	15	Mukiibi et al (1990)

Values in parentheses are percentages.
HA, haemophilia A; HB, haemophilia B; vWD, von Willebrand's disease; NK, not known.
* 1, Whole blood; 2, fresh frozen plasma; 3, cryoprecipitate; 4, clotting factor concentrates; 5, not known.
† 1, Treatment available only in the capital city; 2, treatment available at other major centres; 3, treatment widely available.
‡ Prevalence not calculated because no data from regional centre or small numbers recorded.

Table 9. Prevalence and treatment options of inherited bleeding disorders in South America.

		Prevalence of inherited bleeding disorders						Treatment options		
		Number of patients registered at haemophilia centres								
Country	Reference	HA	HB	vWD	Others or totals	HA : HB	Prevalence/ 100 000 males	Blood products widely used*	24 h emergency service†	Self treatment (%)
Argentina	Di Tomaso (1984)	756 (80)	117 (12)	38 (4)	39 (4)	6.6 : 1	6.52	3, 4	2	18
Brazil	Roisenberg and Morton (1971)	53 (85)	5 (15)	—	—	5.67 : 1	‡	3, 4	2	—
Chile	Prado (1984)	—	—	—	Total = 375§	—	‡	1, 2, 3	1	—
Costa Rica	Rojas (1984)	100 (67)	15 (10)	20 (13)	15 (10)	6.7 : 1	10.65	2, 3, 4	2	4.2
El Salvador	Bloch (1984)	—	—	—	Estimate = 200§	—	‡	1, 2, 3	—	—
Honduras	Salgado (1984)	—	—	—	Total = 25§	—	‡	1, 3	—	—
Nicaragua	Rueda (1984)	26 (96)	1 (4)	—	—	24 : 1	3.15	2, 3	2	60
Peru	Morales (1984)	—	—	—	Total = 36§	—	‡	3, 4	—	—
Uruguay	AHU (1984)	84 (65)	4 (3)	42 (32)	—	21 : 1	6.16	1/2	2/3	8

Values in parentheses are percentages.
HA, haemophilia A; HB, haemophilia B, vWD, von Willebrand's disease.
* 1, Whole blood; 2, fresh frozen plasma; 3, cryoprecipitate; 4, clotting factor concentrates.
† 1, Treatment available only in the capital city; 2, treatment available at other major centres; 3, treatment widely available.
‡ Prevalence not calculated because no data from regional centre or small numbers recorded.
§ Numbers registered at haemophilia centre or estimate.

Table 10. Prevalence and treatment options of inherited bleeding disorders in Asia.

		Prevalence of inherited bleeding disorders							Treatment options		
		Number of patients registered at haemophilia centres									
Country	Reference	HA	HB	vWD	GT or totals	Others	HA:HB	Prevalence 100 000 males	Blood products widely used*	Emergency service†	Home treatment (%)
Jordan	Awidi (1984)	42 (38)	11 (10)	22 (20)	23 (21)	(11)	3:1	4.84	NK	NK	NK
India	Agarwal et al (1981)	171 (39)	52 (12)	74 (17)	42 (10)	103 (22)	2.3:1	‡	2, 3, 4	2	No
Indonesia	Syafei (1984)	—	—	—	Total = 73§	—	—	‡	2, 3	1	No
Iraq	Al Mondhiry (1977)	137 (51)	24 (8.9)	49 (18)	NK	(22)	5.7:1	‡	NK	NK	NK
Korea	Kim et al (1988)	425 (85.3)	73 (14.7)	—	—	—	5.8:1	3.39	3, 4	2	NK
Kuwait	Youssef and Bashir (1984)	—	—	—	Total on Reg. = 43§	—	—	‡	3	1	Limited
Malaysia	Lopez (1984)	172 (82)	20 (9.5)	18 (9)	—	—	8.6:1	3.3	3	1	1.7
Philippines	Gamez (1984)	—	—	—	Total on Reg. = 55§	—	—	‡	2, 3	1	No
Saudi Arabia	Ahmed et al (1988)	15 (44)	—	—	(35)	(5.8)	—	1	NK	NK	NK
Thailand	Isarangkura (1984)	—	—	—	Estimated 1800§	—	—	‡	1, 2, 3, 4	2	No

Values in parentheses are percentages.
HA, haemophilia A; HB, haemophilia B; vWD, von Willebrand's disease; GT, Glanzmann's thrombasthenia; NK, not known.
* 1, Whole blood; 2, fresh frozen plasma; 3, cryoprecipitate; 4, clotting factor concentrates; NK, not known.
† 1, Treatment available only in the capital city; 2, treatment available at other major centres; 3, treatment widely available.
‡ Prevalence not calculated because no data from regional centre or small numbers recorded.
§ Numbers registered at haemophilia centre or estimate.

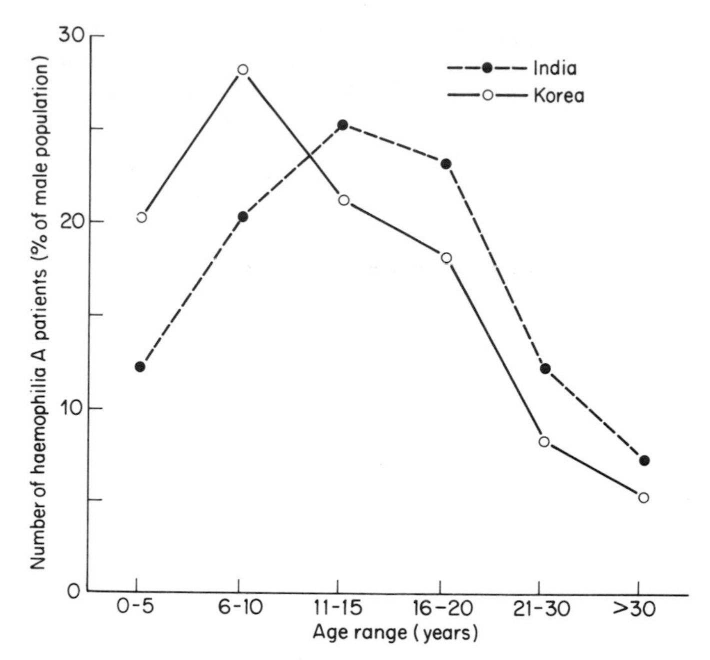

Figure 5. Age distribution of haemophilia A in India and Korea.

This is a reflection of the dire shortcomings of haemophilia care and resembles the desperate predicament of haemophiliacs that existed in the western world in the pretreatment era.

The clinical expression of these disorders is not too different from that described in the West. The main cause of morbidity is haemarthrosis, which is present in two-thirds of the patients (Agarwal et al, 1981; Kasili, 1983; Kim et al, 1988). In many cases arthropathy is far too advanced to be amenable to any form of therapy. At variance with the data from the West is the occurrence of bleeding in the first year of life commonly found in many regions (Agarwal et al, 1981; Kim et al, 1988). The mean age at death depends in part on the proximity of the nearest treatment centre. For example, in Brazil the mean age of death is 15 years in the cities as compared with 10 years for those living in the rural regions (Roisenberg and Morton, 1971).

There is a dearth of data as regards the prevalence of hepatitis B and C and HIV infection amongst haemophiliacs in the developing world. Hepatitis B and C tend to be highly prevalent in these regions and therefore it would not be unreasonable to assume a high prevalence rate amongst haemophiliacs. Studies from India show that the incidence of hepatitis B amongst multitransfused thalassaemics and haemophiliacs is high (22 and 9% respectively) and proportional to the intensity of transfusion (mean unit transfusion is 68 and 24 respectively) (De et al, 1990). However, compared with thalassaemics the incidence of HIV infection is higher amongst haemophiliacs (4.4

versus 0.8%). The explanation of this discrepancy is not obvious but suggests that some of the patients may have been treated with multiple donor pool concentrate at some stage. Those countries that have resorted to the use of American commercial factor VIII concentrates show a relatively higher incidence of HIV infection amongst the recipients (Cohn et al, 1990).

Haemophilia care offered in most developing countries is grossly inadequate. The organized approach to the management of hereditary bleeding disorders in most of these regions has yet to evolve. There are very few developing countries which have resources for providing 24 h haemophilia care. Indeed, in the whole of Africa there are only five countries which provide 24 h haemophilia care, and that only at their regional centres (Essien, 1981; Kasili, 1983; El Shinnawi, 1984; Cohn et al, 1990) (see Table 8). Cryoprecipitate is the most commonly used replacement therapy. There are still a number of countries in which whole blood is used for the replacement of coagulation factors because of lack of facilities for making even fresh plasma, let alone cryoprecipitate. Self-treatment or home treatment remains a dream for most, as only a third of the countries listed in Tables 8–10 provide home treatment. Adverse socioeconomic factors and the prohibitive cost of commercial concentrates will make home therapy impracticable for a long time. Indeed, the best hope for the future of haemophilia care may be with gene therapy.

ACQUIRED DISORDERS OF COAGULATION

Coagulation disorders can be acquired through three major pathological mechanisms: faulty synthesis of coagulation factors, excessive consumption of coagulation factors, or the acquisition of antibodies that inhibit coagulant function. In practice, acquired coagulation disorders are more common than inherited disorders. The causes of acquired defects of haemostatic failure are numerous and are often associated with multisystem disease, particular physiological events such as pregnancy, early infancy or old age, or with drug therapy. The most noteworthy of these are bleeding episodes caused by disseminated intravascular coagulation, snake venoms, vitamin K deficiency and liver disease.

Disseminated intravascular coagulation

Disseminated intravascular coagulation (DIC) is a complicated derangement of the haemostatic system involving the vessel wall, platelets, coagulation cascade, fibrinolytic pathway, coagulation inhibitors, kinin and complement systems. DIC may occur in association with widely differing diseases or clinical states bearing no overt relationship to haemostasis. Whilst the literature is full of single case reports of DIC as a complication of diverse diseases (Table 11), there is, unfortunately, little information regarding the frequency with which DIC may occur in routine hospital practice, and even less for the incidence in the general community. In a

Table 11. Main causes of DIC encountered in clinical practice.

Acute	Subacute	Chronic
Shock	*Leukaemia*	*Metabolic*
Extensive surgical trauma	Acute promyelocytic leukaemia	Liver disease
Burns		Renal disease
Heat stroke		
Infections		*Neoplasia*
Septicaemia		Prostatic carcinoma
Viraemia		
Protozoal (malaria)		
Obstetric disorders		
Septic abortions		Systemic lupus erythematosus, sarcoidosis, allergic vasculitis
Abruptio placentae		
Amniotic fluid embolism		

consecutive necropsy series, 3% of patients were found to have histological evidence of DIC in the absence of clinical suspicion (Kim et al, 1976). Two hospital based studies have reported an incidence of DIC of 1 per 1000 hospital admissions (Siegal et al, 1978; Matsuda and Aoki, 1983). There appears to be little geographical difference in the main aetiological causes of DIC (Table 12), on the basis of three studies from Japan, Israel and the USA (Siegal et al, 1978; Spero et al, 1980; Matsuda and Aoki, 1983). The broad categories of malignancy, surgery and infection account for roughly half of the total patients with DIC in these studies. The infections capable of inducing DIC are numerous (Gram-positive and Gram-negative bacteria, meningococci, chicken pox, malaria) and there may be regional and temporal variation in the importance of a particular infection. Leukaemia accounts for more than 50% of malignancy-induced DIC. In these studies there is only a modest representation of the obstetric causes of DIC. This contrasts with the authors' own clinical experience in which pregnancy is as frequent a cause of DIC as infection or malignancy.

Table 12. Hospital based analysis of DIC.

	Israel*	USA†	Japan‡
Total no. patients with DIC	118	346	503
Incidence	1/1000		1/1000
Aetiological categories (%)			
General infection	39.8	25.7	15.0
Surgery/trauma	23.7	24.3	2.3
Malignancy	6.8	19.1	59.4
Liver disease	4.2	8	5
Obstetric complications	4.2	4	3.7

* From Siegal et al (1978).
† From Spero et al (1980).
‡ From Matsuda and Aoki (1983).

Snake envenomation
(With Alan F. Fleming)

There are over 3000 species of snakes known, but of these only one-sixth are venomous. Venomous snakes belong to five families (Warrell, 1987, 1991).

The Viperidae, or vipers, have long curved fangs which are situated anteriorly, are capable of a wide range of movements, and so are efficient at envenomation. They include *Echis carinatus* (carpet or saw-scale viper), *Bitus arietans* (puff adder), *B. gabonica* (Gaboon viper), *Daboia russelii* (Russell's viper) and the subfamily Crotalinae (rattlesnakes, *Bothrops*, Asian pit vipers).

The Colubridae, or tree snakes, have short, posteriorly situated fangs, capable of only limited movement. Envenomation is unusual and is confined mostly to people who handle the snakes. They include *Dispholidus typus* (boomslang), *Rhabdophis tigrinus* (Japanese keelback or yamakagashi) and *R. subminiatus* (south-east Asian red-necked keelback).

The Atractaspididae, or African burrowing asps (burrowing or mole vipers or adders) have long front fangs and strike sideways.

The Elapidae includes the cobras, kraits, mambas and coral snakes. They have relatively short fangs, anteriorly placed and permanently erect. The venoms are often spat rather than injected.

The Hydrophiidae, which include sea snakes and terrestrial Australasian snakes, also have short, anteriorly placed fangs with limited movement.

Snake venoms may contain up to 20 or more components, and these may have several toxic actions. Many venoms include phospholipase A_2, which can cause presynaptic neurotoxicity, rhabomyolysis, endothelial damage and haemolysis; other components are procoagulants, postsynaptic neurotoxins, cytotoxins, cardiotoxins and potentiators of endogenous substances which increase capillary permeability. Only snake bites causing haemorrhage are discussed here (Table 13; Figure 6), but bleeding cannot be described in isolation from the other effects of envenomation.

Venomous snakes are widely distributed in the world, being found almost everywhere except at above 5000 m altitude, in polar regions and on many islands, such as New Zealand, Pacific islands, Madagascar, western Mediterranean and Atlantic islands, including Ireland and the Caribbean islands. Snake bite is a common and important cause of morbidity and mortality in rural tropical areas. For example, the incidence of death from snake bite, mostly by *D. russelii* is 3.3 per 100 000 population per year in Myanmar (Burma) (Warrell, 1987, 1989). In the Benue valley of north-east Nigeria and in central Benin, snake bites, mostly by *E. carinatus*, have an incidence nearing 500 per 100 000 population per year, account for about one-third of all adult male hospital admissions during the early rains, and carry a mortality of up to 12% (Pugh and Theakston, 1980). People at special risk include hunter-gatherers, in whom snake bite may account for 5% of all adult deaths, in Australia, Papua New Guinea, Thailand, Tanzania and the Amazon basin. Nomadic herdsmen are at risk as they walk through the bush. Farmers experience epidemics of snake bites at the time of harvesting paddy or of the early rains in drier climates: rains bring out small rodents and reptiles, which are the prey of the snakes, at the same time as farmers are digging their fields, often barefoot. Floods can flush out snakes and concentrate both them and humans, leading to epidemics of envenomation. Workers on development projects in jungles are at risk.

Africa

Echis carinatus. The carpet (or saw-scale) viper is the most widely distributed of all the venomous snakes, being found throughout Africa north of the equator, the Middle East, the Indian subcontinent and south-east Asia (Table 13) (Warrell et al, 1977). It is probably the most dangerous snake in the world, accounting for about 23 000 deaths annually in west Africa alone (Pugh and Theakston, 1980).

There is local pain and swelling, which can progress to blistering and necrosis at the site of the bite, but more importantly there is spontaneous systemic bleeding; early sites are tooth sockets and the nose. Blood oozes from venepuncture sites or other recent traumas. Death can follow from intracranial haemorrhage after 1 or 2 days, or from haemorrhagic shock and renal failure after about 1 week. Mortality is 10–20% in patients who attend hospitals but who do not receive appropriate treatment (Warrell et al, 1977).

The blood is incoagulable, which is diagnostic of *E. carinatus* bites in areas where this is common. Levels of fibrinogen and factors V, VIII, II and XIII are low: fibrin degradation products (FDPs) are elevated. Only about 10% have a thrombocytopenia, associated with the severest envenomation, and fibrinolysis is not increased.

Specific treatment is with antivenom; this should be given as soon as

Table 13. Species of snakes commonly responsible for morbidity or death from haemorrhage.

Area	Latin name	Vernacular names
Africa	*Echis carinatus*	Carpet or saw-scale viper
	Bitus arietans	Puff adder
	Naja nigricollis	Spitting cobra
	Dispholidus typus	Boomslang
Asia		
Middle East	*E. carinatus*	Carpet or saw-scale viper
South-east	*Daboia russelii*	Russell's viper
	E. carinatus	Carpet or saw-scale viper
	*Calloselasma rhodostoma**	Malayan pit viper
	Trimeresurus species	Green pit vipers
Australasia	*Notechis scutatus*	Tiger snake
	Oxyuranus scutellatus	Taipan
	Pseudonaja textilis	Eastern brown snake
America		
North	*Crotalus adamanteus*	Eastern diamond-backed rattlesnake
	C. atrox	Western diamond-backed rattlesnake
South	*Bothrops atrox*	Fer-de-lance, barba amirilla
	B. jararaca	Jararaca

* Formerly *Agkistodon rhodostoma*.
From Warrell (1991).

possible but the coagulation defect can be reversed by antivenom several days after the bite. In west Africa the antivenom from the South African Institute for Medical Research (SAIMR) has been shown to be highly effective, but may not be available due to trade sanctions; Pasteur Paris *Echis* antivenom is also reliable in the restoration of the blood coagulation (Warrell et al, 1974; 1980; Pugh and Theakston, 1987).

Bitus arietans. The puff adder is distributed throughout sub-Saharan Africa except in dense forest, and is found also along the African Atlantic seaboard to Morocco, and in western Arabia (Warrell et al, 1975). It is a common snake and a frequent cause of bites and deaths in man and domestic animals.

Within 20 min of a bite, there is local pain and swelling, which are maximal on the second or third day, and may take up to 3 weeks to resolve. These are complicated often by blistering, bullae containing blood-stained fluid, bruising, arterial thrombosis and tissue necrosis. Regional lymph nodes are enlarged and painful. In about half of patients coming for treatment, systemic envenomation leads to hypotension, bradycardia, renal impairment and spontaneous haemorrhage, usually of the gums and nose.

The venom has direct cytotoxic effects on myocardium, the autonomic nervous system, the kidneys and vascular endothelium. Endothelial damage leads to platelet consumption and secondary thrombocytopenia. DIC is unusual, but may occur and be complicated by microangiopathic haemolytic anaemia, with a rapidly falling haemoglobin concentration.

Patients who have extensive local swelling involving half a limb, or systemic envenomation, should be treated with specific polyvalent antivenom, and observed carefully for early signs of circulatory collapse.

The effects of bites from other giant vipers are similar. *B. gabonica* (Gaboon viper) is found throughout sub-Saharan Africa; the venom has anticoagulant action in vitro related to a proteolytic action on fibrinogen (Forbes et al, 1969). *B. nasicornis* (rhinoceros horned viper) is distributed in a belt from west Africa to western Kenya: its venom has multiple effects in vitro on coagulation, fibrinolysis and platelets (MacKay et al, 1970).

Naja nigricollis. The spitting cobra is widespread and common in sub-Saharan Africa, except in the central African forest and temperate South Africa (Warrell et al, 1976). Although it is well known for its ability to spit venom over several metres, and to cause severe inflammation and corneal damage if the venom hits the eye, the snake also bites. The cobra enters homes in search of its prey, including rodents, lizards and other snakes, and human victims are commonly asleep when bitten. Local swelling follows rapidly, often involving a whole limb and progressing to extensive local tissue necrosis. There are not the neurological signs associated with other cobra bites. About one-fifth of patients have spontaneous haemorrhage, which may be the cause of death.

Haematological abnormalities include a failure of clot retraction, due to a platelet defect, probably destruction of platelet actin (thrombasthenin). Procoagulant actions have been demonstrated in vitro, but are probably not important in vivo. There is prolonged whole blood clot lysis about 24 h after the bite, returning to normal in around 1 week. DIC is not a feature, but FDPs can be raised from the fifth day onwards, associated with extensive tissue necrosis. There is activation of the alternative pathway of complement, with depletion of component C3.

Haemorrhage following snake bite in Africa can be characterized by simple tests: failure of whole blood to clot indicates *E. carinatus*; formation of a clot but a failure of clot retraction indicates *N. nigricollis*.

Specific polyvalent antivenoms are not effective in reversing the effects of envenomation by the spitting cobra (Warrell et al, 1976).

Dispholidus typus. The green African tree-snake, the boomslang, is widespread in wooded areas of sub-Saharan Africa except for the central African forest. Its reputation as a dangerous animal is exaggerated, as it is not aggressive and is back-fanged. The few reported cases of envenomation have almost always been in people who keep snakes as pets or otherwise handled snakes. Venom activates thrombin, factors X and XIII, and complement (Figure 6). Spontaneous haemorrhage, which may be extensive, starts 1–2 days after the bite. All laboratory tests are indicative of DIC, which may lead on to microangiopathic haemolytic anaemia and renal failure. There is considerable mortality without treatment, but specific antivenoms are effective.

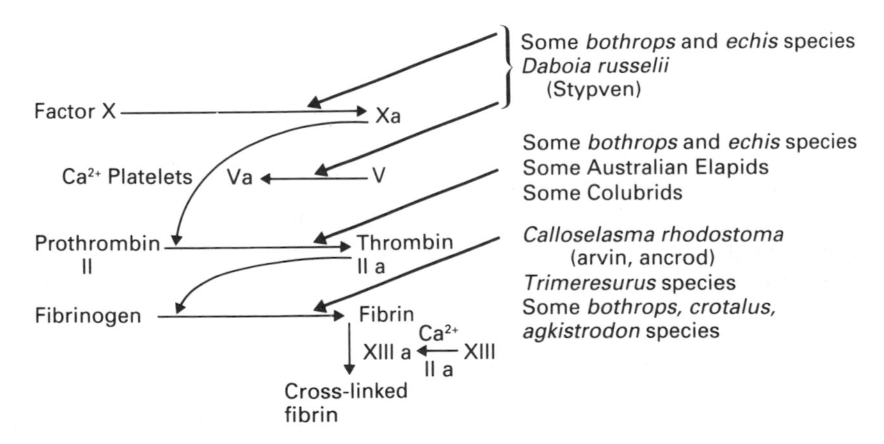

Figure 6. Sites of action of some snake venom procoagulants on the clotting cascade. *C. rhodostoma* was formerly called *Agkistrodon rhodostoma*. *Daboia russelii* was formerly called *Vipera russelli*. The Australian Elapidae are now classified as Hydrophiidae. Reproduced with kind permission of Professor D. A. Warrell.

Asia

D. russelii envenomation is a major health problem in the Indian subcontinent and Burma (Figure 7). The range of *E. carinatus* (see above) includes these areas also, and both the Malayan pit viper (*Calloselasma rhodostoma*) and the green pit vipers (*Trimeresurus* species) are relatively common on the Malaysian peninsula (Table 13).

Daboia russelii. Russell's viper is widely but discontinuously distributed throughout south-east Asia: five subspecies are recognized (Figure 7). Habitats are both in the plains and mountains up to 3000 m. Open land is preferred, especially grasslands and paddy: the jungles are avoided. It is nocturnal; the natural prey include a wide variety of small vertebrates.

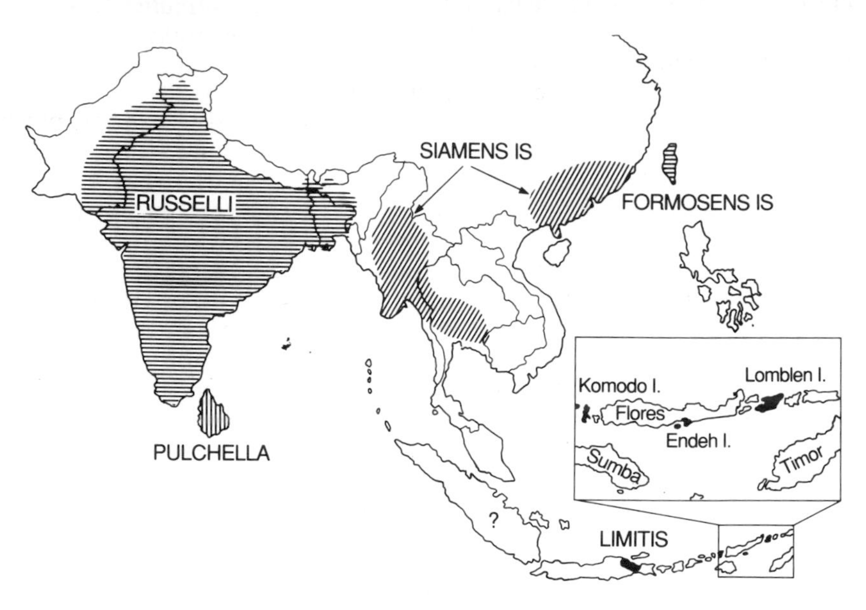

Figure 7. Distribution of the five currently recognized subspecies of *Daboia russelii*. Reproduced from Warrell (1989) with permission.

D. russelii is the most common cause of serious and fatal snake bites in southern India, Sri Lanka and Burma. There are two peaks of incidence, coinciding with the sowing and the harvesting of the rice crop. The incidence of fatal snake bite in Sri Lanka is nearly 6 per 100 000 population per year, of which three-quarters are due to *D. russelii*; incidence in Burma is 3.3 per 100 000 population per year, making this the fifth most common cause of death, of which 70% is due to this viper. It is an important cause of death in the rice-growing areas of Thailand; there are no data from China; it is a lesser problem in Taiwan and Indonesia (Warrell, 1989).

The venom is rich in phospholipase A_2, which is responsible for damage to vascular endothelium, platelet damage, haemolysis, rhabdomyolysis, neurotoxicity, hepatic necrosis, vasodilation, and release by the host of histamine, 5-hydroxytryptamine and other substances increasing capillary permeability. It contains two major procoagulants acting on factors X and V (Figure 6): their activity leads to consumption coagulopathy, DIC with fibrin deposition in the kidneys and other organs, and fibrinolysis.

Around 30% of humans who are bitten do not suffer envenomation. Local symptoms and signs of swelling and painful lymph nodes are generally mild.

Throughout the range of distribution of *D. russelii*, systemic envenomation leads to incoagulable blood, which, with the endothelial and platelet damage, results in spontaneous haemorrhages in the mouth, nose, gastrointestinal tract, conjunctivae, skin and renal tract; intracerebral and subarachnoid haemorrhages are important causes of death. Shock developing early is caused by vasodilation and increased capillary permeability. Late shock may be associated with massive gastrointestinal haemorrhage or acute pituitary-adrenal insufficiency following haemorrhage or infarction. Acute renal failure has as high incidence and mortality.

Other complications show considerable geographical variations, presumably due to differing compositions of the venom. Conjunctival oedema is observed in Burma, acute pituitary insufficiency in Burma and southern India, and rhabdomyolysis and neurotoxicity in Sri Lanka and southern India.

Blood is usually incoagulable: there is extreme hypofibrinogenaemia, severe reductions of factors V, X, XIIIa, and depletion of protein C, antithrombin III, plasminogen and plasmin; FDP levels are very high. There is usually thrombocytopenia and poor platelet aggregation.

Specific antivenom is indicated when there is incoagulable blood, spontaneous haemorrhage, hypotension, shock, neuromyotoxic signs, impaired consciousness, intravascular haemolysis or local swelling involving more than two segments of the bitten limb (Warrell, 1989). Antivenom is effective in the restoration of haemostasis, but does not prevent the development of renal failure, which remains probably the most common cause of death due to the unavailability of dialysis (Myint-Lwin et al, 1985). Chronic pituitary-adrenal insufficiency is a serious late sequela.

Asian pit vipers. Pit vipers are so named from their heat-sensitive pit organs situated behind the nostril. *C. rhodostoma* (Malayan pit viper) is after *D. russelii*, a major cause of snake bite in south-east Asia. There are nine species of *Trimeresurus* (green pit vipers) in Thailand alone: these bite frequently, but usually without serious effects. Envenomation is followed by greater local effects (swelling, pain, enlarged lymph nodes and tissue necrosis) than with *D. russelii*. Haemorrhage may (1) be local, limited to the bitten site, (2) spread up the affected limb, or (3) become generalized.

Venoms contain proteolytic enzymes, for example 'arvin' or 'ancrod' of *C. rhodostoma*, which cleaves fibrinogen, so defribinating the victim within about half an hour (Figure 6). Platelets are damaged and sequestered, and fibrinolysis is activated secondarily, with raised FDPs (Mahasandana et al, 1980; Warrell, 1987, 1991).

Australia

There are about 200 snake bites and an average of 4.5 deaths per year in Australia (Sutherland 1983; Warrell, 1987). The snakes responsible are terrestrial Hydrophiidae, principally *Notachis scutatus*, *Oxyuranus scutellatus* and *Pseudonaja textiles* (Table 13). Venoms cause neurotoxicity, rhabdomyolysis and haemorrhage through the activation of prothrombin

(Figure 6). Antivenom should be given whenever there is pain, or evidence of envenomation, or a bite proven to be by a highly venomous species.

The Americas

Snake bites cause around 200 deaths in Brazil and 100 in Venezuela each year. The important species are rattlesnakes (*Crotalus durissus durissus* and *C. d. terrificus*) and *Bothrops atrox*, *B. asper* and *B. jaracara* (Warrell, 1987) (Table 13). Envenomation by all species causes extensive necrosis; haemorrhage results from cleavage of fibrinopeptide A from fibrinogen, leading to defibrination (Markland, 1976); other complications include intravascular haemolysis, renal failure and neurotoxicity, all features in particular of *C. d. terrificus* envenomation.

In the USA, there are about 7000 venomous snake bites per year, with 9–14 deaths (Parrish, 1980; Warrell, 1987). Most deaths are caused by *C. adamanteus* and *C. atrox* (Table 13). Local signs can be absent or minor: envenomation leads to hypotension and shock; defibrination and haemorrhage are the consequences of splitting fibrinopeptide A from fibrinogen (Markland, 1976).

Antivenom should be given early in all cases of rattlesnake bites, even before there are signs of systemic envenomation.

Caterpillar envenomation

A haemorrhagic syndrome is induced by contact with the caterpillar of a moth, *Lonomia achelous*. This caterpillar, which is covered with long brittle hollow hairs containing the venom, feeds on the leaves of the rubber tree (*Hevia braziliensis*). Hence small outbreaks occur affecting rubber tappers in Brazil. In Venezuela cases also appear sporadically where another food plant is used by the moth. Generalized haemostatic failure follows contact in 7–14 days, with death in severe cases from cerebral haemorrhage. Treatment with fresh frozen plasma or cryoprecipitate is effective in most such cases. The active principles seem to be small glycoproteins which have profibrinolytic and anti-factor XIII properties in vitro (Arocha-Pinango et al, 1988).

Deficiency of vitamin K dependent clotting factors

Primary vitamin K deficiency is uncommon in man because of its widespread distribution in plants and animal tissue and because of endogenous production of vitamin K by the microbiological flora of the normal gut. The normal daily requirement is in the range of only 0.1–0.5 μg/kg for adults and therefore the diet has to be extremely deficient in fat soluble vitamins before vitamin K deficiency occurs. Postsurgical or debilitated patients on fat free diets may develop bleeding problems within 7 to 10 days, particularly if they are also on broad-spectrum antibiotics which eliminate the intestinal bacterial source of vitamin K. Absorption is reduced in coeliac disease and pancreatic insufficiency and absent in patients with complete obstruction of the common bile duct. Liver disease is a frequent cause of a clinically important bleeding tendency. This is because in any form of parenchymal liver disease levels of all vitamin K dependent clotting factors are depressed as part of a general failure of protein synthesis. This results in a prolonged prothrombin time which is often an early indicator of hepatocyte insult. In hepatocellular failure vitamin K supplementation results in only a partial, if any, improvement in the prothrombin time as the ability to utilize the vitamin for post-translational carboxylation is defective. Furthermore, liver disease is associated with other haemostatic defects, including thrombocytopenia, DIC, increased fibrinolysis and dysfibrinogenaemia. Whilst recognized as a common feature of hepatology practice, the geographical incidence of a bleeding tendency in patients with the gamut of liver disorders remains unstudied, but obviously is relatively high in populations in the tropics and elsewhere where there are high rates of transmission of hepatitis viruses and consequently high prevalence of chronic hepatic disease.

In neonates, vitamin K deficiency occurs for several physiological reasons. The placenta transmits lipids poorly and breast milk is a poor source of the vitamin. Furthermore, the gut is sterile during the first days of life. Several distinct bleeding syndromes result (Table 14) (Hathaway, 1987). The exact incidence of early haemorrhagic disease of the newborn (HDN) is unknown. In a survey of 111 pregnant mothers on anticonvulsants, 20 infants had prothrombin levels of less than 20% within 12 h of birth (Deblay et al, 1982). Of these, eight had clinical haemorrhage, which resulted in three deaths and one infant with neurological sequelae.

Estimates of the incidence of classical HDN vary widely from as high as 1.7% in full-term infants (Sutherland et al, 1967) to 0.5% (Lane and Hathaway, 1985). The incidence of bleeding among breast-fed infants who do not receive vitamin K is 15 to 20 times greater than that in infants who receive either cow's milk or formula or vitamin K or both (Sutherland et al, 1967). During the past 10 years it has become apparent that vitamin K deficiency haemorrhage is an important cause of morbidity and mortality in infants older than 1 month (Lane et al, 1983; Verity et al, 1983). In most of these cases of so-called late HDN the infants have been exclusively breast fed, no vitamin K prophylaxis has been given at birth and they present with intracranial bleeding at 1–2 months of age. There is usually no evidence of malabsorption, liver disease or chronic diarrhoea. Whilst the prevalence of late HDN in developing countries is difficult to ascertain, estimates of 1:1200 in England (McNinds et al, 1985) and 3:1000 in Thailand (Hathaway, 1987) have been made. In Japan, where vitamin K prophylaxis was halted, an incidence of late HDN of 1:1700 live births was documented (Motohara et al, 1984), In the USA, where vitamin K prophylaxis is routinely given at birth, cases of late HDN are rarely reported (Lane et al, 1983).

Conclusions on bleeding disorders

Haemophilia of all types is found amongst all nations but there is a relatively higher incidence of serious bleeding disorders recorded in the affluent

Table 14. Clinical features of haemorrhagic disease of the newborn due to vitamin K deficiency.

Clinical syndrome	Age	Common bleeding sites	Cause	Prevention by vitamin K administration at birth	Comments
Early HDN	0–24 h	Cephalohaematoma Intracranial Intrathoracic Intra-abdominal Scalp monitor	1. Maternal drugs Warfarin Anticonvulsants Antituberculous drugs 2. Idiopathic	Not in all instances	Frequently life threatening
Classic HDN	1–7 days	Gastrointestinal Skin Nasal Circumcision	1. Idiopathic 2. Maternal drugs	Yes	Incidence increased in breast-fed neonates and reduced by early formula feeding
Late HDN	1–3 months	Intracranial Skin Gastrointestinal	Idiopathic	Yes	
			Secondary 1. Diarrhoea 2. Malabsorption Cystic fibrosis α_1-antitrypsin deficiency Biliary atresia 3. Prolonged warfarin exposure	Probably no	A cause of intracranial haemorrhage in breast-fed infants 1–3 months of age; may be aggravated by antibiotic administration

From Hathaway (1987), with permission.

regions of the world compared with the poorer countries. This is most probably due to a combination of excessive mortality and under-reporting as a consequence of the lack of treatment and of diagnostic facilities. Comprehensive nationwide data on the incidence and outcome of haemophilia is only available from a few advanced countries. Based on this data, the numbers of haemophiliacs, their quality of life and the amount of treatment material used in their care looks set to rise in the developed countries, despite the tragic setback associated with transmission of the HIV and hepatitis viruses. This trend is also likely to be seen in the developing countries when medical facilities improve, health priorities change, more dedicated medical and paramedical personnel become available and when there is increased public sympathy and funding for haemophilia care.

In regard to acquired bleeding disorders, data of an epidemiological character are hard to find, as most of the published surveys concern the complication rate for a given disease or organ, e.g. liver disease. Nevertheless, acquired haemostatic failure from various causes must, in aggregate, far outnumber the inherited disorders. The consequences of this will be seen at blood bank level in terms of demand for blood component support, which rises inexorably as medical practice intensifies towards salvaging ever sicker patients. A considerable service to the planning of national plasma fractionation and local blood component separation facilities would be provided by epidemiological studies relating demand for haemostatic blood products to general levels of advancing medical and surgical care.

THROMBOTIC DISORDERS

Thrombotic disorders, such as coronary thrombosis, peripheral vascular disease and pulmonary embolus, are collectively implicated in the death of over half of the members of affluent society. As the underdeveloped world makes progress in combating its scourges of infection and malnutrition, thrombosis is rapidly becoming more important. Disabling or fatal thrombotic disease may stem from formation of thrombi within arteries at sites of arterial endothelial damage (e.g. atheroma) or in veins as a consequence of venous stasis and hypercoagulability. Thrombi also can form within the heart chambers, on prosthetic valves or within the microcirculation. Common to both venous and arterial thrombosis are the major factors, identified by Virchow in 1856, which are responsible for modifying the normal haemostatic process so that a thrombus forms. These are the contributions of altered blood flow, altered blood constituents or an abnormality of the vessel wall.

There is an intriguing and as yet unexplained tendency for thrombi to affect certain anatomical regions of the vascular tree with greater frequency than others, and in a given individual to affect some areas far more severely than others. Furthermore, specific risk factors appear to be selectively more important in the development or progression of thrombi. For example, hypertension is particularly associated with the risk of cerebrovascular disease, and heavy cigarette smoking is associated with peripheral vascular disease as well as coronary thrombosis. Clearly the pathogenesis of thrombosis is complex and usually results from the interaction of multiple factors, including a genetic predisposition.

Coronary artery disease

Ischaemic heart disease (IHD) results from the formation in the coronary arteries of atheromas, which act as thrombogenic agents. In most of the industrialized countries IHD is the main cause of death and accounts for nearly 50% of deaths from all causes (Uemura and Pisa, 1985). Even in developing countries IHD takes a steady toll.

The incidence of IHD shows variation on an international scale. The annual incidence varies from 15 per 10 000 in Japan to 198 per 10 000 in Finland (World Health Organization, 1983). Mortality statistics show a similar variation (Figure 8), some of which is undoubtedly due to differences in data collection and diagnostic practice. However, numerous studies using comparable methods have confirmed that real differences exist in the frequency of the disease. In Europe there is an almost threefold difference

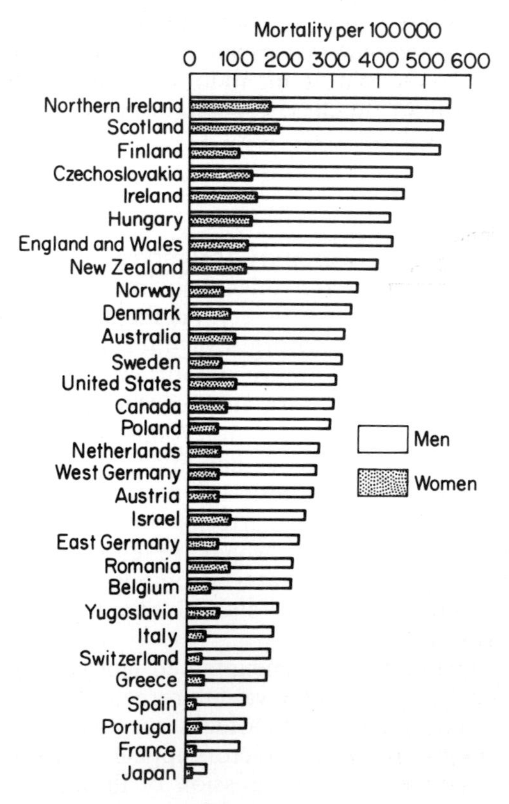

Figure 8. Ischaemic heart disease mortality rates per 100 000 population (1985) of men and women aged 40–69 years, with permission.

between France, Italy and Spain on the one hand and countries such as Finland and Britain on the other. The experience of migrants suggests that the variation between countries is likely to be due mainly to different environmental and behavioural patterns. Thus Japanese migrants to the USA tend to have rates of IHD approaching those of the host country.

In the last 15 years many of the industrialized countries have seen a declining incidence of IHD, the epidemic having reached its peak in the late 1960s. Between 1968 and 1976 the mortality rate in the USA had fallen by about 20% and a similar rate of decline has continued up to the present (Figure 9). The changes that have taken place in Europe during the same period give rise to interesting speculation. The largest increase in IHD mortality have taken place in the Eastern European countries, and the greatest decline in countries which have been actively concerned with population strategies directed towards changes in risk factors. In those countries where total mortality from IHD has decreased, not only have the women participated in this favourable trend but the decline in mortality has been greater among women (Figure 9). In these countries the relative contributions of favourable changes in life-style (such as better diet, less smoking, more physical activity), or of reduction in case fatalities from better and earlier medical intervention, remains unresolved.

Almost all the epidemiological research into the aetiology of IHD has been concentrated on factors which are thought to be directly associated with atherogenesis, such as dietary fat/blood lipid levels. More recent studies on the pathogenesis of IHD have provided good evidence that

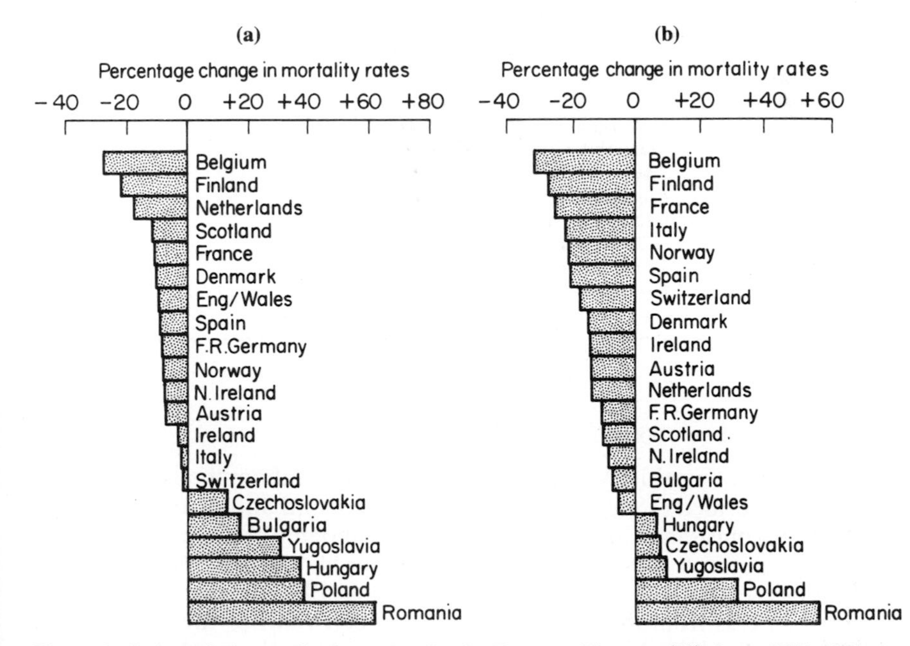

Figure 9. Ischaemic heart disease mortality in Europe. Changes (%) from 1971–1974 to 1981–1984 in **(a)** males and **(b)** females, aged 40–69 years, with permission.

thrombosis within the coronary arteries plays a crucial role in a large number of IHD events (Davies and Thomas, 1985). This, together with large scale surveys of haemostatic variables, has stimulated investigations into the relationship between haemostasis and atherosclerosis. One of the earliest and most extensive of such studies was the Northwick Park Prospective Heart Study (Meade et al, 1980). In this study men who died of cardiovascular disease showed at recruitment significantly higher plasma levels of factor VIIIc and fibrinogen as well as factor VIIc, compared with survivors. This positive correlation between high fibrinogen levels and IHD has been confirmed by three other western studies (Wilhelmsen et al, 1984; Kannel et al, 1985; Stone and Thorpe, 1985). Cross-sectional data from three more studies have found an association between elevated factor VIIc and IHD (Balleisen et al, 1985; Dalaker et al, 1985; Scarabin et al, 1985). Further evidence is provided by international studies comparing communities with marked differences in their incidence of IHD. These studies show a striking difference in the coagulation factor concentration (Table 15) as well as in fibrinolytic activity (Shaper et al, 1966; Dupuy et al, 1978; Meade et al, 1986). These population differences in plasma fibrinogen, factor VIIc and fibrinolytic activity may account for some of the difference in IHD mortality.

Table 15. Mean value of factor VIIc and fibrinogen according to country and race.

Country	Race	Known IHD risk	Number in study	Factor VIIc (%)	Fibrinogen (g/l)
England (London)	Caucasian	High	283	93.3	2.52
	Black	Low	48	84.7	2.51
Scotland (Glasgow)	Caucasian	High	81	94	3.00
Finland (East)	Caucasian	High	45	92	3.62
Czechoslovakia (Prague)	Caucasian	High	101	87	3.48
USA (Minnesota)	Caucasian	High	35	100	2.90
	Japanese	Moderate	37	110	2.43
Japan	Rural Japanese	Low	30	96	2.50
	Urban Japanese	Moderate	34	93	2.23
Gambia	Urban Gambian	Low	54	71	2.90
	Rural Gambian	Low	67	67	2.86
	Urban white expatriate	High	11	112.6	—

Venous thromboembolism

The substantial morbidity produced by venous thromboembolism has been repeatedly verified (Dalen and Alpert, 1975; Bell and Smith, 1982; Hirsh et al, 1986; Rubinstein et al, 1988). Venous thromboembolism manifests itself clinically in three ways: superficial thrombophlebitis (STP); deep vein thrombosis (DVT); and pulmonary embolism (PE). In fact the primary source of PE is from thrombi arising in the deep veins of the lower extremities, usually thrombi which extend into or arise in the popliteal veins or above (Sevitt and Gallagher, 1961; Havig, 1977; Hull et al, 1983). Therefore

PE, a complication of DVT, poses the greatest risk to life (Jones et al, 1986). It is estimated that DVTs result in 300 000–600 000 hospitalizations per year in the USA (Bernstein, 1986); of these patients, 50 000–100 000 die of PE (Dalen and Alpert, 1975; Jones et al, 1986). The majority of these deaths (75–90%) occur within the first few hours (Dalen and Alpert, 1975; Bell and Smith, 1982), offering little time for medical intervention.

The incidence of venous thrombosis in some specific circumstances, such as the postoperative period, has been defined with some degree of precision, but a meaningful assessment of the overall prevalence in the community has been difficult to obtain. From a longitudinal community study it has been estimated that the annual incidence of clinically recognized DVT in the USA is over 250 000, while that of superficial thrombophlebitis is over 123 000 (Coon et al, 1973). Clinical diagnosis of venous thrombosis, however, is notoriously unreliable (Hull et al, 1981) and it is likely that the frequency of venous thrombosis will be considerably underestimated when its detection is based on physical examination alone. The prevalence of venous thrombosis has also been examined in a number of necropsy series. Not surprisingly, in view of the difference in the extent and technique of vein dissection and in the type of patients coming to necropsy, these studies have shown a wide variation (Table 16).

Table 16. Prevalence of venous thrombosis based on necropsy studies.

Reference	*n*	Incidence of thrombosis (%)	Country/region
Gibbs (1957)	253	59	Surrey, England
Roberts (1963)	108	54	Glasgow, Scotland
Havig (1977)	261	72	Oslo, Norway

PE causes an even greater diagnostic problem. Clinical diagnosis and chest radiographs are unreliable and usually result in underdetection of PE. Combined perfusion and ventilation scans seem to be relatively reliable but more complex to perform. For these reasons, perhaps the most accurate, although still very imperfect, values for the frequency of pulmonary embolism are derived from extrapolations based upon necropsy data. The necropsy procedures required, however, tend to be specialized, as routine methods have a relatively low detection rate. Morrell and Dunnill (1968) found pulmonary embolism in 52% of the necropsies in a large series of patients using a specialized technique, as compared with 12% using the routine method. Apart from the differing background of patients coming to necropsy this may be the other reason for the variation in the incidence of PE at necropsy (Table 17). There is disagreement about whether or not the frequency of PE is increasing. There is little doubt that the condition is being reported more frequently (Dupont, 1975; Ruckley, 1975) but this may reflect an increasing awareness on the part of the clinician and an improvement in the diagnostic techniques. Also a pathological, temporal study by the same workers showed no significant difference in the incidence over two

Table 17. Prevalence of pulmonary embolism at necropsy.

Reference	*n*	Incidence of PE (%)	Country/region
Uhland and Goldberg (1964)	981	12	Oregon, USA
Orell (1962)	1076	18	Sweden
Havig (1977)	508	69	Oslo, Norway
Coon 1976 (1964–1974)	4600	12.3	Michigan, USA
Coon and Coller 1959 (1945–1954)	4391	13.6	Michigan, USA

periods covering the years 1945–1955 and 1967–1974 (Coon and Coller, 1959; Coon, 1976).

There is variation in the incidence of DVT after surgery and in association with various medical ailments (Table 18). Similarly, fatal PE has been reported in 4–7% of patients after emergency hip surgery, in 0.3–1.7% of patients after elective hip replacement and 0.1–0.8% of general surgical patients in the USA (Gallus and Hirsh, 1976; Hirsh et al, 1981). The incidence of PE following a myocardial infarction or a stroke is 1–2% and 1–3%, respectively.

Table 18. Incidence of DVT in various medical conditions and postoperatively in western Europe and North America.

	Incidence of DVT (%)	Reference
Surgical procedures		
Patients >40 years undergoing general surgery	25	Bergquist (1983)
Inguinal hernia repair	20–30	Bergquist (1983)
Neurosurgery	9–50	Bergquist (1983)
Surgery following hip fracture	44	Bergquist (1983)
Renal transplantation in a diabetic	40	Bergquist et al (1985)
Thoracic non-cardiac surgery	50	Bergquist (1983)
Aortic aneurysm repair	33	Myhre et al (1974)
Surgery for occlusive aortoiliac disease	12	Myhre et al (1974)
Surgery for varicose veins	12	Lofgren et al (1976)
Medical conditions		
Myocardial infarction	27	Simmons et al (1973)
Strokes (DVT in paralytic leg)	50–70	Warlow et al (1972)

Interestingly there is considerable evidence that geographical variation in the incidence of thromboembolic disease exists. The possible pathogenic factors which have been most frequently offered as an explanation for these differences include altered fibrinolytic activity (Mibashan et al, 1960; Dupuy et al, 1978), dietary elements (Burkitt, 1972) and variations in physique and activity. The incidence of postoperative venous thrombosis varies widely in different parts of the world, suggesting that ethnicity may be a risk factor (Table 19). Against this, however, are studies such as those in South Africa by Joffe (1974) who found a similar incidence of venous thrombosis among those of European, mixed, black African and Indian descent. This implies that any true geographical variation is likely to be environmental rather than genetic.

Table 19. Geographical variation of DVT in surgical patients.

Reference	Race	Medical surgical procedure	No. of patients	Mean age (years)	M:F	Venous thrombosis detected (%)	Method of detection
Atichartakarn et al (1988)	Thai	Hip replacement	50	60s, 70s	2:1	4	Venography
Nillius and Nylander (1979)	Swedish	Hip replacement	134	66	1:2	58	Venography
Cunningham and Yong (1974)	Malaysian	General surgery	68	—	—	12	[^{125} I]fibrinogen scanning
Chumnijarakij and Poshyachinda (1975)	Thai	Abdominal hysterectomy for benign conditions	117	43	—	1.7	[^{125} I]fibrinogen scanning
	Thai	Major pelvic surgery for malignant disease	52	43	—	3.8	
Walsh et al (1974)	English	Abdominal hysterectomy for benign conditions	117	43	—	12	[^{125} I]fibrinogen scanning
	English	Major pelvic surgery for malignant disease	45	56	—	35	
Tso et al (1980)	Chinese	Pelvic surgery for benign conditions	81	—	—	0	[^{125} I]fibrinogen scanning
	Chinese	Pelvic surgery on patients on oral contraceptive	43	—	—	10.5	
	Chinese	Wertheim's hysterectomy for cervical cancer	—	—	—	6.7	
Hassan et al (1974)	Sudanese	Transvesical prostectomy	93	68.7	—	10.7	[^{125} I]fibrinogen scanning
Becker et al (1970)	Swedish	Transvesical prostectomy	187	—	—	21	Venography
Gordon-Smith et al (1972)	English	Retropubic prostectomy	62	>50	—	29	[^{125} I]fibrinogen scanning
Joffe S (1974)	European	Major elective operation	50	—	—	48	[^{125} I]fibrinogen scanning
	Coloured	Major elective operation	34	—	1:1	54	
	Bantu	Major elective operation	10	—	1:4	50	
	Indian	Major elective operation	6	—	6:0	67	

In recent years an increasing number of congenital alterations in blood components have been recognized to endow the affected individual with a marked predisposition to thrombosis, often at an early age. Awareness of these conditions and their identification, both in patients and in other family members, is becoming widespread in the West. The rest of this section reviews the epidemiology of hereditary and acquired haemostatic component alterations implicated in predisposition to venous thromboembolism.

Antithrombin III

Antithrombin III (ATIII) is the plasma glycoprotein which inhibits thrombin factor Xa and, to a lesser extent, factors IXa, XIa and XIIa. The inhibitory activity of ATIII is dramatically accelerated by heparin and some heparan sulphates. The importance of ATIII for the maintenance of the haemostatic balance is illustrated by the fact that an inherited deficiency of ATIII is associated with thromboembolism. In the adult, deficiency of ATIII may be congenital or acquired.

Congenital ATIII deficiency. The first report describing a family with hereditary ATIII deficiency associated with thromboembolism was published in 1965 by Egeberg (Brandt, 1981). Since that initial description an increasing number of families with hereditary deficiency of ATIII have been reported. Specific mutations have been identified in more than 40 families and this has allowed a better understanding of the structure/function relationships of the ATIII molecule. Familial ATIII deficiency is a heterogeneous disorder which has been classified into three main types (Nagy and Losonczy, 1979; Sas, 1988) based on the levels of ATIII measured by three different assays of ATIII expression (Figure 10). Familial ATIII deficiency is inherited as an autosomal dominant disorder. The laboratory abnormality is expressed in approximately half the family members, who are heterozygous, with functional ATIII levels between 40 and 60% of normal control values. Occasional cases have been reported of an affected patient, whose parents have normal ATIII levels, in the absence of a family history of thrombosis. This raises the possibility of spontaneous mutation to an abnormal gene (Winter et al, 1982), as often occurs in other genetic disorders.

The prevalence of ATIII deficiency remains ambiguous due to the absence of appropriately designed studies. The reported prevalence in the literature has varied from 1 in 2000 (Rosenberg, 1975) through 1 in 5000 (Odegaard and Abildgaard, 1978) to 1 in 20 000 (Gladson et al, 1988). The prevalence of ATIII deficiency in a clinic population being investigated for venous thromboembolism is 1.8–3% (Bulter and Ten Cate, 1989; Hirsh et al, 1989). The occurrence of venous thrombosis at a comparatively early age is a characteristic of ATIII deficiency. A recent review of prevalence of hereditary thrombotic disease in patients under 45 years of age with proven venous thrombosis concluded that 20% can be expected to have ATIII, protein C or protein S deficiency (Hirsh et al, 1989). Not all individuals with ATIII deficiency develop thrombosis. However, by the age of 50 about

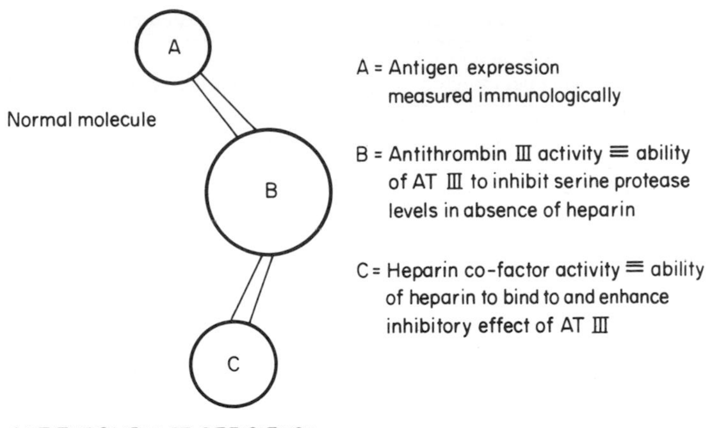

Figure 10. Schematic representation of types of antithrombin III deficiency.

two-thirds of them become symptomatic (Cosgriff et al, 1983), with approximately 50% having their first thrombotic episode in the absence of any obvious predisposing factor. The most frequent site of thrombosis is the deep veins of the legs, sometimes complicated by pulmonary embolism. Thrombosis in unusual sites (for example cerebral veins or mesenteric veins) as well as the other features of ATIII deficiency are summarized in Table 20.

Table 20. Clinical features of ATIII deficiency.

First episode at early age (i.e. under 40 years old)
Family history of venous thromboembolism
Recurrent venous thromboembolism
Unusual site, e.g. cerebral vein, mesenteric vein and renal veins
Thrombosis during pregnancy
'Idiopathic' venous thrombosis
Resistance to heparin therapy
Venous and arterial thrombosis at an early age in homozygotes (type III)

From Hirsh (1989), with permission.

The risk of thromboembolism in those with ATIII deficiency is increased in the presence of other predisposing factors such as surgery, immobility, pregnancy and the use of oral contraceptives. Table 21 details the incidence of venous thromboembolism in many of the kindred described with the three principal types of ATIII deficiency (Hirsh et al, 1989). Even allowing for the

Table 21. Prevalence of ATIII deficiency and thrombosis in kindred with ATIII deficiency.

ATIII deficiency	Family members studied	Deficient	Thrombosis	Thrombosis deficiency rate
Type I	617	260 (42)	136	0.52
Type II	193	105 (54)	57	0.54
Type III	91	51 (56)	3*	0.058

Values in parentheses are percentages.
* Homozygous persons.
From Hirsh (1989), with permission.

very small numbers reported with type III deficiency, its clinical expression clearly differs markedly from that of type I or II deficiency. Homozygotes for type III deficiency are at increased risk of venous thromboembolism during the first decade of life, and arterial thrombosis also occurs.

Acquired ATIII deficiency. Acquired deficiencies of ATIII may result in significant clinical problems (Table 22). With the exception of severe liver disease and DIC, the ATIII levels in these conditions are normally higher than those found in familial ATIII deficiency. However, in aggregate, acquired ATIII deficiency must be many times more prevalent than is familial deficiency of the anticoagulant protein.

Treatment of ATIII deficiency. Lifelong treatment with oral vitamin K antagonist is probably indicated after a first episode of thromboembolism (Cosgriff et al, 1983; Halal et al, 1983). An extensive survey of complete family pedigrees suggests that lifelong treatment with oral anticoagulants in symptom-free ATIII deficient individuals is unlikely to improve survival (Rosendaal et al, 1991). Replacement therapy with ATIII concentrates in both congenital and acquired deficiency states is still undergoing evaluation.

Protein C

Protein C, first named autoprothrombin IIa was purified in 1976 by Stenflo (1976), who called it protein C because it was the third protein to be eluted in ion exchange chromatography. It is now known that this vitamin K dependent glycoprotein is synthesized by the liver and circulates as a double chain plasma zymogen (approximately 5 μ/ml) which is activated by thrombin (Figure 1), in the presence of thrombomodulin. Activated protein C (APC) functions as an anticoagulant by proteolytically inactivating factors Va and VIIIa, the non-enzymatic cofactors of the clotting cascade (Clause and Comp, 1983). The anticoagulant properties of APC are enhanced by protein S. Thus protein C and ATIII are complementary inhibitors, since they inhibit different coagulation factors. There are other antithrombotic properties of protein C in addition to its anticoagulant action, such as stimulation of fibrinolysis.

Table 22. Causes of acquired ATIII deficiency.

Consumption coagulopathy	Liver dysfunction	Renal disease	Malignancies	Malnutrition or gastrointestinal loss	Drugs	Other
DIC (shock, sepsis)	Acute hepatic failure	Nephrotic syndrome	Leukaemia (APL)	Vascular reconstruction, diabetes, age	Oestrogens	Vasculitis
Surgery	Cirrhosis	HUS			Heparin	Infection
Pre-eclampsia	Polytransfused thalassaemia			Protein-calorie deprivation	L-asparaginase	Haemodialysis
	Preterm infants			Inflammatory bowel disease		Plasmapheresis
						Post PCC infusion

HUS, Haemolytic uraemic syndrome; APL, acute promyelocytic leukaemia; PCC, prothrombin complex concentrate.
Adapted from Hathaway (1991), with permission.

Congenital protein C deficiency. The physiological importance of protein C as an anticoagulant is highlighted by the fact that recurrent venous thromboembolism is associated with its inherited deficiency (Horellou et al, 1984). The majority of patients have half-normal levels of protein C and the defect is transmitted from parents to children by both sexes, demonstrating heterozygosity for an autosomal gene with variable penetrance (Griffin et al, 1981). Several families have also been described in which newborn infants have severe, often fatal thrombotic symptoms associated with a very low or unmeasurable plasma protein C. Since their parents have half-normal levels, homozygosity for an abnormal gene is postulated (Tuddenham et al, 1989).

The precise prevalence of isolated hereditary protein C deficiency in various populations is controversial. The prevalence of symptomatic heterozygotes has been estimated to be 1 in 15 000 in a general population by Dutch investigators (Romeo et al, 1987). A recent study of blood donors in St Louis indicated a prevalence as high as 1 in 300 amongst asymptomatic individuals (Miletich et al, 1987). Among patients below the age of 45 years with unexplained venous thrombotic disease, 5–8% are found to be deficient in protein C (Spahn-Attenhofer and von Felten, 1985). Irrespective of whether or not this figure truly reflects the general prevalence of protein C deficiency it is definitely more frequent than ATIII deficiency in the clinic populations.

Bertina et al (1984), using both a functional and an immunological assay for protein C, classified protein C deficiency into types I and II (Table 23).

Table 23. Criteria for the laboratory diagnosis of protein C deficiency.

	Type I	Type II
Protein C activity	↓	↓
Protein C antigen	↓	Normal
Ratio of protein C activity to protein C antigen*	Normal	↓
Ratio of protein C to factor II or X	Low	Low
DIC	Absent	Absent
Chronic liver disease	Absent	Absent

* Must be off oral anticoagulants for at least 2 weeks or stabilized on anticoagulants.
Adapted from Bertina et al (1984).

The majority of protein C deficient patients have a parallel reduction of protein C activity and concentration (type I), whereas subjects with type II have normal protein concentration, but this is inactive. The clinical presentation of homozygous and heterozygous deficiencies are usually quite different. Symptoms of heterozygous protein C deficiency are similar to those for patients with inherited ATIII deficiency (Table 24). However, superficial thrombophlebitis and cerebral haemorrhagic infarction, the latter resulting from cerebral vein thrombosis, seem to be rather peculiar to protein C deficiency (Broekmans, 1985). Another clinical manifestation peculiar to heterozygous protein C deficiency is coumarin-induced skin necrosis characterized by progressive thrombosis in the microcirculation of

Table 24. Clinical manifestations in type I protein C deficiency in comparison with protein S deficiency.

	PS deficiency (%)	PC deficiency (%)
DVT	74	63
Recurrent DVT	77	54
Superficial thrombophlebitis	72	48
Pulmonary embolism	38	40
No venous thromboembolism	—	23

Adapted from Broekmans (1985) and Engesser et al (1987).

the skin. Known risk factors for thrombosis found before the first episode of thrombosis in 54% of the patients in a Dutch–French study (Broekmans et al, 1986) include: pregnancy in 20%, surgery in 15%, immobilization in 9%, oral contraceptives in 7%. In the other 46% of patients the first thrombosis occurred in the absence of a known precipitating condition for thrombosis. Age at the first episode of thrombosis was often between 20 and 30 years in the Dutch heterozygous patients. Of these patients, 50% had thrombosis before the age of 30 years and 80% suffered thrombosis before the age of 40 years (Broekmans, 1985).

Homozygous protein C deficiency, by contrast, manifests itself with dramatic symptoms occurring soon after birth, such as extensive thrombosis of visceral veins or purpura fulminans, often leading to early death if patients are not treated (Tuddenham et al, 1989). However, levels of protein C ranging from 5–16% were found in some homozygous adults with less severe symptoms, suggesting that levels of protein C below 5% are the threshold for the occurrence of life-threatening thrombosis during the neonatal period (Sharon et al, 1986).

Acquired protein C deficiency. This has been found in a number of pathological conditions. Reduced protein C levels have been described in chronic liver disease, in DIC (Takahashi et al, 1983) and in patients with acute respiratory distress syndrome associated with viral pneumonia or sepsis (Mannucci and Vigano, 1982).

Treatment of protein C deficiency. The optimal regimen for the management of patients with thrombosis complicating protein C deficiency, or prophylactic therapy for deficient patients, has not been defined. It is recommended that the initiation of oral anticoagulant therapy should be combined with full doses of heparin in order to minimize the risk of thrombosis in the microcirculation. The value of long-term oral anticoagulants is suggested by the observation of Broekmans et al (1983), who reported recurrences of venous thromboembolism in three patients shortly after withdrawal of the coumarin drug, while four patients who continued anticoagulation therapy remained asymptomatic.

Treatment of homozygotes with neonatal purpura fulminans requires special care and the International Committee on Thrombosis and Haemostasis (ICTH) on protein C recommends administration of fresh frozen plasma (10 ml/kg once or twice daily) for 4–6 weeks, followed by oral anticoagulant treatment (Marlar et al, 1989).

Protein S

Protein S (after Seattle, where it was first purified by Di Scipio in 1977) is a vitamin K dependent glycoprotein which serves as a cofactor for the anticoagulant and profibrinolytic activities of activated protein C (Walker, 1980; DeFouw et al, 1986).

Congenital protein S deficiency. Since protein S acts as a cofactor for the anticoagulant action of activated protein C it could have been predicted by analogy with protein C deficiency that deficiency of protein would result in a predisposition to thrombotic disease. Congenital protein S deficiency resulting in recurrent venous thrombotic disease was first observed in 1984 (Comp et al, 1984), and more cases have been reported since. The prevalence of the deficiency in the general population (1 in 15 000–20 000) and its incidence in patients with juvenile and/or recurrent venous thrombosis are similar to those for protein C deficiency (Gladson et al, 1985; Broekmans et al, 1986). Similar also are the pattern of inheritance (autosomal dominant) and the clinical presentation of the heterozygous deficiency (Table 24). Homozygous protein S deficiency with unmeasurable plasma levels is not associated with the dramatic clinical picture typical of homozygous protein C deficiency, indicating that the levels of protein S needed to avoid life-threatening thrombosis are substantially lower than those for protein C. Coumarin-induced skin necrosis is uncommon in protein S deficient patients.

A study by a Dutch group (Bertina, 1985) found that in the majority (67%) of patients with protein S deficiency the first thrombotic episode occurred without an apparent cause. Known risk factors, when present, were surgery in 6%, immobilization in 11% and the use of an oral contraceptive in 16%. None of the protein S deficient patients experienced a thrombotic episode below the age of 15 years; however, half had experienced one or more thrombotic episodes before they were 25 years old. It was found that a decrease in the plasma protein S level below 0.67 units/ml was associated with a significant risk of venous thromboembolism. The same group screened 37 patients with arterial occlusion presenting before the age of 45 years (Allaart et al, 1990), and identified three patients who were heterozygous for protein S deficiency. Family studies of the relationship of arterial thrombosis and protein S deficiency were less convincing than similar studies for venous thrombosis.

As far as treatment is concerned, vitamin K antagonists are effective in the prevention of further thrombotic episodes. The benefits and risks of long-term anticoagulant treatment, however, need to be assessed.

Acquired protein S deficiency. In liver disease, free protein S antigen is moderately reduced and free PS has significantly reduced specific activity. In DIC, reduced protein S activity occurs due to a redistribution of protein S to the inactive bound form. During warfarin anticoagulation, reduction of free protein S antigen and the appearance of forms with abnormal electrophoretic mobility significantly reduce protein S activity (D'Angelo et al, 1988). In patients with thromboembolic disease a transient protein S deficiency occurs due to the redistribution of the complexed form. Caution should therefore be exercised in diagnosing protein S deficiency in such patients by the use of functional assays. A significant reduction in functional protein S levels occurs in pregnancy and the postpartum period due to a reduction in the total protein S antigen (Comp et al, 1986).

Hence, acquired protein S deficiency is likely to be more common than the congenital form but whether this contributes in any way to morbidity is unknown.

Heparin cofactor II and other rare deficiencies associated with a thrombotic state

A second heparin dependent inhibitor of thrombin, distinct from ATIII was first identified in 1974 and has been characterized as heparin cofactor II (HCII) (Briginshaw and Shanberge, 1974). HCII is a minor inhibitor of thrombin formation in vitro, accounting for a small proportion of the total antithrombin activity of plasma. This fact notwithstanding, several members of two recently described kindreds had venous or arterial thrombotic symptoms associated with half-normal levels of HCII. The frequency of thrombosis in the heterozygote is low and prevalence of the deficiency appears to be around 1% of younger patients with a thromboembolic disorder (Andersson et al, 1987). Acquired deficiencies have been reported in patients with liver disease (Abildgaard and Larsen, 1984) and DIC (Bertina et al, 1985).

In view of the finding that 1% of a normal population had reduced levels of HCII, compatible with heterozygous deficiency, the aetiological role of HCII deficiency in thrombosis is considered unproven at present.

Other deficiencies associated with a thrombotic tendency have been summarized in Table 25.

Conclusions on thrombosis

In contrast to the current state of our knowledge concerning the epidemiology of congenital and acquired bleeding disorders, a great deal of effort has been expended in gathering national and international statistics on thrombosis, particularly arterial thrombosis rates. This work has been directed primarily towards searching for clues as to the pathogenesis of these disorders, the most frequent cause of death in affluent societies, such as those of Europe and North America. Leaving aside the ultimate causes of arterial vessel wall disease, it is clear that the final fatal event is usually a blood clot forming over or near a region of atheromatous plaque. Individuals with raised levels of blood coagulation factors, including fibrinogen, factor VII and factor VIII, have a much higher than average risk of suffering a fatal thrombotic event. Communities with comparatively lower levels of these blood coagulation factors, on the basis of limited data, appear to have a much lower risk of arterial or venous thrombosis. The environmental and

Table 25. Rare inherited thrombotic disorders.

Disorders	Inheritance	Prevalence	Clinical manifestations	Tests					References
				Screening tests					
				PT	PTTK	TCT	BT	Specific assay	
Dysfibrinogenaemia	Autosomal dominant	1% of unexplained juvenile venous thrombosis	1. Majority asymptomatic 2. Approx. 10% bleeding tendency 3. Approx. 10% thrombosis, both venous and arterial	↑	N/↑	↑	N	1. Reptilase time 2. Fibrinogen N/↓	Samama et al (1987)
Plasminogen deficiency	Autosomal dominant	2–3% of unexplained juvenile venous thrombosis*	Recurrent DVT and PE when plasminogen level <45% usually only in propositus	N	N	N	N	1. Prolonged euglobulin lysis time 2. ↓ Plasminogen level or activity	Gladson et al (1985)
Deficiency of tissue plasminogen activator (tPA)	Autosomal dominant	As high as 15% in some studies of juvenile thrombosis	Venous thrombosis in the young (11–28 years)	N	N	N	N	Defective release of tPA with occlusion and DDAVP test	Nilsson et al (1985) Scharrer et al (1986)
Alteration in PAI-1† levels	Acquired >> inherited ? mode of inheritance		Venous thrombosis	N	N	N	N	PAI-1 levels may be ↑ or ↓	Kruithof et al (1988)
Factor VII deficiency	Autosomal with incomplete penetrance	Nine cases reported with thrombosis	Heterozygotes asymptomatic. Homozygotes (levels <10%) usually present with bleeding. Rarely venous thromboembolism	↑	N	N	N	Factor VII assay	Goodnough et al (1983) Shifter et al (1984)
Factor XII deficiency	Autosomal recessive	Less than ten cases reported with thrombosis, including the index case	Both arterial and venous thrombosis	N	↑	N	N	Factor XII assay	Goodnough et al (1983)

PT, prothrombin time; PTTK, activated partial thromboplastin time; TCT, thrombin clotting time; BT, bleeding time.
* Incidence in asymptomatic blood donors = 0.4% (Tait et al, 1991).
† PAI-1 = tPA inhibitor-1.

genetic causes of the variation in blood coagulation factors are beginning to be unravelled by patient epidemiological and molecular genetic research. As the profiles of risk in the population become clearer, so rational intervention to lower that risk can be tested. The role of the epidemiologist in the study of degenerative vascular disease is paramount, affecting as it does such huge numbers of people.

Quite recently a small group of patients has been defined, who suffer early onset of venous thromboembolic disease. Very often a positive family history suggests transmission of an autosomal dominant trait. Gratifyingly for theories of haemostatic control, some of these so-called 'thrombophilias' have proved to be associated with deficiency of a specific protein, such as ATIII, protein C or S. Less satisfying is the realization that, in fact, only a minority of patients with venous thromboembolism have any identifiable defect in their blood and that the majority of people with a reduced level of any putative normal anticoagulant have no symptoms of thrombosis at all. Much better epidemiological data relating to haemostatic variables will be needed to resolve the tangled issue of pathogenesis of 'thrombophilia'.

GENERAL CONCLUSION

It is our earnest hope that the overview provided by this necessarily limited survey will stimulate some interest in our colleagues towards gathering more of the data so badly needed to fill in the gaps, if we are to understand the causes of and propose national measures to ameliorate these prevalent disorders. To paraphrase a saying of the late lamented Tony Mitchell ('For venous thromboembolism we know what to do but we don't care enough, for arterial disease we don't know enough')—for haemophilia we know what to do but we can't afford it, for thrombosis we still don't know much about what causes the problem or what to do about it.

REFERENCES

Abildgaard U & Larsen ML (1984) Assay of dermatan sulfate cofactor (heparin cofactor II) activity in human plasma. *Thrombosis Research* **35:** 257–266.

Agarwal MB, Mehta BC & Bhanotra PC (1981) Classical hemophilia (a study of 236 cases from 212 unrelated families). *Journal of the Association of Physicians of India* **29:** 385–389.

Ahmed MA, Al Sohaibani MO, Al Mohaya SA et al (1988) Inherited bleeding disorders in the Eastern Province of Saudi Arabia. *Acta Haematologica* **79:** 202–206.

AHU (Asociación de Hemofilicos Del Uruguay) (1984) In Schnabel M (ed.) *Status and Atlas of Hemophilia Worldwide*, vol. 295, abstract 2. Uruguay: World Federation of Hemophilia.

AIDS Group of the UK (1986) Prevalence of antibody to HTLV III in haemophiliacs in the United Kingdom. *British Medical Journal* **293:** 175–176.

Allaart CF, Aronson DC, Ryys TH et al (1990) Hereditary protein S deficiency in young adults with arterial occlusive disease. *Thrombosis and Haemostasis* **64(2):** 206–210.

Al Mondhiry HA (1977) Inherited bleeding syndrome in Iraq. *Thrombosis and Haemostasis* **37:** 549–555.

Andersson TR, Larsen ML, Abildgaard U et al (1987) Identification of two distinct heparin cofactors in human plasma. *Thrombosis Research* **4:** 463.

Arocha-Pinango CL, de Bosch NB & Nonel AL (1988) Fibrinolytic and procoagulant agents from a saturnidae moth caterpillar. In *Haemostasis and Animal Venoms* Pirkle H & Markland F Jr (eds) pp 223–240. New York: Dekker.

Atichartakarn V, Pathepchotiwong K, Keorochana S et al (1988) Deep vein thrombosis after surgery among Thai. *Archives of Internal Medicine* **148:** 1349–1353.

Awidi AS (1984) Congenital haemorrhagic disorders in Jordan. *Thrombosis and Haemostasis* **51:** 331–333.

Balleisen L, Bailey J, Epping PH et al (1985) Epidemiological study on factor VII, factor VIII and fibrinogen in an industrial population. I. Baseline data on the relation to age, gender, body weight, smoking, alcohol, pill using and menopause. *Thrombosis and Haemostasis* **54:** 475–479.

Becker J, Borgostom S & Saltzman GF (1970) Occurrence and course of thrombosis following prostatectomy. *Acta Radiologica* **10:** 513–533.

Bell WR & Smith Tl (1982) Current status of pulmonary thromboembolic disease: pathophysiology, diagnosis, prevention and treatment. *American Heart Journal* **103:** 289.

Bergquist D (1983) *Postoperative Thromboembolism. Frequency, Etiology, Prophylaxis.* Berlin: Springer-Verlag.

Bergquist D, Arnodottir M, Bergentz SE et al (1985) Juvenile diabetes mellitus: a risk factor for postoperative thromboembolism. *Acta Medica Scandinavica* **217:** 307–308.

Bernstein MJ (1986) Prevention of venous thrombosis and pulmonary embolism. Office of Medical Applications of Research. NIH. *Journal of the American Medical Association* **256:** 744.

Bertina RM (1985) Hereditary protein S deficiency. *Haemostasis* **15:** 241–246.

Bertina RM, Broekmans AW, Krommenhoek-Van ES et al (1984) The use of a functional and immunological assay for plasma protein C in the study of the heterogeneity of congenital protein C deficiency. *Thrombosis and Haemostasis* **51:** 1–5.

Bertina RM, Von Wijngaarden A, Reinalda-Poot J et al (1985) Determination of plasma protein S—the cofactor of activated protein C. *Thrombosis and Haemostasis* **53:** 268–272.

Biggs R & Rizza CR (1984) *Human Blood Coagulation, Haemostasis and Thrombosis* 3rd edn. Oxford: Blackwell Scientific.

Biggs R, Douglas AS, Macfarlane RG et al (1952) Christmas disease. A condition previously mistaken for haemophilia. *British Medical Journal* **2:** 1378.

Bloch M (1984) Sociedad de Hemofilin de El Salvador. In Schnabel M (ed.) *Status and Atlas of Hemophilia Worldwide*, vol. 87. Uruguay: World Federation of Hemophilia.

Brading S (1990) World Federation of Hemophilia. *Bulletin* **27**.

Brandt P (1981) Observations during the treatment of antithrombin III deficient women with heparin concentrate during pregnancy, parturition and abortion. *Thrombosis Research* **22:** 15–24.

Briginshaw GF & Shanberge JN (1974) Identification of two distinct heparin cofactors in human plasma. *Thrombosis Research* **4:** 463.

Broekmans AW (1985) Hereditary protein C deficiency. *Haemostasis* **15:** 233–240.

Broekmans AW, Veltkamp JJ & Bertina RM (1983) Congenital protein C deficiency and venous thromboembolism. *New England Journal of Medicine* **309:** 340–344.

Broekmans AW, Van der Linden IK, Jansen-Koster Y et al (1986) Prevalence of protein C (PC) and protein S (PS) deficiency in patients with thrombotic disease. *Thrombosis Research* **135** (supplement VI)**:** abstract 268.

Bulter HR & Ten Cate JW (1989) Acquired antithrombin III deficiency. Laboratory diagnosis, incidence, clinical implication and treatment with antithrombin III concentrate. *American Journal of Medicine* **87** (supplement 3b): 445–485.

Burkitt DP (1972) Varicose veins, deep vein thrombosis and haemorrhoids: epidemiology and suggested aetiology. *British Medical Journal* **2:** 536.

Centers for Disease Control (1987) Human immunodeficiency virus infection in the United States. *MMWR* **36:** 801–804.

Chintu C (1976) Haemophilia in Zambian children. *Medical Journal of Zambia* **10:** 77.

Choo QL, Kuo G, Weiner AK et al (1989) Isolation of cDNA clone derived from a blood borne non A, non B viral hepatitis genome. *Science* **244:** 359–361.

Chumnijarakij T & Poshyachinda V (1975) Postoperative thrombosis in Thai women. *Lancet* **i:** 1357–1358.

Clause HL & Comp PC (1983) The regulation of haemostasis: the protein C system. *New England Journal of Medicine* **314:** 1298–1304.

Cohn RJ, MacPhail AP, Hartman E et al (1990) Transfusion-related human immunodeficiency virus in patients with haemophilia in Johannesburg. *South African Medical Journal* **78:** 653–656.

Comp PC, Nixon RR, Cooper MR et al (1984) Familial protein S deficiency is associated with recurrent thrombosis. *Journal of Clinical Investigation* **74:** 2082–2088.

Comp PC, Thurnau GR, Welsh J et al (1986) Functional and immunologic protein S levels are decreased during pregnancy. *Blood* **68:** 881–885.

Coon WW (1976) The spectrum of pulmonary embolism. *Archives of Surgery* **111:** 398–402.

Coon WW & Coller FA (1959) Clinicopathologic correlation in thromboembolism. *Surgery, Gynecology and Obstetrics* **109:** 259–269.

Coon WW, Willis PW & Keller JB (1973) Venous thromboembolism and other venous disease in the Tecumseh community health study. *Circulation* **48:** 839–846.

Cosgriff TM, Bishop DT, Hershgold EJ et al (1983) Familial antithrombin III deficiency: its natural history, genetics, diagnosis and treatment. *Medicine* **62:** 209–219.

Cruz-Coke R & Rivera L (1980) Genetic characteristics of haemophilia A in Chile. *Human Heredity* **30:** 161–170.

Cunningham IG & Yong NK (1974) The incidence of postoperative deep vein thrombosis in Malaysia. *British Journal of Surgery* **61:** 482–483.

Dalaker K, Hjermann I & Prydz H (1985) A novel form of factor VII in plasma from men at risk for cardiovascular disease. *British Journal of Haematology* **61:** 315–322.

Dalen JE & Alpert JS (1975) Natural history of pulmonary embolism. *Progress in Cardiovascular Diseases* **17:** 259–270.

D'Angelo A, Vigano-D'Angelo S, Esmon CT et al (1988) Acquired deficiency of protein S. Protein S activity during oral contraception, in liver disease and in disseminated intravascular coagulation. *Journal of Clinical Investigation* **81:** 1445–1454.

Davies MJ & Thomas AC (1985) Plaque fissuring; the cause of acute myocardial infarction, sudden ischaemic death and crescendo angina. *British Heart Journal* **53:** 363–373.

De M, Banerjee D, Chandra S et al (1990) HBV and HIV seropositivity in multitransfused haemophiliacs and thalassaemics in Eastern India. *Indian Journal of Medical Research* **91:** 63–66.

Deblay MF, Vert P, Andre M et al (1982) Transplacental vitamin K prevents haemorrhagic disease of the infant of epileptic mother. *Lancet* **i:** 1247 (letter).

DeFouw NJ, Haverkate F, Bertina RM et al (1986) The cofactor role of protein S in the acceleration of whole blood clot lysis. *Blood* **67:** 1192–1196.

Di Scipio RG, Hermodson MA, Yates SG et al (1977) A comparison of human prothrombin. factor IX (christmas factor) factor X (stuart factor) and protein S. *Biochemistry* **16:** 698–706.

Di Tomaso R (1984) Fundaci6n de la Hemofilia. In Schnabel M (ed.) *Status and Atlas of Hemophilia Worldwide*, vol. 15. Uruguay: World Federation of Hemophilia.

Dupont PA (1975) The problem of deep venous thrombosis and pulmonary embolism in thromboembolism. Nicolaides AN (ed.), pp 1–9. Lancaster: MTP Press.

Dupuy E, Fleming AF & Caen JP (1978) Platelet function, factor VIII, fibrinogen and fibrinolysis in Nigerians and Europeans in relation to atheroma and thrombosis. *Journal of Clinical Pathology* **31:** 1094–1101.

El Shinnawi (1984) The Egyptian haemophilia Society. In Schnabel M (ed.) *Status and Atlas of Hemophilia Worldwide*, vol. 9. Uruguay: World Federation of Hemophilia.

Engesser L, Broekmans AW, Briet E et al (1987) Hereditary protein S deficiency: clinical manifestations. *Annals of Internal Medicine* **106:** 677–682.

Essien EM (1981) Haemorrhagic disorders part 1: Tropical Africa. *Clinics in Haematology* **10:** 917–932.

Evatt BL, Gomperts ED & McDougal JS (1985) Coincidental appearance of LAV/HTLV III antibodies in haemophiliacs and the onset of AIDS epidemic. *New England Journal of Medicine* **312:** 483–486.

Fletcher ML, Trowell JM, Craske J et al (1983) Non A non B hepatitis after transfusion of factor VIII in infrequently treated patients. *British Medical Journal* **287:** 1754–1757.

Forbes CD, Turpie AG, Ferguson JC et al (1969) Effect of gaboon viper (*Bitus gabonica*) venom on blood coagulation, platelets and the fibrinolytic system. *Journal of Clinical Pathology* **22:** 312–316.

Gallus AS & Hirsh J (1976) Prevention of venous thromboembolism. *Seminars in Thrombosis and Hemostasis* **2:** 232–290.

Gamez LA (1984) For a Philippine Hemophilia Society—a committee. In Schnabel M (ed.) *Status and Atlas of Hemophilia Worldwide*, vol. 225. Uruguay: World Federation of Hemophilia.

Gelfand M (1957) *The Sick African: A Clinical Study* 3rd edn. Cape Town: Juta.

Gibbs NM (1957) Venous thrombosis of the lower limbs with particular reference to bed rest. *British Journal of Surgery* **45:** 209–236.

Gladson CL, Griffin JH, Hach Y et al (1985) The incidence of protein C and protein S deficiency in young thrombotic patients. *Blood* **66** (supplement 1)**:** 350a.

Gladson CL, Scharrer I, Hach V et al (1988) The frequency of type I heterozygous protein S and protein C deficiency in 141 unrelated young patients with venous thrombosis. *Thrombosis and Haemostasis* **59:** 18–22.

Goedert JJ, Biggar RJ, Weirs SN et al (1986) Three year incidence of AIDS in five cohorts of HTLV III infected risk group members. *Science* **231:** 992–995.

Good CM & Kimani VN (1980) Urban traditional medicine. A Nairobi case study. *East African Medical Journal* **57:** 301.

Goodnough LT, Saito H & Ratnoff OD (1983) Thrombosis or myocardial infarction in congenital clotting factor abnormalities and chronic thrombocytopenias: a report of 21 patients and a review of 50 previously reported cases. *Medicine* **62:** 248–255.

Gordon-Smith IC, Hickman JA & El Masri SH (1972) The effect of the fibrinolytic inhibitory and epsilon-aminocaproic acid on the incidence of deep vein thrombosis after prostatectomy. *British Journal of Surgery* **59:** 522–524.

Griffin JH, Evatt B, Zimmerman TS et al (1981) Deficiency of protein C in congenital thrombotic disease. *Journal of Clinical Investigation* **68:** 1370–1373.

Griffiths SB & Lipschitz R (1949) Haemophilia in a South African Bantu: report of a case. *South African Medical Journal* **23:** 720–721.

Halal F, Quenneville G, Laurin S et al (1983) Clinical and genetic aspects of antithrombin III deficiency. *American Journal of Genetics* **14:** 737–750.

Hasiba U, Spero JA & Lewis JH (1977) Chronic liver dysfunction in multitransfused hemophiliac. *Transfusion* **17:** 490–494.

Hassan MA, Rahman EA & Rahman IA (1974) Prostatectomy and deep vein thrombosis in Sudanese patients. *British Journal of Surgery* **61:** 650–652.

Hathaway WE (1987) New insights on vitamin K deficiency. *Hematology/Oncology Clinics of North America* **1**(3)**:** 367–370.

Hathaway WE (1991) Clinical aspects of antithrombin III deficiency. *Seminars in Haematology* **28:** 19–23.

Havig O (1977) Deep vein thrombosis and pulmonary embolism: an autopsy study with multiple regression analysis of possible risk factors. *Acta Chirurgica Scandinavica. Supplementum* **478:** 1–120.

Hay CR, Preston FE, Triger DR et al (1985) Progressive liver disease in haemophilia: an understated problem. *Lancet* **i:** 1495–1498.

Hirsh J (1989) Congenital antithrombin III deficiency: incidence and clinical features. *American Journal of Medicine* **87**(supplement 3B)**:** 34–385.

Hirsh J, Genton E & Hull RD (1981) A practical approach to the prophylaxis of venous thrombosis. In Hirsh J, Genton E & Hull R (eds) *Venous Thromboembolism*, vol. 1, pp 108–121. New York: Grune & Stratton.

Hirsh J, Hull R & Raskob G (1986) Epidemiology and pathogenesis of venous thrombosis. *Journal of the American College of Cardiologists* **8:** 104B–113B.

Hirsh J, Piovella F & Pini M (1989) Congenital antithrombin III deficiency. Incidence and clinical features. *American Journal of Medicine* **87** (supplement 3B)**:** 345–385.

Horellou MH, Conard J, Bertina RM et al (1984) Congenital protein C deficiency and thrombotic disease in nine French families. *British Journal of Medicine* **289:** 1285–1287.

Hull R, Hirsh J, Sackett DL et al (1981) Replacement of venography in suspected venous thrombosis by impedance plethysmography and I^{125} fibrinogen scanning: a less invasive approach. *Annals of Internal Medicine* **94:** 12–15.

Hull R, Hirsh J, Carter CJ et al (1983) Pulmonary angiography ventilation lung scanning and venography for clinically suspected pulmonary embolism with abnormal perfusion scans. *Annals of Internal Medicine* **98:** 891–899.

Ikkala E, Helske T, Myllyla G et al (1982) Changes in life expectancy of patients with severe haemophilia A in Finland in 1930–1979. *British Journal of Haematology* **52:** 7–12.

Isarangkura P (1984) Hemophilia Society of Thailand. In Schnabel M (ed.) *Status and Atlas of Hemophilia Worldwide*, vol. 267. Uruguay: World Federation of Hemophilia.

Joffe SN (1974) Racial incidence of postoperative deep vein thrombosis in South Africa. *British Journal of Surgery* **61:** 982–983.

Johnson RE, Lawrence DN, Evatt BL et al (1985) Acquired immunodeficiency syndrome among patients attending hemophilia treatment centers and mortality experience of hemophilia in the United States. *American Journal of Epidemiology* **121:** 797–810.

Jones TK, Barnes RW & Greenfield LJ (1986) Greenfield vena caval filter: rationale and current indications. *Annals of Thoracic Surgery* **42** (supplement 6): 548.

Kannel WB, Castelli WP & Meeks SL (1985) Fibrinogen and cardiovascular disease. *Abstract of Paper for 34th Annual Scientific Session of the American College of Cardiology*, Anaheim, California.

Karabus CD (1984) South African Haemophilia Foundation. In Schnabel M (ed.) *Status and Atlas of Hemophilia Worldwide*, vol. 241. Uruguay: World Federation of Hemophilia.

Kasili EG (1983) An update on haemophilia and haemophiloid disorders in anglophone African countries. *East African Medical Journal* **50:** 551–558.

Kasper CK & Kipnis SA (1972) Hepatitis and clotting factor concentrates. *Journal of the American Medical Association* **221:** 510.

Khanduri U, Pulimood R, Sudarsanam A et al (1981) Glanzmann's thrombasthenia: a review and report of 42 cases from South India. *Thrombosis and Haemostasis* **46:** 717–721.

Kim ES, Suzuki M, Lie TT et al (1976) Clinically unsuspected disseminated intravascular coagulation (DIC). *American Journal of Clinical Pathology* **66:** 31–39.

Kim KY, Yang CH, Cho MJ et al (1988) Comprehensive clinical and statistical analysis of hemophilia in Korea. *Journal of Korean Medical Science* **3:** 107–115.

Kitonyi GW & Kasili EG (1981) Hereditary bleeding disorder in Kenya. *East African Medical Journal* **58:** 738–747.

Kruithof EK, Gudinchet A & Bachmann F (1988) Plasminogen activator inhibitor 1 and plasminogen activator inhibitor 2 in various disease states. *Thrombosis and Haemostasis* **59:** 7.

Lander JJ, Alter HJ & Purcell RH (1975) Frequency of antibody to hepatitis-associated antigen as measured by a new radioimmunoassay technique. *Journal of Immunology* **106:** 1166–1171.

Lane PA & Hathaway WE (1985) Vitamin K in infancy. *Journal of Pediatrics* **106(3):** 351–359.

Lane PA, Hathaway WE, Githers JH et al (1983) Fatal intracranial hemorrhage in a normal infant secondary to vitamin K deficiency. *Pediatrics* **72:** 562.

Larsson SA (1985) Life expectancy of Swedish haemophiliacs 1831–1980. *British Journal of Haematology* **59:** 593–602.

Levine PH, McVerry BA, Segelman AE et al (1976) Comprehensive health care clinics for hemophiliacs. *Archives of Internal Medicine* **136:** 792–794.

Lofgren EP, Coates HL & O'Brien PE (1976) Clinically suspected pulmonary embolism after vein stripping. *Mayo Clinic Proceedings* **57:** 77.

Lopez G (1984) Haemophilia Society of Malaysia. In Schnabel M (ed.) *Status and Atlas of Hemophilia Worldwide*, vol. 185. Uruguay: World Federation of Hemophilia.

Lothe F (1968) Haemophilia in Uganda: *Transactions of the Royal Society of Tropical Medicine and Hygiene* **62:** 359.

Machin SJ, McVerry BA, Chemsong-Popor R et al (1985) Sero conversion for HTLV III since 1980 in British haemophiliacs. *Lancet* **i:** 336.

MacKay N, Ferguson JC & McNichol GP (1970) Effects of the venom of the rhinoceros horned viper (*Bitus nasicornis*) on blood coagulation, platelet aggregation and fibrinolysis. *Journal of Clinical Pathology* **23:** 789–796.

McNinds AW, Upton C, Samuels M et al (1985) Plasma concentration after oral and intramuscular vitamin K in neonates. *Archives Diseases in Childhood* **60:** 814.

Madhok R & Forbes CD (1990) HIV-1 infections in haemophilia. *Baillière's Clinical Haematology* **3:** 79–101.

Mahasandana S, Rungruxsirivorn Y & Chantarangkul V (1980) Clinical manifestations of bleeding following Russell's viper and green pit viper bites in adults. *Southeast Asian Journal of Tropical Medicine and Hygiene* **11:** 285–293.

Mannucci PM & Vigano S (1982) Deficiency of protein C an inhibitor of blood coagulation. *Lancet* **ii:** 463–466.

Mannucci PM & Tripodi A (1988) Inherited factors in thrombosis. *Blood Reviews* **2:** 27–35.

Mannucci PM, Runi MG, Gringeri A et al (1989) High prevalence of antibody to hepatitis C in multitransfused haemophiliacs with normal aminotransferase. *Blood* **74:** 100a (abstract).

Markland FS (1976) Crotalase. *Methods in Enzymology* **45**(part B): 223–236.

Marlar RA, Montgomery RR & Broekmans AW (1989) Report on the diagnosis and treatment of homozygous protein C deficiency. Report of the Working Party on Homozygous Protein C Deficiency of the ICTH-Subcommittee on Protein C and Protein S. *Thrombosis and Haemostasis* **61:** 529–531.

Matsuda M & Aoki N (1983) Statistics on underlying and causative diseases in DIC in Japan: A cooperative study. *Bibliotheca Haematologica* **43:** 15–22.

Meade TW, North WR, Chakrabarti R et al (1980) Haemostatic function and cardiovascular death: early results of a prospective study. *Lancet* **i:** 1050–1054.

Meade TW, Stirling Y, Thompson SG et al (1986) An international and inter-regional comparison of haemostatic variables in the study of ischaemic heart disease. *International Journal of Epidemiology* **15:** 331–336.

Mibashan R, Nossel HL & Moodie A (1960) Blood coagulation and fibrinolysis in relation to coronary heart disease; a comparative study of normal white men, white men with overt coronary heart disease and normal Bantu men. *British Medical Journal* **1:** 219.

Miletich J, Sherman L & Broze G (1987) Absence of thrombosis in subjects with heterozygous protein C deficiency. *New England Journal of Medicine* **317:** 991–996.

Mohsen B-A M (1984) Association Tunisienne des Hémophiles. In Schnabel M (ed.) *Status and Atlas of Hemophilia Worldwide*, vol. 273. Uruguay: World Federation of Hemophilia.

Morales CC (1984) Asociación Peruana de la Hemofilia. In Schnabel M (ed.) *Status and Atlas of Hemophilia Worldwide*, vol. 221. Uruguay: World Federation of Hemophilia.

Morrell MT & Dunnill MS (1968) The post mortem incidence of pulmonary embolism in a hospital population. *British Journal of Surgery* **55:** 347–352.

Motohara K, Matsukura M, Matsuda I et al (1984) Severe vitamin K deficiency in breast fed infants. *Journal of Pediatrics* **105:** 943.

Mukiibi JM, Paul B, Field SP et al (1990) Haemophilia in Zimbabwe. *Tropical and Geographical Medicine* **42:** 32–36.

Myhre HO, Storen EJ & Ongre A (1974) The incidence of deep venous thrombosis in patients with leg oedema after arterial reconstruction. *Scandinavian Journal of Thoracic and Cardiovascular Surgery* **8:** 73.

Myint-Lwin, Warrell DA Phillips RE et al (1985) Bites by Russell's viper (*Vipera russelli siamensis*) in Burma: haemostatic, vascular and response to treatment. *Lancet* **ii:** 1260–1264.

Nagy I & Losonczy H (1979) Three types of hereditary antithrombin III deficiency. *Thrombosis and Haemostasis* **42:** 187.

Nillius AS & Nylander G (1979) Deep vein thrombosis after total hip replacement: a clinical and phlebographic study. *British Journal of Surgery* **66:** 324–326.

Nilsson IM, Ljungner H & Tengborn L (1985) Two different mechanisms in patients with venous thrombosis and defective fibrinolysis low concentration of plasminogen activator or increased concentration of plasminogen activator inhibitor. *British Medical Journal* **290:** 1453–1455.

O'Brien SJ (1991) Ghetto legacy. *Current Biology* **1:** 209–211.

Odegaard OR & Abildgaard U (1978) Antithrombin III: critical review of assay methods. Significance of variations in health and disease. *Haemostasis* **7:** 127–134.

Omer A & Zadia M (1973) Haemophilia and allied disorders in the Sudan. *British Journal of Haematology* **25:** 69.

Orell SR (1962) The fate and late effects of non-fatal pulmonary emboli. *Acta Medica Scandinavica* **172:** 473–484.

Otto JE (1803) An account of an hemorrhagic disposition existing in certain families. *New York: The Medical Repository* **VI:**1:1.

Parrish HM (1980) *Poisonous Snake Bites in the United States*. New York: Vantage Press.

Patek AJ Jr & Taylor FH (1937) Hemophilia II, some properties of a substance obtained from normal human plasma effective in accelerating the coagulation of hemophilic blood. *Journal of Clinical Investigation* **16:** 113.

Prado RC (1984) Sociedad Chilena de la Hemofilia. In Schnabel M (ed.) *Status and Atlas of Hemophilia Worldwide*, vol. 55. Uruguay: World Federation of Hemophilia.

Preston PE, Triger DR, Underwood JC et al (1978) Percutaneous liver biopsy and chronic liver disease in haemophiliacs. *Lancet* **ii:** 592–594.

Pugh RN & Theakston RD (1980) Incidence and mortality of snake bite in savanna Nigeria. *Lancet* **ii:** 1181–1183.

Pugh RN & Theakston RD (1987) A clinical study of viper bite poisoning. *Annals of Tropical Medicine and Parasitology* **81:** 135–149.

Ramgren O (1962) Haemophilia in Sweden, part 2. *Acta Medica Scandinavica. Supplement* **937s:** 37–60.

Rizza CR & Spooner RJ (1983) Treatment of haemophilia and related disorders in Britain and Northern Ireland during 1976–1980: report on behalf of the directors of haemophilia centres in the United Kingdom. *British Medical Journal* **286:** 929–933.

Rizza CR & Spooner RJ (1992) *UK haemophilia centre directors' national register. Annual returns from 1984–1989.*

Roberts GH (1963) Venous thrombosis in hospital patients, a postmortem study. *Scottish Medical Journal* **8:** 11–15.

Roisenberg I & Morton NE (1971) Genetic aspects of hemophilia A and B in Rio Grande do Sul Brazil. *Human Heredity* **21:** 97–107.

Rojas M (1984) Asociación Costarricense de Hemofilia. In Schnabel M (ed.) *Status and Atlas of Hemophilia Worldwide*, vol. 63. Uruguay: World Federation of Hemophilia.

Romeo G, Hassan HJ, Staempfli S et al (1987) Hereditary thrombophilia: identification of nonsense and missense mutation in the protein C gene. *Proceedings of the National Academy of Sciences of the USA* **84:** 2829–2832.

Rosenberg RD (1975) Action and interaction of antithrombin and heparin. *New England Journal of Medicine* **292:** 146–151.

Rosendaal RF, Varekamp I, Smit C et al (1989) Mortality and causes of death in Dutch haemophiliacs. *British Journal of Haematology* **71:** 71–76.

Rosendaal FR, Heijboer H, Briet E et al (1991) Mortality in hereditary antithrombin III deficiency: 1830 to 1989. *Lancet* **337:** 260–261.

Rosner F (1969) Hemophilia in the Talmud and Rabbinic writings. *Annals of Internal Medicine* **70:** 833.

Rubinstein I, Murray D & Hoffsten V (1988) Fatal pulmonary emboli in hospitalized patients. *Archives of Internal Medicine* **145:** 1425–1426.

Ruckley W (1975) Venous thromboembolic disease. *Journal of the Royal College of Surgeons of Edinburgh* **20:** 10.

Rueda E (1984) Nicaraguan Hemophilia Society. In Schnabel M (ed.) *Status and Atlas of Hemophilia Worldwide*, vol. 207. Uruguay: World Federation of Hemophilia.

Salgado DH (1984) Asociación Hondureña de Hemophilia. In Schnabel M (ed.) *Status and Atlas of Hemophilia Worldwide*, vol. 123. Uruguay: World Federation of Hemophilia.

Samama M, Conard J, Horellou MH et al (1987) Abnormalities of fibrinogen and fibrinolysis in familial thrombosis. *Thrombosis and Haemostasis* **58:** 249.

Sas G (1988) Classification of antithrombin III deficiencies: has a new tower of Babel been built? *Thrombosis and Haemostasis* **60:** 530–531.

Scarabin PY, Bara L, Samama M et al (1985) Further evidence that activated factor VII is related to plasma lipids. *British Journal of Haematology* **61:** 186–187.

Scharrer IM, Wohl RC, Hach V et al (1986) Investigation of a congenital abnormal plasminogen, Frankfurt I and its relationship to thrombosis. *Thrombosis and Haemostasis* **55:** 396–401.

Schimpf K (1986) Liver disease in haemophilia. *Lancet* **i:** 323.

Schulman S & Wiechel B (1984) Hepatitis epidemiology and liver function in hemophiliacs in Sweden. *Acta Medica Scandinavica* **215:** 249–256.

Sevitt S & Gallagher NG (1961) Venous thrombosis and pulmonary embolism: a clinico-pathologic study in injured and burned patients. *British Journal of Surgery* **48:** 475–482.

Shaper AG, Jones KW, Kyobe J et al (1966) Fibrinolysis in relation to body fatness, serum lipids and coronary heart disease in African and Asian men in Uganda. *Journal of Atherosclerosis Research* **6:** 313–327.

Sharon C, Tirindelli MC, Mannucci PM et al (1986) Homozygous protein C deficiency with moderately severe clinical symptoms. *Thrombosis Research* **41:** 483–488.

Shifter T, Machtey I & Creter D (1984) Thromboembolism in congenital factor VII deficiency. *Acta Haematologica* **71:** 60–62.
Siegal T, Seligsohn U, Aghai E et al (1978) Clinical and laboratory aspects of disseminated intravascular coagulation (DIC): a study of 118 cases. *Thrombosis and Haemostasis* **39:** 122–134.
Simmons AV, Sheppard MA & Cox AF (1973) Deep venous thrombosis after myocardial infarction. Predisposing factors. *British Heart Journal* **35:** 623.
Sjoln KE (1960) *Haemophilic Disease in Denmark*. Oxford: Blackwell Scientific.
Spahn-Attenhofer CH & von Felten A (1985) Coagulation studies in 100 consecutive patients with severe thromboembolic disease to identify an increased risk of rethrombosis. *Thrombosis and Haemostasis* **54:** 234 (abstract).
Spero J, Lewis J & Hasiba U (1980) Disseminated intravascular coagulation. Finding in 346 patients. *Thrombosis and Haemostasis* **43:** 28.
Stenflo J (1976) A new vitamin K-dependent protein: purification from bovine plasma and preliminary characterisations. *Journal of Biological Chemistry* **251:** 355–363.
Stone MC & Thorpe JM (1985) Plasma fibrinogen: a major coronary risk factor. *Journal of the Royal College of General Practitioners* **35:** 565–569.
Sutherland JM, Glueck HI & Gleser G (1967) Haemorrhagic disease of the newborn: Breast feeding as a necessary factor in the pathogenesis. *American Journal of Diseases of Children* **113:** 524.
Sutherland SK (1983) *Australian Animal Toxins. The Creatures, Their Toxins and Care of the Poisoned Patient*. Melbourne: Oxford University Press.
Syafei (1984) Indonesian hemophilia society. In Schnabel M (ed.) *Status and Atlas of Hemophilia Worldwide*, vol. 145. Uruguay: World Federation of Hemophilia.
Tait RS, Walker ID, Islam SI et al (1991) Plasminogen levels and putative prevalence of deficiency in 4,500 blood donors. *British Journal of Haematology* **77**(supplement 1)**:** 10 (abstract).
Takahashi H, Takakuwa E, Yoshino N et al (1983) Protein C levels in disseminated intravascular coagulation and thrombotic thrombocytopenic purpura: its correlation with other coagulation parameters. *Thrombosis and Haemostasis* **54:** 445–449.
Trowell HC (1941) A case of haemophilia in a Muganda. *East African Medical Journal* **17:** 464.
Tso SC, Wong V, Chan V et al (1980) Deep vein thrombosis and changes in coagulation and fibrinolysis after gynaecological operations in Chinese: the effect of oral contraceptives and malignant disease. *British Journal of Haematology* **46:** 603–612.
Tucker J, Ludlam CA, Craig A et al (1985) HTLV III infections associated with glandular fever like illness in haemophiliacs. *Lancet* **i:** 585.
Tuddenham EG, Takase T, Thomas AE et al (1989) Homozygous protein C deficiency with delayed onset of symptoms at 7 to 10 months. *Thrombosis Research* **53:** 475–484.
Uemura K & Pisa Z (1985) Recent trends in cardiovascular disease mortality in 27 industrialised countries. *World Health Statistics Quarterly* **138:** 142–162.
Uhland H & Goldberg (1964) Pulmonary embolism: a commonly missed clinical entity. *Diseases of the Chest* **45:** 533–536.
Vehar GA, Keyt B, Eaton D et al (1984) Structure of human factor VIII. *Nature* **312:** 337–342.
Verity CM, Carswell F & Scott GL (1983) Vitamin K deficiency causing infantile intracranial haemorrhage after the neonatal period. *Lancet* **i:** 1439 (letter).
Walker FJ (1980) Regulation of activated protein C by a new protein. *Journal of Biological Chemistry* **255:** 5521–5524.
Walsh JJ, Bonnar J & Wright FW (1974) A study of pulmonary embolism and deep vein thrombosis after major gynaecological surgery using labelled fibrinogen: phlebography and lung scanning. *Journal of Obstetrics and Gynaecology of the British Commonwealth* **81:** 311–316.
Warlow C, Ogston D & Douglas AS (1972) Venous thrombosis following strokes. *Lancet* **i:** 1305.
Warrell DA (1987) Venoms and toxins of animal and plants. In Weatherall DJ, Ledingham JG & Warrell DA (eds) *Oxford Textbook of Medicine* 2nd edn, vol. 6, pp 66–67. Oxford: Oxford University Press.
Warrell DA (1989) Snake venoms in science and clinical medicine. 1. Russell's viper: biology, venom and treatment of bites. *Transactions of the Royal Society of Tropical Medicine and Hygiene* **83:** 732–740.

Warrell DA (1991) Snakes. In Strickland GT (ed.) *Hunter's Tropical Medicine* 7th edn, pp 877–888. Philadelphia: WB Saunders.

Warrell DA, Davidson NMcD, Omerod LD et al (1974) Bites by the saw-scaled or carpet viper (*Echis carinatus*): trial of two specific antivenoms. *British Medical Journal* **iv:** 437–440.

Warrell DA, Omerod LD & Davidson NMcD (1975) Bites by puff-adder (*Bitus arietans*) in Nigeria, and value of antivenom. *British Medical Journal* **iv:** 697–700.

Warrell DA Omerod LD & Davidson NMcD et al (1976) Necrosis, haemorrhage and complement depletion following bites by the spitting cobra (*Naja nigricollis*). *Quarterly Journal of Medicine* **45:** 1–22.

Warrell DA, Davidson NMcD, Greenwood BM et al (1977) Poisoning by bites of the saw-scaled or carpet viper (*Echis carinatus*) in Nigeria. *Quarterly Journal of Medicine* **46:** 33–62.

Warrell DA, Warrell MJ, Edgar W et al (1980) Comparison of Pasteur and Behringwerke antivenoms in envenoming by the carpet viper (*Echis carinatus*). *British Medical Journal* **i:** 607–609.

Wilhelmsen L, Svardsudd K, Korsan Bengtson K et al (1984) Fibrinogen as a risk for stroke and myocardial infarction. *New England Journal of Medicine* **311:** 501–555.

Williams IC (1976) Bleeding disorder in three male siblings. *East African Medical Journal* **53:** 651.

Winter JH, Fenech A, Ridley W et al (1982) Familial antithrombin III deficiency. *Quarterly Journal of Medicine* **51:** 373–395.

Wintrobe MM, Lee GR, Boggs DR et al (1974) *Clinical Haematology* 7th edn, p 1158. Philadelphia: Lea & Febiger.

World Health Organization (1972) Inherited blood clotting disorders. Report of a WHO Scientific Group. *World Health Organization Technical Report Series* **504:** 1–15.

World Health Organization (1983) Multifactoral trial in the prevention of coronary heart disease, incidence and mortality results. *European Heart Journal* **4:** 141–147.

Youssef AH & Bashir A (1984) Kuwait Hemophila Society. In Schnabel M (ed.) *Status and Atlas of Hemophilia Worldwide*, vol. 179. Uruguay: World Federation of Hemophilia.

7

Platelets and platelet disorders in Africa

E. M. ESSIEN

The blood platelet is functionally a very dynamic cell. Although its role in haemostasis has received the greatest attention, it is becoming increasingly clear that the circulating platelet plays significant roles in many other aspects of vertebrate biology. These include its involvement in the regulation of growth, angiogenesis and determination of vasomotor tone, among other functions. This chapter will concentrate, however, on the haemostatic aspects of the circulating platelet in man in the tropical African environment and the response to some prevalent infections. For its role in other diseases, for example cardiovascular diseases, diabetes mellitus, malignancy and different haematological disorders, the reader is referred to several existing excellent texts and reviews.

Platelets are derived from mature megakaryocytes by a process of cytoplasmic fragmentation following formation and subsequent widening of the demarcation membrane system (DMS) during megakaryocyte maturation. The platelets are subsequently shed by a mechanism finally involving constriction of the DMS stalk attached to the megakaryocyte cytoplasm, and up to 4000 platelets may be released from each mature megakaryocyte (Federeko and Lichtman, 1982). The circulating blood platelet has a normal lifespan of 8–10 days, including its period of temporary rest in the splenic platelet pool. The normal spleen may accommodate up to about one-third of the total viable platelets in the pool (Shulman and Jordan, 1982); the size of the pool increases in splenomegaly and may give rise to thrombocytopenia, in some instances without concomitant hypersplenism.

Platelet structure

The circulating platelet is a small, disc-shaped non-nucleated blood cell, whose volume varies, depending on the method of its isolation, in the range $6 \pm 0.2\,\mu m^3$ (Karpatkin, 1969). Viable platelets usually exist in either a non-activated (Figure 1) or an activated state (Figures 2 and 3).

In the non-activated state, the platelet surface appears smooth, although closer study reveals tiny indentations which are openings from the interior of the platelet to its surface. These openings, unique to the platelet among blood cells, are connected to the open canalicular system (OCS) within the cell (Hovic, 1968; White, 1971).

Baillière's Clinical Haematology—
Vol. 5, No. 2, April 1992
ISBN 0–7020–1627–6

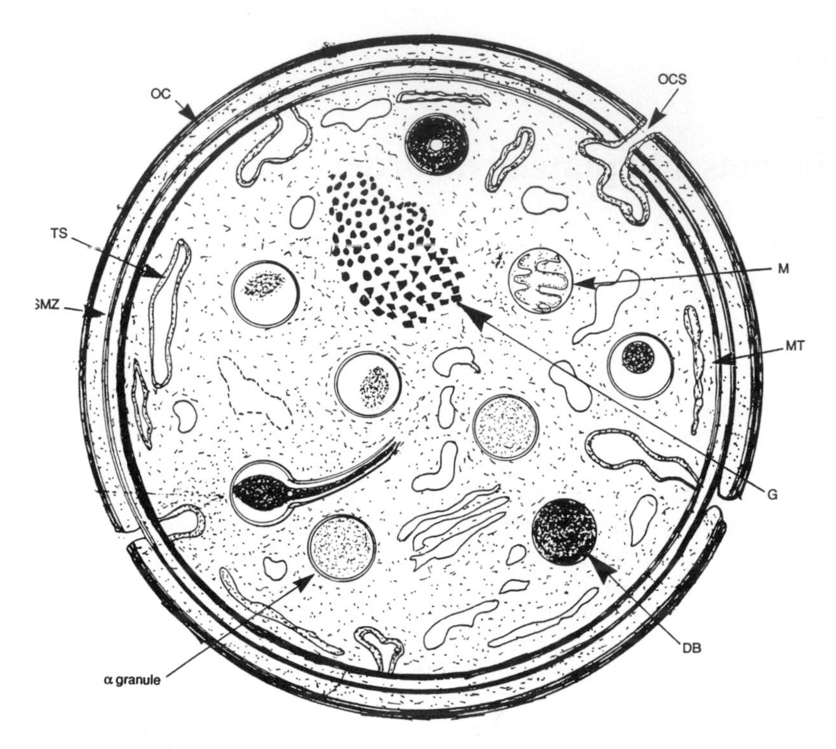

Figure 1. Diagram of a resting platelet showing internal structures. DB, dense body; G, glycogen granules; M, mitochondria; MT, circumferential band of microtubules; OC, outer coat; OCS, open surface canalicular connecting system; SMZ, submembrane zone; TS, tubular system. (Modified from White and Gerrard, 1982).

Peripheral zone of the platelet

A cross-sectional view of the resting platelet (see Figure 1) at the equator shows from the outside inwards: (1) a wall consisting of an exterior coat (glycocalyx) of about 2×10^{-7}µm thick; (2) a typical unit membrane; and (3) an immediate submembrane zone made up of 8–24 filaments, each of which is composed of short actin fibres cross-linked by actin-binding protein (White, 1969; Gerrard and White, 1976). The filaments, although associated with the membrane glycoproteins (Gp) or integrins, such as GpIb-IX complex and GpIa-IIa receptors, are responsible for keeping other structures away from direct contact with the internal platelet cell wall. The glycocalyx, the unit membrane and the sub-membrane filaments, together with the immediate layer of blood plasma surrounding each platelet (sometimes called the 'atmosphere plasmatique' (Roskam, 1923)), constitute the platelet peripheral zone.

The plasma environment surrounding each circulating platelet contains other blood cells with which platelets may interact, and several chemical substances such as fibronectin, fibrinogen, other blood coagulation factors

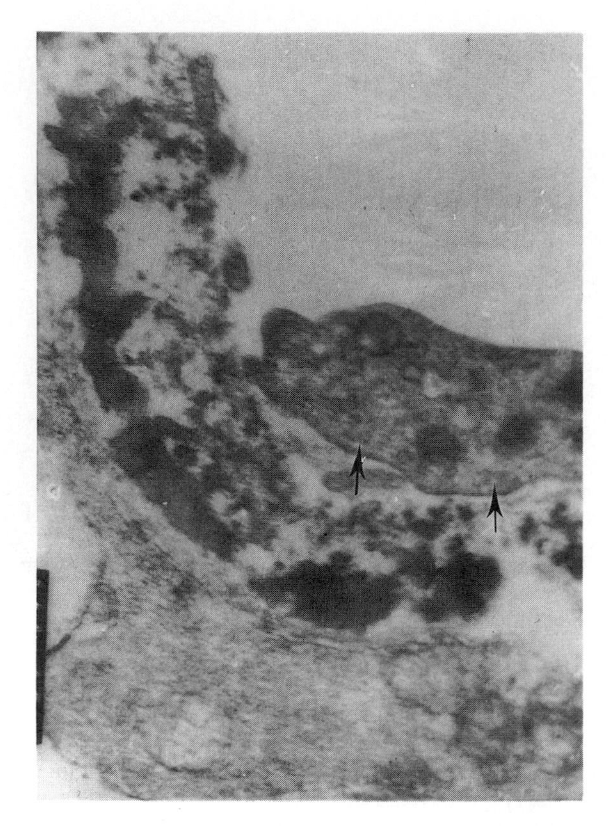

Figure 2. Transmission electron micrograph showing part of a platelet lying on and adapting to the shape of the inner surface of a damaged rabbit thoracic aorta. Arrows show points of contact between the platelet and the damaged surface. (Magnification × 8250.)

as well as other plasma proteins. These frequently exert significant immediate or potential effects on the platelet. If activated platelets are present in the vicinity, their secreted proteins and other chemical substances (see below) will also be present in this environment. Therefore, the plasma region immediately surrounding the glycocalyx is usually regarded as an extension of the platelet external wall.

Internal structure

Resting platelets. Deep to the platelet wall, as defined above, is a ring of 8–24 circumferential microtubules, each $2.5 \times 10^{-7}\mu m$ in diameter and made up of 12–15 sub-filaments, the latter composed of tubulin protein (see Figure 1) (White and Gerrard, 1982). These microtubules are cross-linked in a net-work pattern by actin-binding protein (ABP), and form part of the platelet cytoskeleton. Another major component of the cytoskeleton is actin, which forms 15–20% of the platelet total protein. Other important components

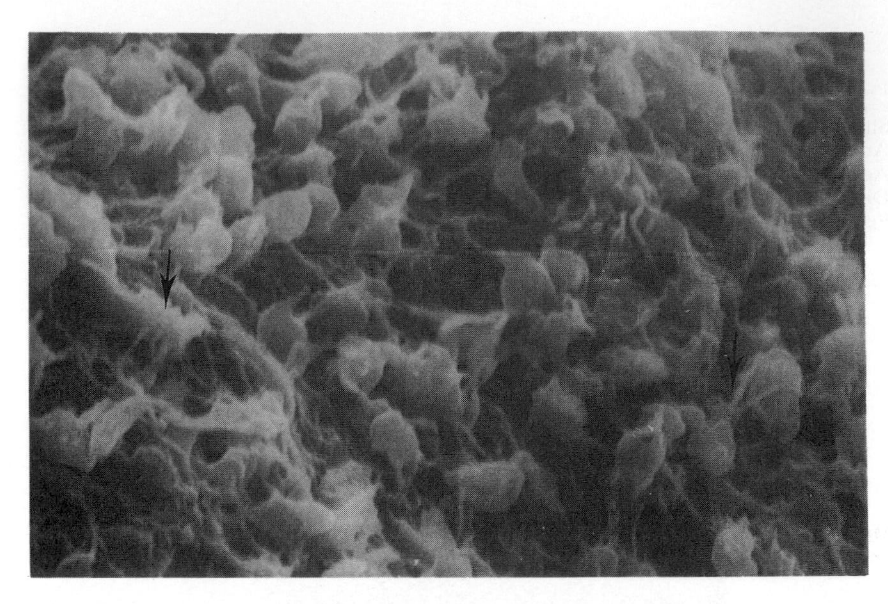

Figure 3. Electron micrograph of platelets on the inner surface of a damaged rabbit thoracic aorta. Note the shape change manifested by the platelets, and the pseudopodia with which the platelets adhere to the surface and to each other. (Magnification ×24 000; reduced to 75% on reproduction.)

include: α-actinin, tropomyosin, profilin, gelsolin, talin, vinculin and spectrin (Fox, 1987).

Dispersed within the cytoplasm of each platelet are a number of structures and substances which are vital to platelet function and survival (see Figure 1). These include α-granules, dense bodies, mitochondria, glycogen storage granules and the network of OCS, whose lining and structure are similar to, and continuous with the components of the platelet cell wall. There is, in addition, the dense tubular system (DTS), a distinct system of channels derived from the rough endoplasmic reticulum of the megakaryocyte. The DTS is closely associated with the circumferential microtubules. However, both communication systems, the OCS and DTS, though distinct are in close apposition to each other and are involved in ionic (especially Ca^{2+}) transfer to the exterior.

Activated platelets. When platelets are activated, either on interaction with agonists (including thrombin, adenosine diphosphate (ADP), adrenaline, ionophore A 23187, hirudin, collagen, serotonin or arachidonate and its products such as thromboxane A_2 (TXA_2)), or on contact with damaged vascular endothelium or sub-endothelium, there follows a sequence of both morphological and biochemical changes. These usually manifest as shape change, adhesion and aggregation (see Figure 2). A result of the activation is that the platelets secrete their contents into the surrounding medium (Tables 1 and 2).

Table 1. Summary of features of resting platelet and changes on its activation.

Feature	Resting platelet	Activated platelet
Shape	Discoid	Discoid shape lost
Actin polymerization	?	Burst
Actin filament content (%)	40–50	100
Distribution	Loose network	+++
Periphery	Few	?
Centre	Loose network	Rings around centralized granules
Profilactin	Associated	Dissociated
Filopodia	Nil	++ in bundles
Actin in filopodia	Scanty	++
Myosin distribution	Uniform	Concentrated around centralized granules
Myosin phosphorylation (%)	10	100
Tropomyosin distribution	Diffuse	Concentrated in filopodia
Actin-binding protein	Diffuse	Concentrated in filopodia
α-Actinin	Diffuse	Concentrated in filopodia
Protein 4.1	?	Concentrated in submembranous arrays in filopodia
Membrane skeleton	Intact	Dispersed

Table 2. Some important secretory proteins from activated platelets.

Thrombogenic promoting proteins
Adenosine diphosphate (ADP)
Adenosine triphosphate (ATP)
Thromboxane A_2 (TXA_2)
von Willebrand's factor (vWF)
Platelet factor 4 (PF_4)
Thrombospondin
Platelet activating factor (PAF)
Elastase
Endoglycosidase
Proteins which increase vasomotor tone
Platelet derived growth factor (PDGF)*
Serotonin (5-HT)
Vasopressin
PAF*
TXA_2 (in human coronary arteries)
Growth modulators
PDGF†
Transforming growth factor β (TGF-β)†

Some substances are cell adherence promoters, e.g. PDGF, PAF, TGF-β, and are also produced by vascular endothelial cells.
* Also promote cell adherence.
† Also produced by vascular endothelial cells.

Platelet shape change and centralization of internal structures and contents are the major morphological features characteristic of an activated platelet. The details and mechanisms of these changes have been extensively reviewed (Hovic, 1968; Mustard and Packham, 1970; White and Gerrard, 1982; Lasslo, 1984) (see Table 1).

The normal platelet count in different populations

The normal platelet count in adult European populations has been established at $150–400 \times 10^9$/l (Dacie and Lewis, 1975). However, the lower limit of the normal platelet count in adult African populations has been established at 100×10^9/l, with a normal range of $100–300 \times 10^9$/l (Essien et al, 1973; Dupuy et al, 1978; Gill et al, 1979; Ukaejiofor et al, 1979; Mukiibi et al, 1981; Onwukeme and Uguru, 1990; O. Akinyanju, personal communication; A. A. Lawal et al, personal communication). In Nigerian neonates, a normal platelet count of $59–490 \times 10^9$/l was obtained (Effiong et al, 1976) and was reported as being comparable to the values obtained in neonates from other populations (Aballi et al, 1968).

The reasons for these relatively lower normal figures in adults are not clear. A suggestion was that the finding might be related to the factors of poor nutrition and high prevalence of infection due to the socioeconomic circumstances of the subjects studied (Essien et al, 1973): this was disputed (O. Akinyanju, personal communication). Another suggestion was that the high prevalence of relative 'splenomegaly' due to recurrent malaria, with a resultant enlarged splenic platelet pool, might account for the observation. These suggestions, amongst others, have not, to my knowledge, been resolved.

Platelet function

The circulating platelet plays a critical role in haemostasis and significant roles in tissue repair. It also contributes to body defence. The critical role of platelets in providing balanced haemostasis becomes evident when purpura manifests in thrombocytopenic states, irrespective of their causes. Thrombocytopenia is defined as a state of reduced circulating platelet count in blood below the normal level (see above). It may be mild, moderate or severe; typical purpuric bleeding, with or without ecchymosis, very frequently occurs in severe thrombocytopenia, and may occur, usually without ecchymosis, in moderate thrombocytopenia.

The mechanism of bleeding in thrombocytopenia is fairly well known. It has been suggested that breaks in the vascular endothelial lining frequently occur in vivo, but blood seepage through such damaged sites is readily prevented by prompt platelet responses, which include platelet shape change, adhesion, secretion, aggregation and the formation of an unstable platelet plug (Packham and Mustard, 1984), subsequently stabilized by fibrin strands formed around the plug through platelet coagulant activity (Walsh, 1974). These changes are initiated by platelet contact with the damaged site where, as a result of the damage, the normal electrostatic forces between the platelet and the vascular endothelium are disrupted, and direct contact between the circulating platelet and the damaged site occur. As a result of such contact, the platelet is activated, changes its shape to assume that of the damaged site and adheres through exposed receptors (see Table 3 and Figure 2). Within 30 seconds of such contact and activation, there is rapid centralization of platelet contents and secretion of some of them into the platelet environment (see Table 2). Other platelets within the vicinity react in a similar fashion to the chemical substances (such as ADP, serotonin and TXA_2), or to the exposed submembrane structures (e.g. collagen), and form the platelet aggregates and plug on the damaged site: the haemorrhage is thus arrested. Later, clot lysis removes the plug. In thrombocytopenia, the number of circulating platelets is inadequate to perform these functions.

Table 3. Some platelet and platelet-related adhesion proteins.

Platelet glycoproteins	Integrins	Extracellular protein substrate
Gp1b/IX	?	von Willebrand factor (vWF)
GpIV	?	Thrombospondin (TSP)
GpIa–IIa	$\alpha_2\beta_1$	Collagen
GpIc–IIa	$\alpha_5\beta_1$	Fibronectin
GpIc–IIa	$\alpha_6\beta_1$	Laminin
GpII6–IIIa	$\alpha_{II6}\beta_3$	F6/FN/vWF/VN/TSP/Coll
GpII6–IIIa	$\alpha_v\beta_3$	F6/FN/vWF/TSP

Repair of the damaged vasculature is promoted by, among other substances, the platelet secretory proteins, platelet derived growth factor (PDGF) (Ross et al, 1986; Schwartz et al, 1986; Sjolund et al, 1988), which is a powerful mitogen, and transforming growth factor-β (TGF-β) (Roberts et al, 1985; Assoian and Sporn, 1986; Majack, 1987). PDGF and TGF-β are also released from activated vascular endothelial cells (Dicorleto and Bowen-Pope, 1983) and smooth muscle cells (Rabinovitch and Turner-Gomes, 1989). TGF-β also inhibits vascular smooth muscle cell proliferation in appropriate circumstances (Roberts et al, 1985), thus exhibiting modelling and modulating roles in tissue repair. These latter actions have longer-term effects and are designed to secure not only vascular repair but also its recovery from accidents (Barrett and Benditt, 1987).

As summarized above, the role of platelets in health involves not only vital normal haemostatic functions, but also promotion of tissue growth and angiogenesis, roles that can all be deranged.

CIRCULATING PLATELETS IN AFRICANS IN THE TROPICAL ENVIRONMENT

In the tropical African environment, the scanty evidence available indicates that environmental factors frequently affect some aspects of normal platelet function in man. These factors include infections, such as malaria, a situation that is now complicated by the recent onset of the phenomenon of chloroquine resistance in *Plasmodium falciparum*: This has exacerbated the burden of malaria. There is also the more recent onset of the human immunodeficiency virus (HIV) pandemic. Another important factor is the abject poverty and malnutrition that are widespread in the continent, made worse in some areas by unfavourable climatic conditions like drought or flooding, and unstable sociopolitical situations. These factors and their effects have been exacerbated by the downturn in the world economy of the last one and a half decades (The Challenge to the South, 1990). Some effects of the latter situation include worsening malnutrition, with the attendant disturbances in the immune system and resultant increased susceptibility to different infections of the population in general. HIV infection at present appears to affect some regions of Africa and black Africans more severely than other world regions and other populations. The reason for this include poverty, malnutrition and their associated health and social effects (Konotey-Ahulu, 1989). Therefore, this section will examine in greater detail the respective effects of the interactions between the circulating blood platelet and the malaria parasite, as well as those between the platelet and HIV infection, including the acquired immunodeficiency syndrome (AIDS).

The circulating platelet and malaria parasite

Following Maslova's early observation that platelets were reduced in the peripheral blood of patients with acute malaria (Maslova, 1924), it is now generally accepted that the circulating platelet is *regularly* affected during acute malaria infection in man or in experimental infections in animals, (Essien et al, 1979; Inyang et al, 1987a; Essien, 1989). Splenomegaly is a regular feature in chronic malaria infection. It may be complicated by hypersplenism, but it frequently occurs without such complication. Non-hypersplenic splenomegaly may sometimes result in severe thrombocytopenia, as a result of the enlarged splenic platelet pool; however, thrombocytopenia occurs more frequently in hypersplenism. The question of detailed platelet changes in chronic malaria infection with splenomegaly has, as far as I am aware, not been fully addressed. The discussions below, however, refer to platelet dysfunction in acute malaria infection.

Platelet count in acute malaria

During acute malaria infection in man, the blood platelet count is regularly reduced and reaches thrombocytopenic levels (i.e. $<100\times10^9/l$) in only a minority of cases of people normally resident in holoendemic areas, including infants aged 2 years and below (Essien and Oruamabo, 1976; Essien et al, 1979; E. M. Essien and M. I. Ebhota, unpublished observations; A. A. Lawal, unpublished observations). Other reports, however, usually based on studies involving small numbers of cases (25–40 cases) of non-immune subjects who visited malarial zones, have stated that thrombocytopenia, often severe, occurs regularly in acute malaria infection in man (Dennis et al, 1967; Beale et al, 1972; Horstmann et al, 1981; Kueh and Yeo, 1982; Perrin et al, 1982).

In a study of 202 cases, including 105 children aged 4 months to 12 years, the mean platelet count of $132.0 \times 10^9/l \pm 61.6 \times 10^3$ was significantly lower than the count of $234.0 \times 10^9/l \pm 94.0 \times 10^3$ ($t = 6.496$; $P < 0.001$) in the same subjects 12 days after day 0, including days of treatment with chloroquine sulphate. Severe thrombocytopenia (platelet count $< 50 \times 10^9/l$) was observed in only 5% of our cases with *P. falciparum* infection (Essien et al, 1979) and in experimental infection of animals with *P. bergei bergei* (Essien et al, 1984; Inyang et al, 1987a). (Chloroquine resistance was not detected until about a decade later in the hospital where the above study was carried out.) However, in that series and in subsequent observations over the years, we have confirmed the earlier observation that thrombocytopenia, severe or moderate (Table 4), occurred relatively infrequently in cases of acute *P. falciparum* malaria, as well as in infection with other plasmodium species. By contrast, a reduced platelet count, usually above thrombocytopenic levels, is a regular feature of acute human malarial infection (Essien et al, 1979; E. M. Essien, unpublished observations).

Table 4. Relationship between platelet count ($\times 10^9/l$) and malaria parasitaemia graded as 1+ to 3+.

	Pre-treatment			Post-treatment		
	1+	2+	3+	1+	2+	3+
$\bar{x}$	118.46	142.8	102.5	231.23	195.1	257.75
SE	12.95	16.43	20.8	20.8	18.69	57.1

n = 105; $\bar{x}$ = mean; SE = Standard error of mean; 1+ to 3+ = degree of parasitaemia.
From Essien et al (1979) with permission.

Although reports from different groups have indicated that the incidence of severe thrombocytopenia varies between 66–97% (see earlier references) and about 5% (Essien et al, 1979; B. Lawal et al, personal communication), the reasons for this wide disparity remain unclear. One reason may be due to the imprecise definition of the term 'severe thrombocytopenia', as used in the different reports. It is clear from our reports and those of others that bleeding episodes occur relatively rarely in acute malaria infection. As is suggested in our studies, this may be due to: (1) the fact that platelets are usually only mildly reduced in such infection; and (2) there is normally in vivo platelet activation during the infection, and this most likely compensates functionally for the reduced platelet numbers. These questions require closer re-examination.

Other disorders of platelet function in acute malaria

In vitro platelet hypersensitivity to exogenous ADP and adrenaline has been described in acute human (Essien and Ebhota, 1981) and experimental animal (Inyang et al, 1987a) malarial infections. Inhibition respectively of

Table 5. Platelet aggregation following interaction of washed normal platelets with *P. falciparum* infected red blood cells (RBCs).

Incubation time (minutes)	Aggregation (%) With control RBCs	With infected RBCs	*n*	*P*	*t*
1.0	22.2 ± 18.3	94.1 ± 4.3	11(10)	<0.005	12.13
2.0	18.4 ± 4.2	91.1 ± 11.3	8	<0.005	11.17
5.0	17.5 ± 8.7	92.8 ± 5.5	9(8)	<0.005	21.00

n = no. of experiments (including numbers in parentheses). Students *t* test was used in the statistical computations.
From Inyang (1986) and the University of Ibadan with permission.

Note. Blood samples, and washed platelets obtained therefrom, were obtained from healthy volunteers (Mustard et al, 1972; Kinlough-Rathbone et al, 1976). The platelets were incubated with agitation at 37°C in a waterbath with washed *P. falciparum* infected red blood cells in culture (Trager & Jensen) for 1, 2 or 5 minutes before the platelets were separated by differential centrifugation and tested for aggregation. For controls, aliquots of the washed red blood cells used to feed the parasites were mixed with equivalent volumes of the washed platelets and treated as for infected red blood cells.

ADP, thrombin or TXA_2 showed that 57–72% of the hypersensitivity reaction was due to these substances, which were produced by, or followed interactions between, the circulating platelet and *P. falciparum* infected red blood cells. These changes were demonstrated in an elegant in vitro model (Inyang, 1986; Inyang et al, 1987b) (Table 5); the hypersensitivity was transferable to fresh platelets within 1, 2 or 5 minutes of interaction between washed *P. falciparum* infected red blood cells and washed normal platelets. In vivo, the platelet activation was associated with increased platelet lysis, as shown by enhanced loss of platelet lactate dehydrogenase (LDH) activity, as well as increased secretions of the platelet-specific proteins β-thromboglobulin (β-TG) and platelet factor 4 (PF_4) (Essien and Ebhota, 1983). Enhanced platelet production of TXA_2 has also been described, the latter being associated with delayed (by about 48 hours) but enhanced production of prostacyclin, probably by neointima (Essien et al, 1984). Shortening of platelet life-span to about 2.9 days has also been reported in human infection with *P. falciparum* (Skudowitz et al,1973), and with *P. bergei* in Wistar rats to about 2.01 days (normal 4.3 days) (Inyang, 1986). Another feature observed was reduction, by up to 36–62%, of the total platelet sialic acid content (Inyang, 1986; A. L. Inyang et al, unpublished data). It had earlier been shown that when total platelet sialic acid was reduced by >10% of its normal value, such platelets were rapidly cleared from the circulation (Greenberg et al, 1975). However, if the reduction was between 8 and 10%, such platelets exhibit hypersensitivity to agonists. The relationship between loss of membrane sialic acid and blood cell senescence in normal states remains controversial with respect to red cells, where the question has been extensively examined (Aminoff, 1988; Bosman and Kay, 1988; Schlepper-

Schäfer and Kolb-Bachofen, 1988), and may be equally controversial with respect to platelets. However, the evidence presented in the study by Inyang and associates (Inyang, 1986; A. L. Inyang et al, unpublished data) demonstrated a strong relationship between the extent of reduction of the total platelet membrane sialic acid and the density of malarial parasitaemia in rats. A similar relationship was also established between reduction in total platelet sialic acid content and platelet recovery in platelet survival studies. It has been suggested from the above findings that reduction in total platelet sialic acid in acute *P. falciparum* infection in man or experimental infection in animals (Essien, 1989) is a mechanism for the lowered platelet counts, which may result in severe thrombocytopenia in some cases. The details of the processes involved in such changes remain to be fully clarified.

Thrombocytopenia in HIV infection and AIDS

The spectrum of the pathology and pathophysiology of the HIV pandemic and AIDS is still unfolding. With respect to changes affecting the megakaryocyte or the circulating platelet, information is relatively scanty. Transient mild thrombocytopenia has been reported during the acute phase of HIV infection before antibodies develop (Cooper et al, 1985). However, the problem has been studied only occasionally elsewhere, and as far as I am aware, it has not been examined in the African environment. In Africa, it would be compounded by other more frequent and easily detectable causes of mild thrombocytopenia, such as acute malarial infection. The discussion below concerns patients with established HIV infection and/or AIDS.

It has been reported that among 26 British homosexual men who were HIV infected but symptom-free, the platelet count in each was normal. By contrast, among a small group of 13 asymptomatic HIV-positive homosexual men in New York, USA, thrombocytopenia was often observed (Karpatkin, 1990). Thrombocytopenia was also recorded among 8% of patients with AIDS-related complex (ARC) and in 30% of AIDS patients (Murphy et al, 1987). The reasons for the differences observed in these reports are not clear because, as far as possible, overt causes of thrombocytopenia were excluded in the studies. Determinations of some platelet parameters, such as platelet survival time, splenic transit time and blood flow as well as other criteria, gave normal results in each group. Platelet survival time was, however, markedly shortened to 1 day in the patient group compared with 8–10 days in normal controls (Bel-Ali et al, 1987). With respect to the mechanisms of the thrombocytopenia in the affected groups, it was found that platelet bound immunoglobulin (Ig)G, complement C_3C_4 and circulating immune complexes were elevated among the US group of homosexual men and intravenous drug users (IVDUs), when compared with levels in patients with classical acute thrombocytopenic purpura. It was also found that 50% of the immune complexes bound to platelets or to megakaryocytes comprised anti-HIV and anti-idiotype fractions. Normal levels of these parameters were observed in samples from IVDUs and male homosexuals who were HIV-1 negative and had normal platelet counts (Karpatkin, 1990). It was suggested that platelets to which such complexes are bound are damaged and then destroyed, and that this results in thrombocytopenia. Similarly, megakaryocytes with bound complexes are damaged, with resultant ineffective thrombopoiesis (Karpatkin, 1990).

Some haematological parameters have been examined in three African patients, who were seen and treated for different haematological problems between 1982 and 1990 in two Nigerian University Hospitals, and found to be HIV-2 seropositive (patients 1–3, Table 6). Four patients (nos 4–7, Table 6) presented primarily with ARC or AIDS. Two of the three haematological patients (nos 1 and 3) were thrombocytopenic, both as a result of aplastic

Table 6. Summary of data on African patients with haematological disorders primarily but found to be HIV seropositive (nos 1–3), or with HIV-related disease (nos 4–7).

Patient no.	Age	Sex	Initial PCV	WBC ($\times 10^9$/l)	Platelets ($\times 10^9$/l)	IgG (g/l)	IgA (g/l)	IgM (g/l)	Immune complex (mg/100ml)	HIV
1	73	M	0.26	5.2	59	9.75	1.89	1.58	54.27	2
2	32	M	0.17	4.4	141	13.50	2.43	2.00	83.76	2
3	26	F	0.24	1.6	50	10.50	2.16	1.16	46.2	2
4	34	M	0.26	3.0	<10	—	—	—	—	1
5	38	M	0.25	5.9	100	—	—	—	—	1
6	40	M	0.27	2.5	120	—	—	—	—	?1
7	26	F	0.25	2.7	140	—	—	—	—	
Normal*	—	—	0.42 ± 0.5(F) 0.47 ± 0.7(M)	4–10	100–300					

PCV, Packed cell volume or haematocrit; WBC, Total white cell count; M, male; F, female.
* See Essien et al, 1973; Ukaejiofor et al, 1979.
—, no data available.

anaemia which could not be attributed to HIV infection, as far as it was possible to ascertain. The serum immune complexes in the three haematological patients were elevated, but the specificity of the complexes was not determined. With respect to the group of patients (nos 4–7, Table 6) who presented primarily with ARC or AIDS, the platelet counts were essentially in the normal range for the environment in three, and one patient had a severe thrombocytopenia. Their serum immunoglobulins and immune complexes were not determined. Thus, in this small group of HIV-infected patients, some of whom were already thrombocytopenic due to primary haematological disorders, thrombocytopenia occurred in about 30%. Anaemia of a considerable degree was observed among the entire group of seven patients, while about 60% of them were leucopenic. It would appear from this very preliminary data that HIV infection has increased unduly the burden of an already high frequency of anaemia in the population, and has also increased the frequency of leucopenia, but has had only a marginal effect on platelet counts. It is considered essential that a detailed study of the haematological status of HIV infected persons in Africa should be undertaken urgently.

Idiopathic thrombocytopenic purpura in African children

Acute idiopathic thrombocytopenic purpura (ITP), excluding onyalai, is reportedly rare among Africans. For instance, in a study of ITP among African children, the incidence was 0.01% (Lewis and Essien, 1975), which was significantly lower ($P<0.001$) than the 0.18% incidence reported in other populations (Doan et al, 1960). In addition to the relative rarity of the disorder, moderate splenomegaly in 38% and anaemia in 76% of patients were two other features reported among the Africans (Lewis and Essien, 1975). These two features would have constituted contraindications to making the diagnosis of ITP if they were found among European and north American patients. These features, however, reflected the influence on disease manifestation of environmental factors such as a high prevalence of malaria, other parasitic diseases and bacterial infections, as well as malnutrition. For instance, the environment in which the African ITP patients lived is holoendemic for malaria, which could have contributed to or caused the splenomegaly. Similarly anaemia could have been caused either by malaria, other infections or malnutrition. It is suggested that the presence of splenomegaly and anaemia in patients who satisfy other criteria, do not constitute contraindications to making a diagnosis of ITP in environments where such features are common.

SUMMARY

Blood platelets, which are known to play important roles in normal vertebrate biology, are influenced by a variety of factors, the majority of which are acquired. In this chapter, attention is drawn to the need to re-examine one of the old accepted values in haematology, the normal platelet count. In addition, effects of some environmental factors, such as malarial parasitaemia, on both platelet count and platelet function are fully discussed. Similarly, the effects of HIV on platelets, as well as on other haematological parameters, in the African environment are described briefly. The urgent need is stressed for careful evaluation of the impact of HIV on the total disease burden in the population.

In addition, the effect of environmental factors on the manifestations of some clinical features, e.g. splenomegaly and anaemia, in acute idiopathic thrombocytopenic purpura are highlighted. It is suggested that in such environments, the presence of these features do not constitute contraindications to making the diagnosis when other criteria are met.

Acknowledgements

I thank the following for assistance with the preparation of this manuscript: Professor I. Akinsete, Head of the Haematology Department of the Lagos University Teaching Hospital (LUTH) for data on some HIV and AIDS/ARC patients; the Consultants in the Haematology Department, University College Hospital (UCH), Ibadan, for assistance with other HIV positive patients; Mr I. Saliu for carrying out the HIV tests. Dr I. Okpala, Senior Registrar in Haematology Department, UCH, Ibadan, made helpful criticisms. Dr S. L. Salimonu, Head of the Immunology Unit, Department of Chemical Pathology, UCH, Ibadan, kindly determined the immunoglobulins and immune complexes. Mr S. J. P. Umobong of the National Institute for Medical Research (NIMR), Yaba, Lagos, kindly typed the manuscript.

REFERENCES

Aballi, AJ, Puapondh Y & Desposite F (1968) Platelet counts in thriving premature infants. *Pediatrics* **42:** 685–689.

Aminoff D (1988) The role of sialoglyco-conjugates in the aging and sequestration of red cells from circulation. *Blood Cell* **4:** 229–257.

Assoian RK & Sporn MB (1986) Type B transforming growth factor in human platelets release during platelet degranulation and action on smooth muscle cells. *Journal of Cell Biology* **102:** 1217–1223.

Barrett TB & Benditt EP (1987) Sis (platelet derived growth factor B-chain) gene transcript levels are elevated in human atherosclerotic lesions compared to normal artery. *Proceedings of the National Academy of Sciences of the USA* **84:** 1099–1103.

Beale PF, Cormack JD & Oldrey TBN (1972) Thrombocytopenia in malaria with immunoglobulin (IgM) changes. *British Medical Journal* **1:** 345–349.

Bel-Ali Z, Dufour V & Najeen Y (1987) Platelet kinetics in human immunodeficiency virus induced thrombocytopenia. *American Journal of Hematology* **26:** 299–304.

Bosman GJ & Kay MM (1988) Erythrocyte aging: a comparison of model systems for simulating cellular aging in vitro. *Blood Cell* **14:** 19–46.

Cooper DA, Maclean P, Finlayson R et al (1985) Acute AIDS retrovirus infection. Definition of a clinical illness associated with seroconversion. *Lancet* **i:** 537–540.

Dacie JV & Lewis SM (1975) *Practical Haematology*, pp 21–67. Edinburgh: Churchill Livingstone.

Dennis LH, Eichelbeger JW, Inman MM & Conrad ME (1967) Depletion of coagulation factors in drug-resistant *Plasmodium falciparum* malaria. *Blood* **29:** 713–721.

Dicorleto PE & Bowen-Pope DF (1983) Cultured endothelial cells produce a platelet derived growth factor-like protein. *Proceedings of the National Academy of Sciences of the USA* **80:** 1919–1923.

Doan CA, Bouroncle BA & Wiseman BK (1960) Idiopathic and secondary thrombocytopenic purpura: clinical study and evaluation of 381 cases over a period of 28 years. *Annals of Internal Medicine* **53:** 861–876.

Dupuy E, Fleming AF & Caen JP (1978) Platelet function, factor VIII, fibrinogen and fibrinolysis in Nigerians and Europeans in relation to atheroma and thrombosis. *Journal of Clinical Pathology* **31:** 1094–1101.

Effiong CE, Usanga EA & Mellits ED (1976) Platelet counts in healthy full-term Nigerian neonates. *Tropical and Geographical Medicine* **28:** 329–332.

Essien EM (1989) The circulating platelet in acute malaria infection: medical hypothesis. *British Journal of Haematology* **72:** 589–590.

Essien EM & Ebhota MI (1981) Platelet hypersensitivity in acute malaria (*Plasmodium falciparum*) infection in man. *Thrombosis and Haemostasis* **46:** 547–549.

Essien EM & Ebhota MI (1983) Platelet secretory activities in acute malaria (*Plasmodium falciparum*) infection. *Acta Haematologica* **70:** 183–188.

Essien EM & Oruamabo RS (1976) Depression of platelet count during acute *Plasmodium falciparum* malaria infection. *Nigerian Journal of Paediatrics* **3:** 69–70.

Essien EM, Usanga EA & Ayeni O (1973) The normal platelet count and platelet factor-3 availability in some Nigerian population groups. *Scandinavian Journal of Haematology* **10:** 378–383.

Essien EM, Adekunle CO & Oruamabo RS (1979) Effect of acute *Plasmodium falciparum* infection on platelet count in man. *Nigerian Journal of Medical Science* **1:** 59–63.

Essien EM, Arnout J, Deckmyn H, Vermylen J & Verstraete M (1984) Blood changes and enhanced thromboxane B_2 and 6-keto-prostaglandin production in acute *Plasmodium bergei* infection in hamsters. *Thrombosis and Haemostasis* **51:** 363–365.

Federeko ME & Lichtman MA (1982) Megakaryocyte structure maturation and ecology. In Colman RW, Hirsh J, Marder UJ & Salzman EW (eds) *Hemostasis and Thrombosis: Basic Principles and Clinical Practice*, pp 210–236. Philadelphia: Lippincott.

Fox JEB (1987) The platelet cytoskeleton. In Verstraete M, Vermylen J, Lijneu R & Arnout J (eds) *Thrombosis and Haemostasis*, pp 175–225. Leuven: Leuven University Press.

Gerrard JM & White JG (1976) The structure and function of platelets with emphasis on their contractile nature. In Iochim HL (ed.) *Pathology Annual*, pp 31–58. New York: Appleton–Century–Crofts.

Gill GV, England A & Marshal C (1979) Low platelet counts in Zambians. *Transactions of the Royal Society for Tropical Medicine and Hygiene* **73:** 111–112.

Greenberg I, Packham MA, Cazenave J-P, Reimers H-J & Mustard JF (1975) Effects on platelet function of removal of platelet sialic acid by neuraminidase. *Laboratory Investigation* **32:** 476–484.

Horstmann RD, Dietrich M, Bienzle U & Rashe H (1981) Malaria-induced thrombocytopenia. *Blut* **42:** 157–164.

Hovic T (1968) The ultrastructure of blood platelets in normal and abnormal states. *Series Haematologica* **1:** 3–64.

Inyang AL (1986) *Platelet changes in experimental malaria*. PhD thesis, University of Ibadan, Nigeria.

Inyang AL, Okpako DT & Essien EM (1987a) Platelet reactions in acute *Plasmodium bergei* infection in Swiss albino mice. *Haematologica* **20:** 101–108.

Inyang AL, Sodeinde O, Okpako DT & Essien EM (1987b) Platelet reaction after interaction with cultured *Plasmodium falciparum* infected erythrocytes. *British Journal of Haematology* **66:** 375–378.

Karpatkin S (1969) Heterogeneity of human platelets. I: Metabolic and kinetic evidence suggestive of young and old platelets. *Journal of Clinical Investigation* **48:** 1073–1082.

Karpatkin S (1990) HIV-1 related thrombocytopenia. In Colman RW & Rao RK (eds) *Hematology/Oncology Clinics of North America: Platelets in Health and Disease*, pp 193–219. Philadelphia: W. B. Saunders.

Kinlough-Rathbone RL, Packham MA, Perry DW & Mustard JF (1976) Isolation of platelets: centrifugation and washing techniques. In Day HJ, Holmsen H & Zucker MB (eds) *Platelet Function Testing*, pp 50–55. DHEW Publication No. (NIH) 78–1087, US Department of Health, Education and Welfare.

Konotey-Ahulu FID (1989) *What is AIDS?* pp 112–131. Tetteh-A'Domeno.

Kueh YK & Yeo KL (1982) Haematological alterations in acute malaria. *Scandinavian Journal of Haematology* **29:** 147–152.

Lasslo A (1984) Blood platelet function, medicinal agents and other chemical entities. *Federation Proceedings* **43:** 1382–1389.

Lewis MJ & Essien EM (1975) Idiopathic thrombocytopenia in Nigerian children. *Nigerian Journal of Paediatrics* **2:** 9–15.

Majak RA (1987) Beta type transforming growth factor specifies organizational behaviour in vascular smooth muscle cell cultures. *Journal of Cell Biology* **105:** 465–471.

Maslova AN (1924) The changes in quantity of blood platelets (Bizzozero) and the velocity of coagulation of the blood in malaria. *Journal of Tropical Medicine* (Moscow) **3:** 7–14.

Mukiibi JM, Okelo GBA & Kanja C (1981) Platelet counts in normal Kenyan adults. *East African Medical Journal* **58:** 136–139.

Murphy MF, Metcalfe P & Waters AH (1987) Incidence and mechanism of neutropenia and thrombocytopenia in patients with human immunodeficiency virus infection. *British Journal of Haematology* **66:** 337–340.

Mustard JF & Packham M (1970) Factors influencing platelet function: adhesion, release and aggregation. *Pharmacological Reviews* **22:** 97–170.

Mustard JF, Perry DW, Ardlie NG & Packham MA (1972) Preparation of suspensions of washed platelets from humans. *British Journal of Haematology* **22:** 193.

Onwukeme KE & Ugura VE (1990) Haematological values in pregnancy in Jos. *West African Journal of Medicine* **9:** 70–75.

Packham MA & Mustard JF (1984) Normal and abnormal platelet activity. In Lasslo A (ed.) *Blood Platelet Function and Medicinal Chemistry*, pp 61–128. New York: Elsevier.

Perrin LH, Lindsay JM & Miescher PA (1982) The hematology of malaria in man. *Seminars in Hematology* **19:** 70–82.

Rabinovitch M & Turner-Gomes SO (1989) Platelet-endothelial factors. *Advances in Pediatrics* **36:** 91–116.

Roberts AB, Anzano MA, Wekefield LM et al (1985) Type B transforming growth: a bifunctional regulator of cellular growth. *Proceedings of the National Academy of Sciences of the USA* **82:** 119–123.

Roskam J (1923) Contribution a l'étude de la physiologie normale et pathologique du globulin. *Archives Internationales de Physiologie* **20:** 241–330.

Ross R, Raines EW & Bowen-Pope DF (1986) The biology of platelet derived growth factor. *Cell* **46:** 155–169.

Schlepper-Schäfer J & Kolb-Bachofen V (1988) Red cell aging results in a change of cell surface carbohydrate epitopes allowing for recognition by galactose-specific receptors of rat liver macrophages. *Blood Cell* **14:** 259–274.

Schwartz SM, Campbell GR & Campbell JH (1986) Replication of smooth muscle cells in vascular disease. *Circulation Research* **58:** 427–444.

Shulman NR & Jordan JV (1982) Platelet dynamics. In Colman RW, Hirsh J, Marder JV & Salzman EW (eds) *Hemostasis and Thrombosis: Basic Principles and Clinical Practice*, pp 237–258. Philadelphia: Lippincott.

Sjolund M, Hedin U, Sejersen T et al (1988) Arterial smooth muscle cells express platelet-derived growth factor (PDGF) A-chain in RNA, secrete a PDGF-like mitogen, and bind exogenous PDGF in a phenotype and growth state-dependent manner. *Journal of Cell Biology* **106:** 403–413.

Skudowitz RB, Katz J, Lurie A, Levin L & Metz J (1973) Mechanisms of thrombocytopenia in malignant tertian malaria. *British Medical Journal* **ii:** 515–517.

The Challenge to the South (1990) The Report of the South Commission. Oxford: Oxford University Press.

Ukaejiofor EO, Isaacs-Sodeye WA, Adigun S & Ipadeola A (1979) Normal haematological values in adult Nigerians. *Nigerian Medical Journal* **9:** 117–119.

Walsh PN (1974) Platelet coagulant activities and haemostasis: an hypothesis. *Blood* **43:** 597–605.

White JG (1969) The submembrane filaments of blood platelets. *American Journal of Pathology* **56:** 267–277.

White JG (1971) Platelet morphology. In Johnson SA (ed.) *The Circulating Platelet*, pp 45–121. New York: Academic Press.

White JG & Gerrard JM (1982) Anatomy and structural organization of the platelet. In Colman RW, Hirsch J, Marder VJ & Salzman EW (eds) *Hemostasis and Thrombosis: Basic Principles and Clinical Practice*, pp 343–363. Philadelphia: Lippincott.

8

Onyalai

PETER B. HESSELING

HISTORICAL INTRODUCTION

Wellman (1904) first recorded onyalai amongst inhabitants of the Benguella District, Angola: 'Hemorrhagic Bulla (native name onyalai)—A common and very treacherous disease greatly feared by the natives. Considered by them very fatal. I was once disposed to treat the native view very lightly, but after seeing cases die from it in a few hours from the beginning of an attack, I revised my notion. The bullae may be small and affect only the surface of the body, or occur only on the tongue, soft palate or buccal mucous membrane. When large and involving the oesophagus and pharynx, they may cause trouble, but when you get them in the brain, its membranes or even in the important abdominal viscera, death often results. The size of the bullae varies markedly, ranging from that of a split pea to that of a half-crown piece.' In the same year Massey (1904) published three case reports, excluded bilharzia and malaria as the cause, and commented on the tendency of the bullae to recur. He suggested treatment with bicarbonate of soda and cod liver oil. The word onyalai is still used by the Kimbundu tribe who inhabit central and western Angola to describe the disease; literally translated it means a blood blister. The terms 'ondjito' and 'omukotta' in Ovambo (Gildenhuys, 1974), 'madambwe' in Kavango (M. Fisch, personal communication) and 'chilopa' and 'akembu' in Zambia (Gilkes, 1934) are true synonyms for onyalai.

Marked thrombocytopenia at the onset of disease was first noted by Blackie (1937), and the presence of serum IgG and IgM platelet antibodies was recorded by Brink et al (1981).

CLINICAL FINDINGS

The clinical hallmark of onyalai is the sudden appearance in previously healthy people of haemorrhagic trabeculated bullae on the mucous membranes of the mouth, tongue or palate and, less frequently, the skin (Figure 1). In severe cases the whole buccal cavity and tongue appear to be a fungating haemorrhagic mass. Patients have halitosis, and typically they sit in bed with a blood- and saliva-filled container in the hand. The teeth and

ISBN 0–7020–1627–6

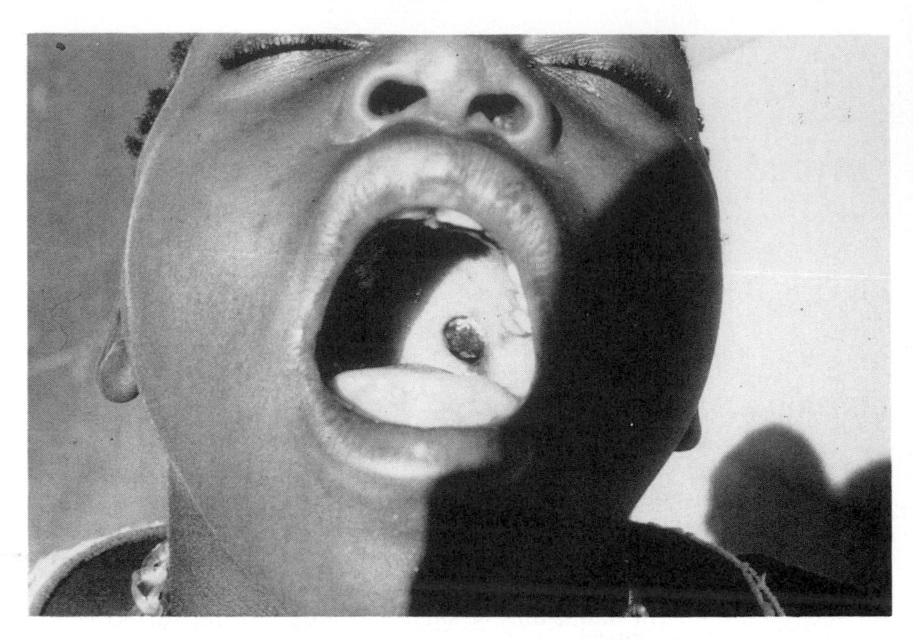

Figure 1. Haemorrhagic bullae on palate.

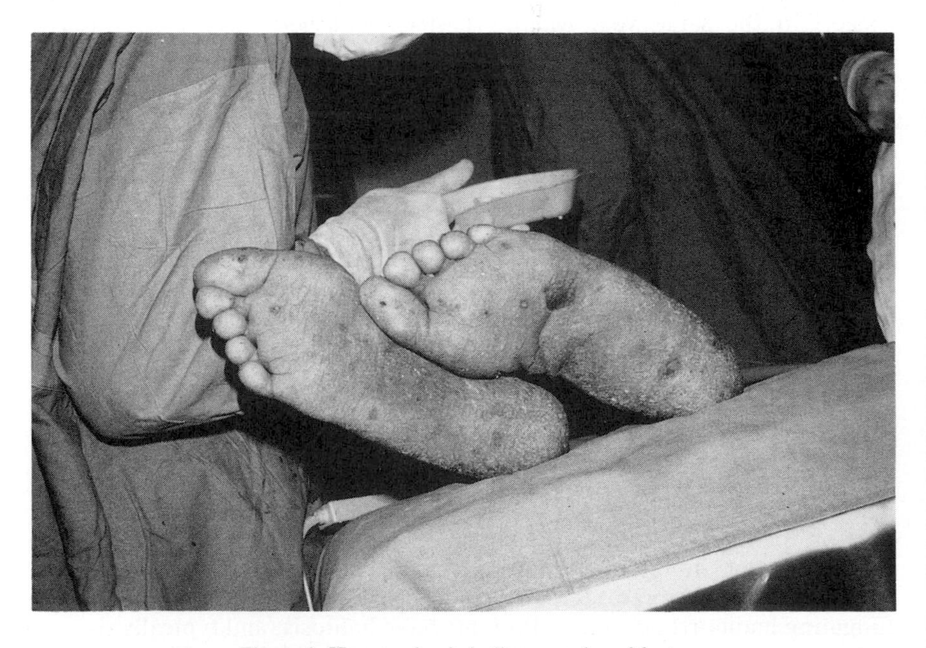

Figure 2. Haemorrhagic bullae on soles of feet.

gums are normal in appearance. Epistaxis, which may be severe, is often present on admission. Petechiae and ecchymoses are easily overlooked in dark skinned patients. Likewise, bullae on the soles of the feet (Figure 2) may be missed easily without proper cleaning of the feet in patients who normally go barefoot. Bleeding from the gastrointestinal and genitourinary tract may be present at the onset of symptoms, but more commonly manifests after the appearance of the bullae. Intracranial haemorrhage in the acute phase presents with typical neurological signs. A short history of vague prodromal signs such as headache, malaise, abdominal discomfort and generalized aches has been recorded in some of the patients (Gilkes, 1934; Gelfand, 1943; Squires, 1950; Barss, 1976). The occasional presence of pyrexia was noted as a prodromal sign and was considered to be a favourable prognostic sign in the acute phase by Gilkes (1934), but this has not been substantiated by subsequent reports. The diagnosis of onyalai should be based on the presence of haemorrhagic bullae and the criteria for the diagnosis of idiopathic thrombocytopenic purpura (ITP), as proposed by Wiseman et al (1940). The relative frequency of the various signs and symptoms, which were observed in 103 patients at presentation, is listed in Table 1 (Hesseling, 1987). Epistaxis was present in about half, and skin petechiae and/or ecchymosis in only a quarter of the patients. Blood loss in the acute phase from persistently bleeding bullae in the mouth, epistaxis and gastrointestinal bleeding may cause haemorrhagic shock. In a series of 40 patients observed in hospital for 21 days, 22 patients required a total of 92 units of blood (1–16 units per patient) in the acute phase to maintain the haemoglobin above 10 g/dl (Hesseling et al, 1986a). The median duration of active haemorrhage was found to be 8 days, ranging from 1 to 118 days in 612 patients (Hesseling, 1990). The risk for cerebral haemorrhage in 103 patients was 2% on admission (Table 1) and 4% after a limited period of observation. The mean haemoglobin was 10.3 g/dl (range 2.2–15.6 g/dl) and the mean platelet value was 22×10^9/l (range $1–85 \times 19^9$/l) on admission of the same 103 patients. The natural course of onyalai is characterized by the disappearance of clinical haemorrhage in survivors. Seventeen of 21 patients (81%) who were followed up at 2-monthly intervals for 1 year after an acute attack gave a history of a documented previous episode of onyalai or had a

Table 1. Signs and symptoms at presentation in 103 Namibian patients with onyalai.

Signs/symptoms	Number of patients
Haemorrhagic bullae	
Oronasopharynx	103
Skin	11
Epistaxis	53
Skin petechiae/ecchymoses	23
Eye subconjunctival/scleral	17
Melaena/haematemesis	16
Haematuria (no schistosomiasis)	12
Vaginal bleeding ($n = 60$)	9
CNS haemorrhage	2

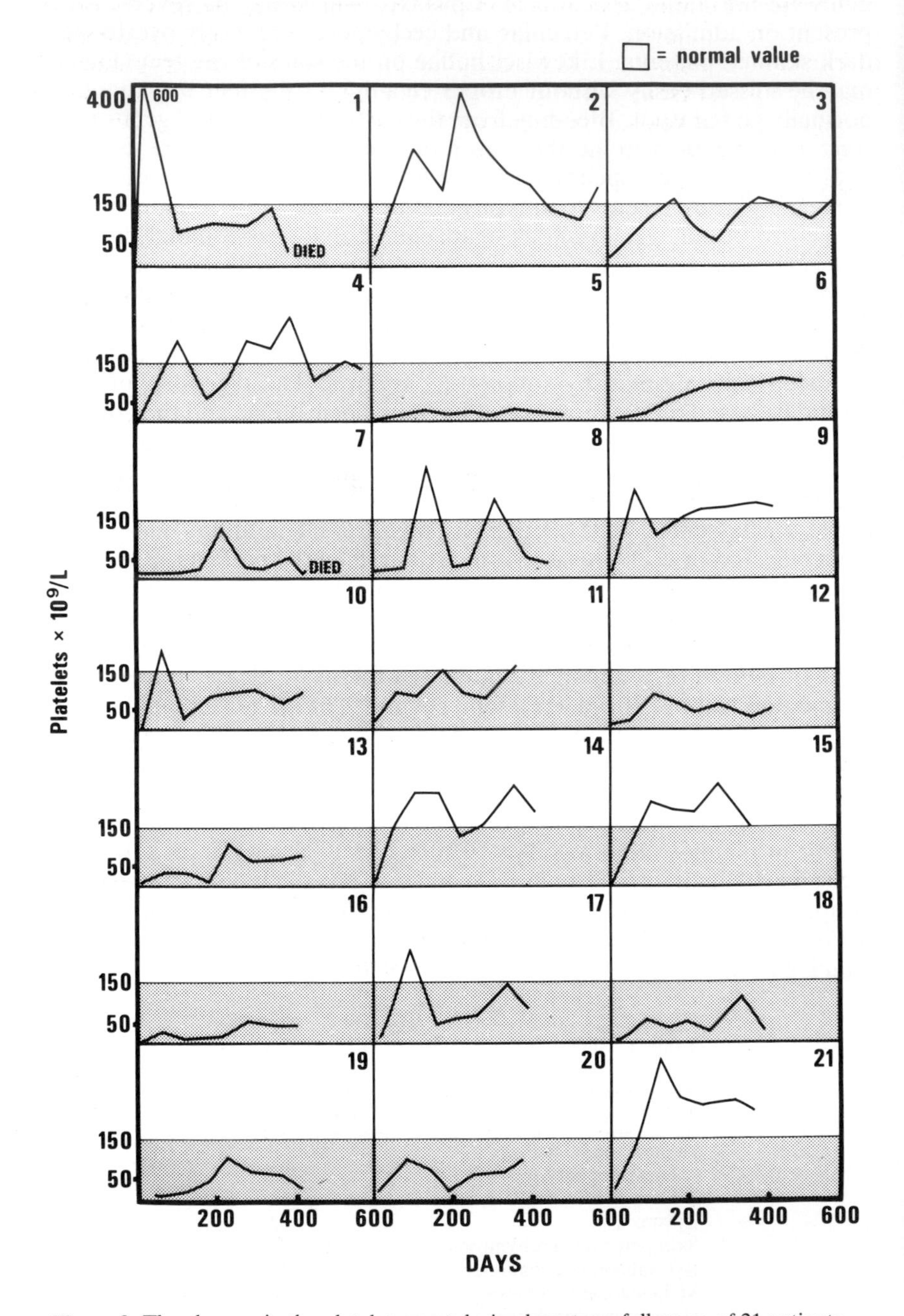

Figure 3. The changes in the platelet count during long-term follow-up of 21 patients.

recurrence of clinical disease. However, asymptomatic thrombocytopenia persists in the majority of patients (Figure 3) (Hesseling, 1983). The chances of clinical remission and normalization of the platelet count is better in patients after a first attack (Stein and Miller, 1943), and also if the patient is younger than 18 years at the time of the first attack (Hesseling, 1983).

EPIDEMIOLOGY

Geography

Onyalai is limited to some African populations inhabiting the central plateau of Africa, within a zone extending from the equator to 30° south latitude (Figure 4). The localities indicated in Figure 4 represent all the reports in the literature which appear to comply with the clinical (earlier reports) and laboratory criteria for the diagnosis of onyalai. A close scrutiny

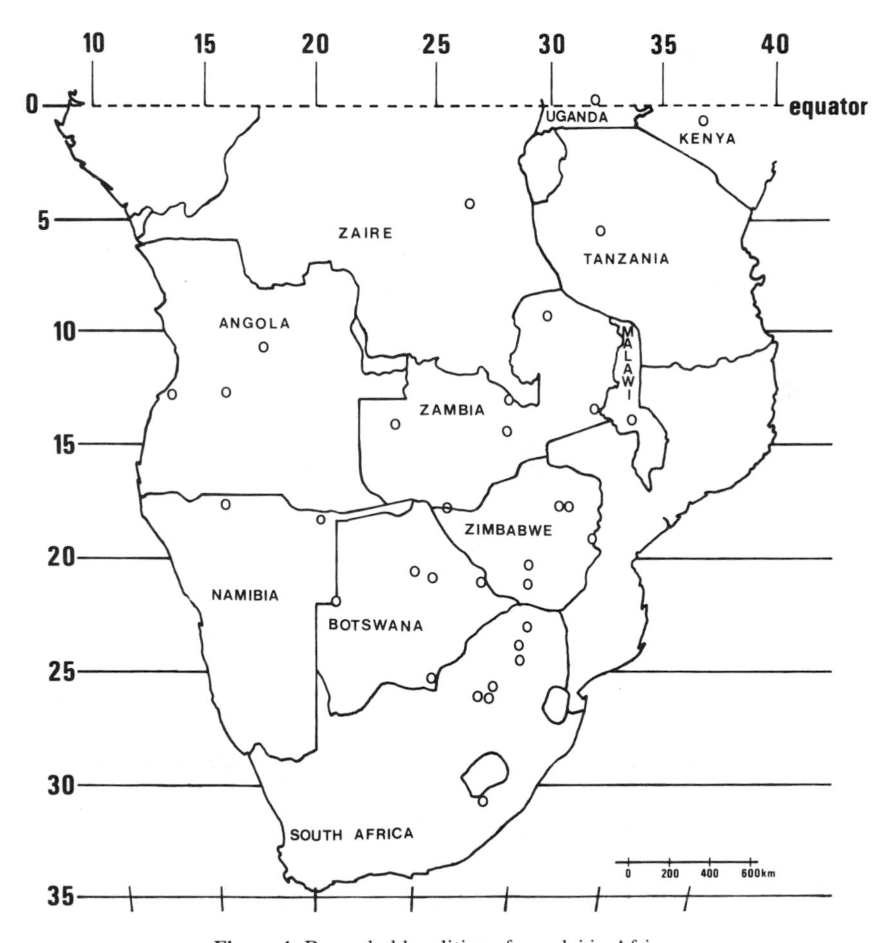

Figure 4. Recorded localities of onyalai in Africa.

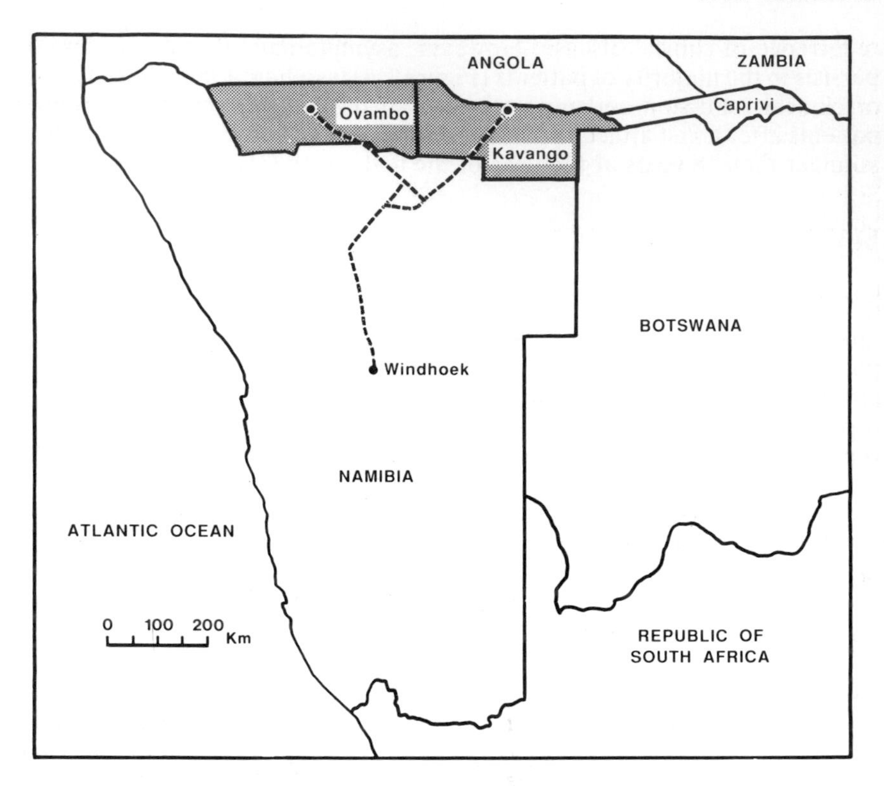

Figure 5. Map to illustrate locality of Kavango and Ovambo.

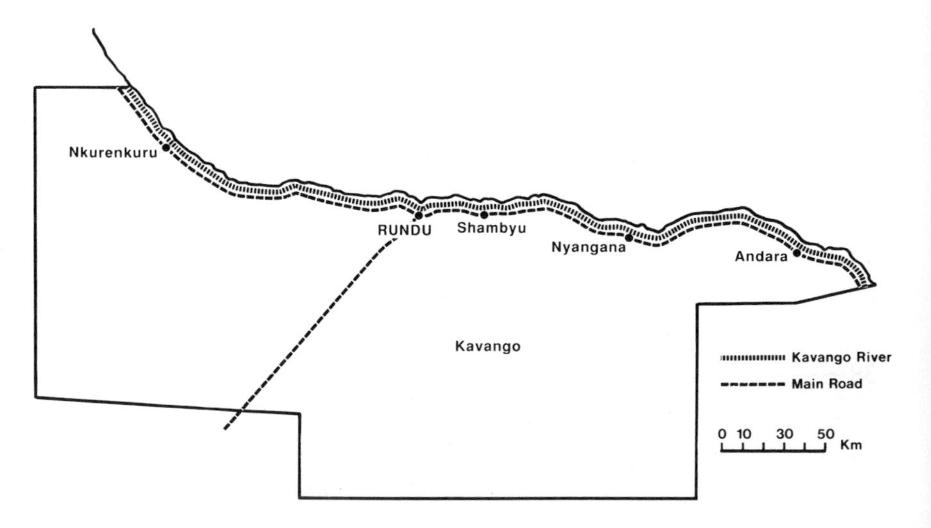

Figure 6. Major hospitals in Kavango.

of the few recorded cases of onyalai amongst non-African patients reveals that these patients had underlying systemic disease, or had been treated with drugs known to cause haemorrhagic bullae, or that the reports contained inadequate clinical and haematological data to satisfy the previously stated criteria for the diagnosis of onyalai (Stein and Miller, 1943; Gear et al, 1944; Strangway and Strangway, 1949; Lewis and Lurie, 1953; Gelfand, 1954; Shee, 1961). Although cases of classical ITP have not been documented amongst the Namibian African populations who develop onyalai, African patients in Kenya develop classical ITP without haemorrhagic bullae (Mukiibi and Kyobe, 1982; Almeida and Kasili, 1983). Metz et al (1958) recorded a 75% incidence of haemorrhagic bullae in 60 African patients treated for acute ITP in Johannesburg. Many of these patients probably came from neighbouring countries to work on the gold mines. Goldin and Gelfand (1980) described 13 cases of ITP from Zimbabwe, of whom three had typical haemorrhagic bullae. Gildenhuys (1974) noted in his thesis on the disease profile of the Ovambo population in Namibia, in which he described onyalai, that he had never encountered classical ITP. The author has likewise never observed a patient with ITP amongst the Kavango population of Namibia.

Onyalai appears to be a disappearing disease entity in the Republic of South Africa and Zimbabwe. The last report quoting South African patients by Edginton et al (1972) briefly describes 15 patients belonging to the Pedi tribe at Jane Furse Hospital in the Transvaal province. An enquiry to this hospital at the time of writing revealed that the last documented case of onyalai was seen in 1975. The authors point out that these patients lived in a rural area, had all first consulted a traditional healer and were illiterate. Wicks (1972), in his case report from Zimbabwe, mentions that medical practitioners in the rural areas of Mashona Land now rarely see the disease, whereas it was commonly encountered before. Only two patients were diagnosed at Harare Hospital in Zimbabwe between 1977 and 1979 (Goldin and Gelfand, 1980). Squires (1943), in his report of 52 patients from Botswana, illustrated the geographical distribution of onyalai between Lobatsi and Francistown. In another report (Squires, 1950) the same author described 106 cases of onyalai. The present-day incidence of onyalai in Botswana is unknown. Barss (1976) stated that onyalai was seen fairly frequently in Central Angola, and warned against overdiagnosis in patients with simple epistaxis and other causes for bleeding. He emphasized the importance of meticulous technique when the platelet count was assessed with microscopy. The ravages of war in Angola, political instability, limited government health funding, medical manpower shortage and limited peripheral laboratory services in the countries where onyalai was known to occur, must have hampered research and the collection of health statistics. This may have caused underreporting of the condition.

Onyalai is still encountered commonly in the northern Kavango and Ovambo territories of Namibia, and in southern Angola (Figures 5 and 6). No current information is available about the present-day prevalence in Botswana and Zambia, and it is hoped that this report will elicit such information.

The explanation for the 'contracting' geographical distribution appears to be linked to a changing life-style of the populations. Onyalai still occurs in rural populations who maintain a traditional diet and way of life, but disappears with urbanization and westernization. The possible aetiological link with the diet will be discussed later.

Incidence in Namibia

The incidence of onyalai in the Kavango territory in the north-east of Namibia was recorded prospectively at every health service point during a 12-month period starting in February 1981. This territory extends over 49 000 km^2 and had about 101 000 inhabitants, living mainly within walking distance of the river at the time (Figure 6). The 153 patients who were registered represented a minimum incidence of one case per 660 inhabitants per annum (Hesseling, 1983). Onyalai accounted for 612 (1.2%) out of 51 253 admissions to the regional hospital in this territory between 1981 and 1988, with the annual relative frequency varying between 0.96 and 1.66% of all admissions. The lowest admission rate was during the dry season, from June to August, and the highest admission rate in March to May, at the end of the rainy season, which precedes the new millet harvest in June. However, the difference in seasonal incidence did not achieve statistical significance (Hesseling, 1990). The numbers of patients with onyalai who were admitted to the four major mission hospitals in Kavango (Nkurenkuru, Sambyu, Nyangana, Andara) and Rundu State Hospital for the years 1971 to 1980 were obtained from the hospital admission registers (Table 2; Figure 6) (Hesseling, 1983). These figures confirm a high frequency of onyalai in the Kavango territory over the past two decades.

Table 2. Onyalai: recorded frequency in the main hospitals of Kavango, 1971–1980.

Hospital	1971	1972	1973	1974	1975	1976	1977	1978	1979	1980
Rundu	NA	NA	NA	8	30	23	10	38	50	43
Nyangana	NA	NA	NA	NA	NA	4	23	12	11	17
Sambyu	14	17	9	13	7	5	9	9	4	11
Andara	NA	NA	NA	NA	10	6	20	19	7	5
Nkurenkuru	NA	NA	19	26	10	15	9	16	25	13
Total						53	71	94	97	89

NA, not available.

The only other area in Namibia where onyalai is commonly encountered is the more populous central northern Ovambo territory (see Figure 5). Gildenhuys (1974) refers to old health reports for the Ovambo territory, and quotes figures of 704 cases in 1950, 570 cases in 1952, and 674 cases in 1956. I have not been able to relocate these official reports in order to assess the diagnostic criteria which were applied. Gildenhuys (1974) did record between 14 and 21 admissions per annum of well-documented cases of onyalai to Oshakati Hospital between 1969 and 1972. At the present time, onyalai is still a common disease in Ovambo, according to personal accounts of doctors who are working there, but the exact incidence is unknown.

Age and sex

Onyalai affects all age groups but with 50% of cases presenting before the age of 20 years (Table 3); the male:female ratio is 4:6. The youngest recorded case was an infant of 6 months (Hesseling, 1987). Neonates born to mothers with onyalai appear clinically normal and have normal platelet counts at birth (Gilbert, 1943; Lewis and Lurie, 1953; Hesseling, 1985), in contrast to infants born to mothers with chronic ITP who have a 33% risk of thrombocytopenia at birth (Kaplan et al, 1990).

Table 3. Age distribution of patients with onyalai at Rundu Hospital, 1981–1988.

Age (years)	Number
0–10	127 (28.2)
11–20	109 (24.2)
21–30	66 (14.6)
31–40	48 (10.6)
41–50	46 (10.2)
51–60	31 (6.9)
61–70	18 (4.0)
71+	6 (1.3)
Total	451

Values in parentheses are percentages.

Genetic factors

A family history is uncommon, although the occurrence of onyalai in more than one family member and in members of the same household has been recorded (Mense, 1906; Gilkes, 1934; Squires, 1943; Gelfand, 1944; Lewis and Lurie, 1953). There has never been an epidemic of onyalai, and only rarely does more than one case at a time occur in a village. Onyalai in Namibia is limited to the Kavango and Ovambo population groups, who inhabit the central, northern and north-eastern part of the country. The Koisan (collective term for inhabitants of Bushman and Hottentot descent), Herero and Himba peoples do not develop onyalai. Likewise, the disease is not encountered in missionaries from western Europe who have lived in the area for decades, or amongst other inhabitants of European descent. Gildenhuys (1974) pointed out that all the populations subject to onyalai had a common dietary pattern, namely the cultivation and use of millet as a staple diet. This will be discussed further under aetiology.

AETIOLOGY

Traditional beliefs and medicine

The Mrewa tribe in Zimbabwe believed that onyalai followed the eating or drinking from utensils contaminated by the saliva of a patient, or of a person who had recovered from the disease (Morris, 1934). The Kwangali tribe in

Kavango also use separate drinking and eating vessels when they have onyalai (R. Shekapukela, personal communication), and the Kuanyama tribe in Ovambo believe that the disease is contagious (S. Amadhila, personal communication). Although Gear et al (1944) ascribed three cases of onyalai to the use of traditional medicine, the consensus of opinion is that this is not an aetiological factor (Gelfand, 1948; Squires, 1950). It is nevertheless true to the present day that a large percentage of patients in northern Namibia (personal observation) and patients in southern Africa (Edginton et al, 1972) will consult a traditional healer first when they take ill.

Nutritional factors

Many authors have commented on the well-nourished state of patients and that the disease was not related to periods of famine (Massey, 1904; Wellman, 1907; Gilkes, 1934; Squires, 1950; Gelfand, 1954). Ascorbic acid deficiency was postulated by Strangway and Strangway (1949), who also claimed therapeutic success with oral and intravenously administered lemon juice. However, they did state in the same article that the urinary vitamin C excretion of patients was normal. The ascorbic acid content of the liver is normal in onyalai (Gear, 1938).

The staple diet of the inhabitants of Namibia and Angola who develop onyalai is millet, and sorghum or maize in some other populations with a high prevalence of onyalai (Strangway and Strangway, 1949; Edginton et al, 1972; Gildenhuys, 1974). McDonald (1952) was the last to report on a series of patients (36) who lived in a periurban environment, that of Johannesburg. Edginton et al (1972) commented that onyalai was much more prevalent in rural areas, and suggested the possible aetiological role of an environmental agent with specific effects on the platelets or megakaryocytes. Many of the inhabitants of Windhoek, the capital of Namibia, originate from areas to the north with a high prevalence of onyalai, but have of necessity changed their traditional way of life. Onyalai is seen rarely in the Windhoek state hospitals. Likewise, Ovambo long-term contract workers at the diamond mines on the Namibian west coast, who are provided with ample non-traditional meals and a sophisticated western environment, do not develop onyalai. These observations point to a link between the traditional way of life (possibly diet) and onyalai.

Gildenhuys (1974), who observed heavy growths of moulds on millet in the large reed storage baskets used in Ovamboland, questioned the role of mycotoxins in the aetiology. Four species of fungi which were isolated from the granary of a household of a patient with onyalai caused a haemorrhagic tendency and death when fed to New Hampshire day-old chicks and Wistar-derived rats. One of these fungi, *Phoma sorghina*, was also isolated from fresh samples of millet and grain sorghum in Ovamboland at harvest time, from millet, sorghum and peanuts in Mozambique, and grain sorghum obtained from the household of a patient with onyalai in the northern Transvaal (Rabie et al, 1975). Three other observations provide indirect evidence of an environmental aetiological factor, such as a mycotoxin: women who traditionally cultivate the lands and harvest, pound and cook the millet, sorghum or maize have a higher incidence of onyalai; the bullae are limited anatomically to the oropharynx stretching as far down as the uvula, and occasionally on the skin (Gilkes, 1934; Morris, 1934; Gear, 1938; Gelfand, 1944; personal observation at post mortem); the level of serum IgG platelet antibodies was significantly raised in 58 family and household members of five patients with onyalai compared with controls (Hesseling, 1983).

Infectious agents

The geographical distribution of onyalai in Africa falls within the 'malaria belt'. Acute *Plasmodium falciparum* malaria may be associated with thrombocytopenia which recovers after schizontocidal treatment (Horstmann et al, 1981), and also with the presence of IgG and IgM serum platelet antibodies (Louw et al, 1982). However, malarial parasites have never been observed in the peripheral blood of any of the patients with onyalai. Although the highest incidence of onyalai in the Kavango area coincides with the peak malaria season, the incidence is not statistically different from the incidence in other months. Morris (1934) succinctly remarked on the isolated incidents of the disease and the absence of spread to contacts, even in the crowded conditions of a gaol. No serological evidence of rickettsioses, leptospirosis, brucellosis (Wessels et al, 1986) and human T-cell leukaemia virus 1 (HTLV-1) infection (Van der Riet et al, 1984) has been found.

Immunological findings

Laufer (1953) proposed that onyalai was an allergic disease of the capillaries. Platelet survival in onyalai as measured with ^{51}Cr was markedly shortened and associated with a rise in radioactivity, mainly over the spleen, in four patients. Attempts to demonstrate a humoral thrombocytopenia-inducing factor in two of these patients failed however (Lurie et al, 1969).

Normal numbers of megakaryocytes in the bone marrow and a normal myelogram have been recorded repeatedly (Gear, 1938; Stein and Miller, 1943; Lewis and Lurie, 1953). IgG platelet antibodies were demonstrated in the serum of 23 out of 24 and IgM platelet antibodies in 18 of the same 24 patients with onyalai by Brink et al (1981), using the indirect platelet suspension immunofluorescence test (PSIFT) (Von dem Borne et al, 1978). These findings were subsequently confirmed with the indirect and direct PSIFT (Hesseling, 1983). Platelet-associated IgG (PAIgG) antibodies were measured (General Diagnostics ELISA platelet antibody assay) in the serum of 49 patients with onyalai, 10 patients with leprosy and 57 pregnant women, all from the Kavango territory in Namibia. Thirty-one patients with onyalai (63.2%) showed a raised PAIgG level (more than 109 ng IgG/10^7 platelets). None of the pregnant women or leprosy patients had a raised PAIgG (P. B. Hesseling and R. C. Cooper, unpublished observations).

McMillan et al (1987) assayed plasma autoantibodies against the platelet glycoprotein (GP) IIb/IIIa complex in 59 patients with chronic ITP, with an immunobead and microtitre-well assay using radioactive iodine-labelled anti-GP monoclonal antibodies. GPIIb/IIIa autoantibodies were noted in 21 patients (36%), GPIb autoantibodies in 11 patients (19%), and both GPIb and GPIIb/IIIa autoantibodies in 2 patients (3%). The same technique was applied to plasma of 14 personally verified cases of onyalai. In 12 (86%) patients, GPIIb/IIIa autoantibodies were demonstrated at a level exceeding three standard deviations compared with healthy controls, whilst no patients with onyalai demonstrated GPIb autoantibodies (B. Lawal et al, unpublished observations). The GPIIb/IIIa complex performs a key role in platelet aggregation by acting as a receptor for the adhesive fibrinogen, fibronectin and von Willebrand factors (Plow et al, 1985; Ruggeri et al, 1986). There is therefore a clear difference in the autoantibody response between chronic ITP and onyalai as measured with the same technique. This difference may explain in part why patients with onyalai bleed much more severely than patients with ITP.

Serum immunoglobulin IgA, IgG and IgM levels, complement fractions C3 and C4, total serum complement, circulating immune complex estimations and antinuclear antibody titres do not differ significantly in patients with onyalai and appropriate controls (Hesseling et al, 1986a). Brink et al (1981) measured serum platelet antibodies in children with ITP and patients with onyalai with the indirect PSIFT. In ITP a statistically significant association between platelet IgG antibody levels and the platelet count was noted and the recovery in the platelet count was associated with a decrease in antibody levels after 14–25 days. In patients with onyalai, IgG and IgM antibodies were present with equal frequency. Antibody levels did not decrease commensurate with the increase in the platelet count at day 14. The difference in immune response between patients under 14 years with ITP and patients with onyalai was statistically significant ($P<0.05$) using the Student *t* test.

HAEMATOPATHOLOGY

Profound thrombocytopenia is present in all the patients. Excessive blood loss in the acute phase of the disease is a cardinal feature and may be associated with a precipitous decline in the haemoglobin level. The total and differential white cell count is normal. The bone marrow is essentially within normal limits, with normal or increased megakaryocyte activity. Erythroid hyperplasia occurs in patients who have suffered marked blood loss. A prolonged bleeding time, increased capillary fragility, defective clot retraction and defective prothrombin consumption all illustrate the classical defects associated with thrombocytopenia (Stein and Miller, 1943). The platelets are morphologically normal when examined by scanning electron microscopy (S. Wolf-Coote and P. B. Hesseling, unpublished observations).

The findings at autopsy have been recorded by Gilkes (1934), Morris (1934), Blackie (1937), Gelfand (1943) and Stein and Miller (1943), and also observed by the author in two patients. The outstanding macroscopical pathological feature is the presence of oval or circular umbilicated trabeculated vesicles, which are filled with blood and restricted to the skin and the mucous membranes of the nose and oral cavity, extending as far down as the epiglottis. Petechial and larger haemorrhages may be present in the skin and visible internally in all the endothelial and serosal surfaces. Frank haemorrhage may occur in any organ, including the brain.

TREATMENT

The primary aim on admission should be to prevent unnecessary morbidity and mortality due to haemorrhagic shock. The policy of transfusing patients with whole blood whenever the haemoglobin dropped below 10 g/dl resulted in a decline in the mortality rate from 9.8% for 508 cases recorded in the English literature until 1980 (Hesseling, 1983) to 2.78% for 612 patients admitted to Rundu Hospital between 1981 and 1988 in the acute phase of the disease (Hesseling, 1990). The second objective is to improve the platelet count in order to minimize bleeding and to reduce the risk of cerebral haemorrhage, which caused four deaths (3.9%) amongst 103 patients during a first or subsequent episode of acute onyalai (Hesseling, 1987). Thirdly, general measures such as antiseptic mouthwashes and vitamin supplements improve the condition of the oral mucosa. Treatment with progesterone derivates, as used in contraception, may prevent severe menorrhagia in parous females who remain thrombocytopenic. In assessing the merits of the therapeutic interventions which are aimed at raising the platelet count, the natural tendency of a better recovery rate in the platelet count in young patients and in patients who suffer a first attack should be borne in mind. It is, however, difficult to justify a conservative treatment approach if the high risk of haemorrhagic shock and cerebral haemorrhage in the acute phase is taken into account.

Traditional healers are often consulted before the patient turns to modern medicine. The Mbukushu tribe in Kavango uses a remedy made from the bark and roots of the shivi tree, *Guibourtia coleosperma*, and the roots of the ironwood tree, *Ziziphus mucronata* (M. Fisch, personal communication). The Angoni tribe in Zimbabwe scald the roots of the mupungulila bush and then use the water as a mouthwash (Morris, 1934). In Angola the plants *Geigera wellmani* Hutch and a species of the plant *Albizzia* were employed by the local inhabitants (Wellman, 1907). An old Kwangali herbalist near Rundu, Namibia provided me with leaves of the mpeke tree, subsequently identified as the small sourplum, *Ximenia americana*. These are rubbed into a powder when dry and added to water for a short while, after which the extract is applied to the nose and oral cavity of patients with onyalai. Seeds of this tree are used elsewhere in Africa to tan leather.

The therapeutic effects of prednisolone, vincristine sulphate, splenectomy and low and high dose intravenous gammaglobulin have been investigated. In a prospective randomized trial, oral prednisolone at a dose of $3\,mg\,kg^{-1}\,day^{-1}$ was administered to 14 patients for 7 days after admission, whilst two other groups of 14 patients each were treated with ascorbic acid (as a placebo) and low dose intravenous gammaglobulin respectively. The outcome and change in the platelet count at weekly intervals was monitored for 3 weeks. No statistical difference was found between the three treatment groups (Hesseling et al, 1984a).

A splenectomy was performed in four adults with a history of repeated attacks of severe haemorrhage and who again had active bleeding which was difficult to control. A 14-year-old boy with one to three documented annual attacks in the preceding 6 years was also splenectomized. All the patients responded with a rise in the platelet count and cessation of haemorrhage within 24 hours. During a follow-up period of between 280 and 544 days, all the patients achieved a normal platelet count, which was sustained in three of the patients. However, two patients died at 280 days and 330 days, respectively, from haemorrhagic shock or cerebral haemorrhage during a clinical recurrence (Hesseling et al, 1984b). There is only one other brief mention of a splenectomy in two patients (Lurie et al, 1969).

The therapeutic effect of vincristine sulphate was assessed in a randomized trial in 40 patients sequentially admitted for acute onyalai. Of the 40 patients who remained thrombocytopenic or who were still bleeding actively 7 days after admission, 20 were randomized to receive either a vincristine sulphate bolus of 1.5 mg/m^2 or an equivalent volume of normal saline intravenously on days 8 and 15 respectively. Five out of ten patients who received vincristine achieved a platelet count of more than $100 \times 10^9/l$ on day 22, compared with two of the ten patients who received placebo. The numbers were small and the difference was not statistically significant (Hesseling et al, 1986b). The therapeutic effect of high dose immunoglobulin (Sandoglobulin), as reported by Imbach et al (1981) in ITP, was investigated in four patients admitted with onyalai. Immunoglobulin was infused on three successive days at a cumulative dose of 2 g/kg body weight. Clinical bleeding stopped within 3 days in all the patients. This was followed by a rise in the platelet count which was maintained over a 10–22-day follow-up period (Hesseling, 1991). These findings need to be confirmed in a larger number of patients with a longer follow-up period. The cost of intravenous gammaglobulin puts this therapy beyond the reach of the majority of patients with onyalai, who live in developing countries with limited financial and medical resources.

SUMMARY

Onyalai is an acquired form of immune thrombocytopenia which differs clinically, epidemiologically and immunologically from idiopathic thrombocytopenic purpura (Table 4). The clinical hallmark is haemorrhagic bullae on the mucosa of the oronasopharynx. Haemorrhage from ruptured bullae, epistaxis or gastrointestinal bleeding is severe and may cause shock and death. The disease is limited to some black populations of central southern Africa, with a recorded incidence of one per 660 inhabitants per year in the Kavango territory of Namibia. The majority of patients demonstrate both IgG and IgM serum platelet antibodies and serum platelet glycoprotein IIb/IIIa autoantibodies. Chronic thrombocytopenia often ensues and recurrent episodes of clinical bleeding are common. Treatment directed at the

Table 4. Major differences between onyalai and ITP.

	Onyalai	ITP
1.	Limited to Africa between the equator and 30° south latitude	Ubiquitous
2.	Restricted to some negroid populations	Affects all ethnic groups
3.	Incidence 151/100 000 per annum	Incidence 6–11/100 000 per annum (Newland, 1987)
4.	Linked to traditional diet and life-style	Not linked to cultural habits
5.	Haemorrhagic bullae a clinical hallmark	Haemorrhagic bullae rarely present
6.	Newborns of affected mothers have normal platelet counts	Newborns of mothers have a 33% risk of thrombocytopenia
7.	Seldom responds to corticosteroid therapy	Often responds to corticosteroid therapy
8.	Majority of patients require blood transfusion(s)	Minority of patients require blood transfusions
9.	IgM and IgG platelet antibodies in serum	Mainly IgG platelet antibodies in serum
10.	GPIIb/IIIa platelet autoantibodies in serum in 86%	GPIIb/IIIa platelet autoantibodies in serum in 36%
11.	GPIb platelet autoantibodies absent in serum	GPIb platelet autoantibodies sometimes present in serum
12.	Recorded average mortality rate in the acute phase 9.8% until 1983	Mortality rate below 1% in acute phase
13.	Aetiology unknown	Viral disease may precipitate.

prevention of haemorrhagic shock reduced the mortality rate in the acute phase from 9.8 to 2.8%. Standard dose prednisolone does not increase the platelet count. Vincristine sulphate may benefit some patients and splenectomy is indicated in patients with severe uncontrollable haemorrhage. High dose intravenous gammaglobulin may be followed by a rise in the platelet count and cessation of haemorrhage. The aetiology is unknown. The possible aetiological role of mycotoxins from contaminated millet, sorghum or maize requires further investigation.

Acknowledgements

I thank the Ministry of Health, Namibia, for providing access to all their facilities, and Ms J. Barnes and Ms W. Visser for assistance with the preparation of the manuscript.

REFERENCES

Almeida BM & Kasili EG (1983) Childhood idiopathic thrombocytopenic purpura at the Kenyatta National Hospital, Nairobi. *East African Medical Journal* **60:** 432–437.

Barss P (1976) Diagnosis and management of onyalai. *Tropical Doctor* **6:** 50–53.

Blackie WK (1937) Onyalai: a review. *Transactions of the Royal Society of Tropical Medicine and Hygiene* **31:** 207–226.

Brink S, Hesseling PB, Amadhila S & Visser HS (1981) Platelet antibodies in immune thrombocytopenic purpura and onyalai. *South African Medical Journal* **59:** 855–858.

Edginton ME, Hodkins J & Seftel HC (1972) Disease patterns in a South African rural Bantu population. *South African Medical Journal* **46:** 968–976.

Gear J (1938) Onyalai: a form of purpura occurring in tropical Africa. Report of cases occurring in South Africa. *South African Medical Journal* **12:** 632–637.

Gear JHS, Yeo RM & Bodenstein JC (1944) The aetiology of onyalai. *South African Medical Journal* **18:** 265–266.
Gelfand M (1943) Onyalai. *Clinical Proceedings* **2:** 281–286.
Gelfand M (1944) The haemorrhagic bulla in onyalai. *Clinical Proceedings* **3:** 255–259.
Gelfand M (1948) A few of the rarer diseases seen in Africa. *East African Medical Journal* **25:** 447–453.
Gelfand M (1954) Onyalai: a clinical study. *Transactions of the Royal Society of Tropical Medicine and Hygiene* **48:** 353–359.
Gilbert B (1943) Onyalai: a tropical condition characterized by haemorrhages: its gynaecological aspects. *Journal of Obstetrics and Gynaecology of the British Empire* **50:** 437–439.
Gildenhuys J (1974) *Die siekteprofiel van die Ovambo en 'n oorsig van die belangrikste voorkomingsmaatreëls*. MD thesis, University of Pretoria, pp 289–307.
Gilkes HA (1934) Two little-known diseases of Northern Rhodesia: onyalai and chiufa. *Transactions of the Royal Society of Tropical Medicine and Hygiene* **27:** 491–498.
Goldin R & Gelfand M (1980) Idiopathic thrombocytopenic purpura and onyalai in Zimbabwean Africans. *Central African Journal of Medicine* **26:** 236–239.
Hesseling PB (1983) *Onyalai: an epidemiological study*. MD thesis, University of Stellenbosch.
Hesseling PB (1985) Onyalai in pregnancy. Effects on the mother and the newborn. *South African Medical Journal* **67:** 252–253.
Hesseling PB (1987) Onyalai in Namibia. Clinical manifestations, haematological findings, course and management of 103 patients in the Kavango territory. *Transactions of the Royal Society of Tropical Medicine and Hygiene* **81:** 193–196.
Hesseling PB (1990) Onyalai at Rundu, Namibia 1981–1988: age, sex, morbidity, mortality and seasonal variation of 612 hospitalized patients. *Transactions of the Royal Society of Tropical Medicine and Hygiene* **84:** 605–607.
Hesseling PB (1991) High dose immunoglobulin therapy in four patients with onyalai. *Transactions of the Royal Society of Tropical Medicine and Hygiene* **85:** 131–132.
Hesseling PB, Girdle-Brown B & Smit J (1984a) Onyalai: treatment with prednisolone, intravenous gammaglobulin and ascorbic acid. *South African Medical Journal* **66:** 917–918.
Hesseling PB, Oosthuizen E, Pretorius L, Swart A & Steynberg J (1984b) Splenectomy in onyalai. *South African Medical Journal* **66:** 580–582.
Hesseling PB, Cooper RC & Girdle-Brown B (1986a) Serum immunoglobulin and complement values in onyalai: comparison with Black, San and White inhabitants of Kavango, SWA/Namibia. *South African Medical Journal* **70:** 203–205.
Hesseling PB, Girdle-Brown B & Smit J (1986b) Onyalai: therapeutic effects of vincristine sulphate. A prospective randomised trial in 40 patients in Kavango, Namibia. *South African Medical Journal* **70:** 201–202.
Horstmann RD, Dietrich M, Bienzle U & Rosche H (1981) Malaria-induced thrombocytopenia. *Blut* **42:** 157–164.
Imbach P, d'Apuzzo V, Hirt A et al (1981) High-dose intravenous gammaglobulin for idiopathic thrombocytopenic purpura in childhood. *Lancet* **i:** 1228–1231.
Kaplan C, Daffos F, Forestier F et al (1990) Fetal platelet counts in thrombocytopenic pregnancy. *Lancet* **336:** 972–982.
Laufer WE (1953) Onyalai. *South African Medical Journal* **27:** 657–659.
Lewis SM & Lurie A (1953) Onyalai: a clinical and laboratory survey. *Journal of Tropical Medicine and Hygiene* **56:** 281–289.
Louw W, Stevens K & Nel J (1982) Platelet antibodies in malaria. *Internist* **3:** 15.
Lurie A, Katz J, Ludwin SK, Seftel HC & Metz J (1969) Platelet life-span and sites of platelet sequestration in onyalai. *British Medical Journal* **4:** 146–148.
McDonald AP (1952) *Aspekte van plaatjiegetalle in gesondheid in Onyalai en ander siekteto-estande by die Bantoe*. MD thesis, University of Pretoria.
McMillan R, Tani P, Millard F et al (1987) Platelet-associated and plasma anti-glycoprotein autoantibodies in chronic ITP. *Blood* **70:** 1040–1045.
Massey AY (1904) Onyalai: a disease of Central Africa. *Journal of Tropical Medicine* **7:** 269–270.
Mense C (1906) *Einige wenig bekannte Krankheitsbilder. Handbuch der Tropenkrankheiten 3*, 789 pp. Leipzig: Barth.
Metz J, Kramer S & Cassel R (1958) Acute idiopathic thrombocytopenia in the Bantu. *South African Journal of Medical Science* **23:** 93–100.

Morris RM (1934) Onyalai in Southern Rhodesia. *Native Affairs Department Annual (Salisbury)* **12:** 17–19.
Mukiibi JM & Kyobe J (1982) Chronic idiopathic thrombocytopenic purpura (ITP) in Kenyan Africans. *Journal of Tropical Medicine and Hygiene* **85:** 165–168.
Newland AC (1987) Idiopathic thrombocytopenic purpura and IgG. A review. *Journal of Infection* **15** (supplement 1)**:** 14–49.
Plow EF, Piersbacher MD, Ruoslahti E, Marguerie G & Ginsberg MH (1985) The effect of Arg-Gly-Asp-containing peptides on fibrinogen and Von Willebrand binding to platelets. *Proceedings of the National Academy of Sciences of the USA* **81:** 8057–8061.
Rabie CJ, Van Rensburg SJ, Van der Watt JJ & Lübben A (1975) Onyalai: the possible involvement of a mycotoxin produced by *Phoma sorghina* in the aetiology. *South African Medical Journal* **49:** 1647–1650.
Ruggeri ZM, Houghton RA, Russel SR & Zimmerman TS (1986) Inhibition of platelet function with synthetic peptides designed to be high affinity antagonists of fibrinogen binding to platelets. *Proceedings of the National Academy of Sciences of the USA* **83:** 5708–5712.
Shee JC (1961) Onyalai in an elderly European woman. *Transactions of the Royal Society of Tropical Medicine and Hygiene* **55:** 239–241.
Squires BT (1943) A further note on onyalai in the Bechuanaland Protectorate. *South African Medical Journal* **17:** 292–293.
Squires BT (1950) Onyalai in the Bechuanaland Protectorate. *Transactions of the Royal Society of Tropical Medicine and Hygiene* **43:** 667–672.
Stein HB & Miller E (1943) Acute thrombocytopenic purpura associated with haemorrhagic bullae with special reference to onyalai. *South African Journal of Medical Science* **8:** 1–24.
Strangway WE & Strangway AK (1949) Ascorbic acid deficiency in the African disease onyalai. *Archives of Internal Medicine* **83:** 372–376.
Van der Riet F de St J, Allan BR & Hesseling PB (1984) Antibodies to human T-cell leukaemia virus protein P24 in healthy and diseased persons in SWA/Namibia. *South African Medical Journal* **66:** 515–516.
Von dem Borne AEGKr, Verheugt FWA, Oosterhof F et al (1978) A simple immunofluorescence test for the detection of platelet antibodies. *British Journal of Haematology* **39:** 195–207.
Wellman FC (1904) Brief conspectus of the tropical diseases common in the Highlands of West Central Africa. *Journal of Tropical Medicine* **7:** 52–56.
Wellman FC (1907) Report on a peculiar disease of tropical Africa called 'onyalai'. *Boston Medical and Surgical Journal* **157:** 365–367.
Wessels G, Hesseling PB & Cooper RC (1986) Q Fever, OX19, OX2 and leptospirosis antibodies in patients with onyalai and in negroid, bushman and white inhabitants of Kavango, Namibia. *Transactions of the Royal Society of Tropical Medicine and Hygiene* **80:** 847–848.
Wicks ACB (1972) Onyalai—a disappearing disease entity. A case report and review of the literature. *Central African Journal of Medicine* **18:** 93–97.
Wiseman BK, Doan CA & Wilson SJ (1940) The present status of thrombocytopenic purpura with special reference to diagnosis and treatment. *Journal of the American Medical Association* **115:** 8–14.

9

Epidemiology of aplastic anaemia

EDWARD COLIN GORDON-SMITH
SURAPOL ISSARAGRISIL

Acquired aplastic anaemia is a rare disorder of bone marrow function, of unknown pathogenesis and disputed aetiology. It is possible that there is heterogeneity in the pathogenesis of the aplasia between cases, even when the cause is thought to be the same, though this hypothesis stems perhaps more from ignorance of the many probable factors which lead to bone marrow failure, rather than positive evidence of important differences between individual cases. The requirement for accurate information about the epidemiology of aplastic anaemia arises from the suspicion that the disease can be caused by drugs or chemicals used in ordinary medical, industrial or domestic practice. Since there are no tests to confirm or refute such an association in any individual case, suspicion can only be converted into evidence by accurate epidemiological studies. The word 'evidence' is deliberately chosen to highlight the often litigious aspects of aplastic anaemia when a causative agent is assumed, and to indicate that scientific evidence and legal evidence are not necessarily the same thing. In this chapter we examine the geographic distribution of aplastic anaemia, its incidence and the epidemiological association with drugs, chemicals and viruses.

Definition

One of the difficulties in determining the incidence of aplastic anaemia has been the imprecision of criteria for diagnosis. Diagnosis requires the presence of pancytopenia in the peripheral blood together with hypocellularity of the bone marrow where normal haemopoietic tissue is replaced by fat cells. Negative criteria include the absence of abnormal cells in peripheral blood and in the bone marrow, absence of major dysplastic features in the bone marrow, a negative Ham's test and no evidence of exposure to cytotoxic drugs or radiation which would produce an inevitable aplasia. Unfortunately, such straightforward criteria may not always be fulfilled. Variations in presentation may affect the apparent incidence of aplasia both upwards and downwards. Aplastic anaemia may present as a single cytopenia (most commonly amegakaryocytic thrombocytopenia) or may be associated with a patchily cellular marrow (Lewis, 1965) with so called 'hot pockets' (Kansu and Erslev, 1976): these may deceive if only a

Baillière's Clinical Haematology—
Vol. 5, No. 2, April 1992
ISBN 0-7020-1627-6

single marrow is taken, either by excluding the true cases of aplastic anaemia or, more commonly, leading to the inclusion of cases of pancytopenia which are associated with myelodysplastic syndromes (MDS) rather than aplastic anaemia (IAAAS, 1987). Furthermore, aplastic anaemia is an evolving or unstable disease. In the early stages it appears to be a failure of haemopoiesis with depressed proliferation and differentiation from all haemopoietic stem cells, and such recovery as does occur is polyclonal. Clonal evolution to paroxysmal nocturnal haemoglobinuria (Josten et al, 1991) MDS or acute leukaemia may also take place, perhaps in as many as 25–40% of cases over a 10-year period (de Planque et al, 1988; Tichelli et al, 1988). Such difficulties in diagnosis should be borne in mind when trying to assess the incidence of aplastic anaemia in different populations from the published literature, particularly where retrospective studies relying on death certificates and medical records have been carried out.

The major prospective studies on the epidemiology of aplastic anaemia which have been carried out recently, the IAAAS (1986) and the French Cooperative Group study (Mary et al, 1990), have used strict criteria for the inclusion of cases coinciding with the original definition given above. The exclusion of cases where the diagnosis is doubtful has probably led to an underestimate of the true incidence.

Geography of aplastic anaemia

The incidence of aplastic anaemia is generally held to be several times higher in the Far East, including China, Japan, Thailand and the Indian subcontinent, compared with Europe and the United States. This belief is based on observations of hospital practice and, as will be appreciated from the introduction, firm data on incidence is difficult to obtain, so that the differences may not be as great as generally assumed. Studies from Africa (Mukiibi et al, 1987) suggest that the disease is at least as common as in Europe.

WESTERN EUROPE AND THE USA

The practice of haematology, the diagnostic services available and the recording of cases of aplastic anaemia make western Europe and the USA relatively uniform through their common practices for purposes of epidemiology. The environment of these areas, the exposure to viruses (as measured by the prevalence of hepatitis B in blood donors for example) and the controls for the prescription of drugs suggest that the populations may be considered to have comparable risk factors also, or at least measurable risk factors. The overall genetic pools of the white populations in each region are likely to be similar and allow some limited conclusions to be drawn from observing individual rates in other groups with different gene pools. Thus, differences in the incidence of aplastic anaemia of Chinese, Japanese and south-eastern Asian populations living in the USA or Europe, compared with the same populations living in the regions of origin, could help to indicate the relative importance of environmental factors and genetic susceptibility in the pathogenesis of the disease.

Incidence

Retrospective studies

Early attempts to establish the incidence of aplastic anaemia concentrated on the association of the disease with exposure to drugs, in particular Atabrine (quinacrine, mepacrine) (Custer, 1946) and chloramphenicol (Wallerstein et al, 1969). This type of association will be considered later. One of the earliest population-based attempts to determine incidence in Europe was made by Böttiger and Westerholm (1972) in Sweden. This study was also designed to investigate the incidence of drug-induced aplastic anaemia (and agranulocytosis) in the Uppsala region of Sweden, but suffered from the disadvantage that bone marrow biopsies were not employed in the diagnosis and many patients probably had MDS, particularly in the older age group. The reported incidence of 13 cases per million of the population per annum is now considered to be an overestimate (IAAAS, 1987). The survey covered a 5-year period in a relatively stable population, and it is interesting to note that the incidence of aplastic anaemia (including the MDS cases) and agranulocytosis seems to have remained constant over that period despite considerable changes in prescribing habits, notably the sharp drop in the use of chloramphenicol. A study carried out in Israel during the 5-year period 1961–1965 (Modan et al, 1975) showed an incidence of 7.1 per million in males and 8.7 per million in females throughout the country. The study was conducted to test the suggestion that Jews were less sensitive to the development of chloramphenicol-induced aplasia than non-Jewish populations. In the event, an association with chloramphenicol was present in about 25% of these cases, similar to that in other chloramphenicol studies of that time from the USA (Smick et al, 1964; Wallerstein et al, 1969).

In a retrospective study of severe aplastic anaemia occurring in children under the age of 15 years in Denmark, Clausen (1986) estimated an incidence of 2.2 per million over the 15-year period 1967–1982. During this period 39 children were diagnosed as having severe aplastic anaemia, three of these having constitutional aplasia. Rather higher incidences of aplasia in the total population have been reported from the USA. Szklo and colleagues (1985), using medical records and death certificates to calculate the incidence of aplastic anaemia in an urban population of Baltimore, identified 118 cases of acquired aplastic anaemia from all ethnic groups in the 8-year period 1970–1978 and found an incidence of just over 6 per million of the population per year in the white population. In a neighbouring 'more rural' setting, Linet and colleagues (1989) found an incidence of 8.5 per million per year, also in the white population: the period covered by this study was 1970–1981 and it should be noted that the total number of aplastic cases on which the incidence rates are based was only 20, compared with 94 from the urban Baltimore population. The very small number of cases seen when relatively small populations are studied detracts from the reliability of such incidence rates, particularly as the rural study was based on an observation of a 'cluster' of cases, which would already bias the sample towards a falsely high incidence (Linet et al, 1985).

Prospective studies

Prospective studies based on large populations should provide a better estimate of the disease. Problems of reporting and verifying cases still remain. The IAAAS (1986) examined the incidence of aplastic anaemia from varied populations throughout Europe and Israel, with a total population of 20.5 million, in the 4-year period 1980–1984. Not all the centres in the study took part throughout the whole period, but allowance was made for this. A total number of 168 cases of aplastic anaemia were identified during this time, giving an incidence of 2.2 per million per year calculated as a population weighted average of the age- and sex-standardized region-specific rates. Between regions in this study, the annual incidence rate varied from 0.6 to 3.1 per million. In the French epidemiological study (Mary et al, 1990) an attempt was made to identify all cases of aplastic anaemia in the country during the 3-year period 1984–1987. Of 292 cases recorded, 250 were confirmed as having aplastic anaemia. The population of France during this period was estimated from the national census, with population increase projections being taken into account: the population studied was just over 55 million, and the overall incidence of aplastic anaemia was estimated to be 1.51 per million per annum. In the UK, a prospective study was carried out by the Leukaemia Research Fund Centre for Clinical Epidemiology as part of a more detailed survey of the incidence of leukaemia in defined areas of the UK. Between 1985 and 1990, 181 cases were identified (R. A. Cartwright, personal communication). The data are somewhat crude and the cases have not all been verified. The population studied numbered just over 15 million, giving an incidence of about 2.4 per million per annum. The results of published series from Europe and the USA are shown in Table 1.

Age distribution

A number of attempts have been made to estimate the incidence of aplastic anaemia at different age groups in European and American populations. In Böttiger and Westerholm's study (1972), the annual incidence rose from 4 per million in the under 25 age group, to 74 per million in the population aged more than 70 years. The very steep rise in incidence from 11 per million in patients under 65 probably reflects the inclusion of patients with MDS in the older age group. In the Baltimore study (Szklo et al, 1985), amongst the white male population, there was an incidence around 4 per million in the under 20 age group, falling to 0.5 per million between 20 and 40 and rising again over 60 to around 25 per million per year. As mentioned above, Clausen in Denmark (1986) found an annual incidence of 2.2 cases per million children. In the South Carolina study (Linet et al, 1989), again there was a higher annual incidence of 9.7 per million in white males aged between

Table 1. Studies on the incidence of aplastic anaemia from USA and Europe.

Type of study	Study period	Region	Source of cases	No. of cases	Combined incidence $\times 10^6$/year	Incidence $\times 10^6$/year Male	Incidence $\times 10^6$/year Female	Reference
Retrospective	1961–65	Israel	MR	93	7.8	7.1	8.7	Modan et al (1975)
	1964–68	Sweden	MR/CR	80	13.0	13.0	13.0	Böttiger and Westerholm (1972)
	1970–78	Baltimore, USA	MR/DC	94 (Whites)	~6.0	7.0	6.1	Szklo et al (1985)
	1970–81	South Carolina, USA	MR/DC	20 (Whites)	11.7	5.4	—	Linet et al (1989)
	1971–78	Northern Region, UK	MR	172	6.6	4.2	10.3	Davies and Walker (1986)
Prospective	1980–84	Parts of Europe and Israel	MR	168	2.2			IAAAS (1986)
	1984–87	France	MR/E	250	1.4	1.6	1.3	Mary et al (1990)
	1985	Parts of UK	MR/E	49	2.3	1.4	3.2	Cartwright et al (1988)
	1985–90	Parts of UK	MR/E	181	2.4	—	—	R. A. Cartwright (personal communication)

CR, computer record; DC, death certificate; E, enquiry; MR, medical records.

10 and 20, falling in the next two decades to 2.8 per million and rising in those over 60 to 43.5 per million. The trends in both the Baltimore and the South Carolina series were much more marked in males than in females. The French study (Mary et al, 1990) likewise found a bimodal distribution of aplastic anaemia more marked in males than females: the annual incidence rose from 1.34 per million below the age of 15 to 2.38 per million in those aged 15–29, fell to below 1 per million between the ages of 30 and 60, and rose again in old age to 2.18 per million. In the UK study (R. A. Cartwright, personal communication), an incidence of 1.5 per million of the population may be calculated for patients less than 20 years old, falling markedly between 20 and 60, with a rise in the older age group. In this study the difference between male and female is less pronounced. Combining the results from all these studies in a consensus fashion suggests that there is a bimodal distribution of aplastic anaemia, with one peak somewhere between the ages of 10 and 25, a trough between the ages of 30 and 60, and a further rise which may be exponential in the older age group. It will be appreciated that difficulties in diagnosis increase also with age.

Male : female ratios

The effect of the sex of the patient on the incidence of aplastic anaemia in Europe and the USA has been assessed in most published studies and has produced somewhat conflicting results. The study of Böttiger and Westerholm (1972) showed no difference in the sex distribution of aplastic anaemia in Sweden, but the study in Israel by Modan et al (1975) showed a slight preponderance of females (male 7.1 and female 8.7 per million per annum). In the UK study there was also a slight preponderance of females, mainly in the older age groups, but adjustment had not been made for alterations of the sex ratio of this older group. Clausen (1986) found a preponderance of males in the under 15 age group (males 23, females 13), whereas both the American studies showed a higher incidence in white males compared with white females, though the difference was much greater in the South Carolina study (Linet et al, 1989) than in Baltimore (Szklo et al, 1985). In the French study (Mary et al, 1990) the number of cases overall were equal between the sexes, but again in the age distribution young males had almost 1.5 times the incidence of young females.

Effects of ethnic origin

Data are somewhat limited for making an assessment of race upon the incidence of aplastic anaemia. The two American studies quoted (Szklo et al, 1985; Linet et al, 1986) suggested that white males had a higher incidence than non-white males in both studies, but that non-white females had a higher incidence than white females. However, the number of non-white males recorded in each group was very low and it would be injudicious to draw too many conclusions from such an observation. In the European studies attempts have been made to determine whether Jewish people have a higher incidence of aplastic anaemia compared with the non-Jewish population (Modan et al, 1975; IAAAS, 1986), and in neither report has there been any convincing evidence of a difference between the two groups. Differences between groups which were found in the IAAAS study (1986), between Budapest and other European centres included in the study, probably reflect the difficulties of low numbers, since only three cases were reported in Budapest during this period, a rate of just over one case per annum.

Role of drugs in aetiology

There are no tests available which demonstrate that a particular drug or agent is responsible for aplastic anaemia in any individual case. The implication of drugs in the aetiology of aplastic anaemia depends on observations which properly fall into the realm of epidemiology. The probability that a drug is involved increases if the drug was the only one administered, if it was taken within 6 months of the presentation of the aplasia, if the patient had been exposed to the drug before and if other cases have been reported. Perhaps the best study of drug-related aplasia was that conducted on American soldiers taking Atabrine as malarial prophylaxis during World War II (Custer, 1946). He was able to show clearly the increase in cases of aplastic anaemia in soldiers who had received Atabrine, particularly when good discipline had made sure the drug was taken, compared with those who had not. This study was possible because a very large number of otherwise healthy people were exposed to a single agent. With most associations these factors do not hold true; for example, most patients who take non-steroidal anti-inflammatory drugs (NSAIDs) and develop aplastic anaemia have an underlying connective tissue disease, often rheumatoid arthritis, for which they took the NSAID in the first place. If an association does exist between the NSAIDs and aplasia, it may hold true only for patients with an underlying systemic disease of this type. Such observations may detract from the conclusions derived from even the best case-controlled studies of the disease.

The association of chloramphenicol with aplastic anaemia also indicates the importance of proper epidemiological studies. It was predicted, on the basis of the similarity of chemical structure between chloramphenicol and amidopyrine, that chloramphenicol would produce blood dyscrasias (Smadel, 1949) and the first case of aplastic anaemia was reported in 1950 in a patient who received a prolonged course of the drug (Rich et al, 1950). Many further reports of the association followed, including some in which low doses of chloramphenicol preceded the onset of aplasia (Cone and Abelson, 1952). This observation led to the idea that the development of aplastic anaemia is independent of the dose of chloramphenicol which is administered, and indeed cases of aplastic anaemia have been recorded following the administration of chloramphenicol as eye drops or eye ointment (Fraunfelder et al, 1982). However, review of the world literature makes the association of aplastic anaemia with chloramphenicol eye drops somewhat difficult to sustain. Fewer than 20 cases are documented covering the 40 years since chloramphenicol was introduced. Some of the cases where clinical details are given render the temporal association between eye drops and the onset of aplasia not very convincing, and there is no denominator of the number of chloramphenicol eye drop or ointment prescriptions given over this period of time. It may be that the incidence of aplastic anaemia is not higher in this group of patients than in the general population, or may be only marginally so. An attempt was made to estimate the effect of chloramphenicol on the incidence of aplastic anaemia in California (Smick et al, 1964). In this study 138 deaths due to aplastic anaemia were identified, of which 30 (22%) gave a history of exposure to chloramphenicol. These authors put the risk of developing aplastic anaemia following exposure to chloramphenicol as 1:60 000 compared with between 1:24 500 and 1:40 800 given in an earlier study (Wallerstein et al, 1969). An earlier study had found that 47% of aplastic anaemia cases were associated with chloramphenicol use (Welch et al, 1954). It is also interesting that the overall rate of death from aplastic anaemia in California between 1949 and 1961 remained constant at about 4.5 per million per year over this whole period, despite an enormous increase and then a fall in sales of chloramphenicol during that time. These studies led to a great reduction in the use of chloramphenicol throughout Europe and the USA. Thus the two case-controlled studies (IAAAS, 1986; Linet et al, 1989) record only one case of chloramphenicol-induced aplastic anaemia. Williams and colleagues (1973) found that in their population of patients with aplastic anaemia there was a significant history of re-exposure to chloramphenicol preceding the onset of aplastic anaemia.

The chloramphenicol story illustrates the role of anecdote in the epidemiology. A suggestion that chloramphenicol-induced aplastic anaemia was unknown in south America (Aladjem, 1969) produced the swift response that, at least in Colombia, it was 'not rare at all' (Sarasti, 1970) and furthermore that the incidence had 'decreased sharply' when chloramphenicol sales were controlled (Ghitis, 1970). Unfortunately, none of the observations were controlled. An incidence of 6.0 per million was found in a study based on a defined area of Buenos Aires (Aggio et al, 1988), similar to European and American rates (Table 1).

The IAAAS (1986) study examined exposure to drugs in the 180 days before hospital admission for aplastic anaemia. Case controls were matched as closely as possible for age and sex and were hospital patients admitted at approximately the same time as each aplastic anaemia patient. No normal controls were used. In this study, indomethacin, diclofenac and butazones were found to have an increased risk of promoting aplastic anaemia. The study from Baltimore (Linet et al, 1989) failed to show any association with drug exposure, probably because small numbers (59) of newly diagnosed cases were studied. They were matched with 59 normal controls for age, sex and location by random digit dialling. No study in Europe or the USA has yet shown any clear-cut change in the incidence of aplastic anaemia with time, despite the introduction, exploitation and reduction in the use of a whole variety of drugs thought to be associated with its aetiology.

Occupational and domestic exposures

There have been only two case-controlled studies of aplastic anaemia in which occupational exposure has been taken into account. The study by Linet et al (1989) found that exposure to paint, either through occupation or domestic use, was six times more common in patients with aplastic anaemia than in the controls. Exposure to benzene also seemed to have an increased risk ratio. Wang and Grufferman (1981) failed to find any excess exposure to pesticides in patients with aplastic anaemia compared with their case controls, and no such association was found in the Baltimore study (Szklo et al, 1985). Despite the failure to demonstrate an excess risk associated with exposure to organochlorine pesticides, case reports continue to suggest that there may be such an association (Rugman and Cosstick, 1990). γ-Hexachlorocyclohexane (γ-benzenehexachloride, lindane) and pentachlorophenol, agents used in preservation of wood, are the most commonly implicated. γ-Hexachlorocyclohexane was also used to treat children with lice, but there have been no excess reports of aplastic anaemia following this type of exposure, although concerns have been expressed (Wilkinson, 1988). The argument for the association of γ-hexachlorocyclohexane with the aetiology of aplastic anaemia thus lacks controlled epidemiological evidence and is based on the temporal association in individual cases and the accumulation of reports of the association.

In a study of shoe workers heavily exposed to benzene in Italy, there were seven cases of aplastic anaemia (six males and one female) during the period studied, 1959–1984 (Paci et al, 1989), compared with an expected incidence of 0.38. In the same study, six cases of leukaemia were observed compared with 1.5 expected. A high rate of leukaemia had also been found in Turkey amongst those workers exposed to benzene (Aksoy et al, 1974; Aksoy and Erdem, 1978), although aplastic anaemia was not recorded in excess.

Virus infections

Virus infections frequently produce transient cytopenia (Baranski and Young, 1987), sometimes in a predictable fashion, for example the reticulocytopenia produced by parvovirus B19. Numerous case reports suggest that rarely a virus infection may be followed by the development of aplastic anaemia (Young and Mortimer, 1984). The majority of cases indicate an association with hepatitis (Hagler et al, 1975). It is interesting that in this study there was a high incidence of both hepatitis-like illness and exposure to chloramphenicol prior to the aplasia, supporting a view that aplastic anaemia may represent a 'multiple hit' disorder. The case control study from Baltimore (Linet et al, 1989) also found an excess exposure to virus infection in aplastic anaemia patients compared with controls, although the nature of the virus infection was not identified. The most common type of hepatitis infections reported are non-A, non-B infections but hepatitis C does not appear to be a major cause despite interesting findings in liver transplant patients in the USA (Tzakis et al, 1988), not observed in the UK (Forbes et al, 1989).

APLASTIC ANAEMIA IN THE FAR EAST

There is a widespread belief that aplastic anaemia is more common in the Far East than in the West (Aoki et al, 1978; Young et al, 1986). This belief is based mainly on the number of patients seen annually in Asian hospitals compared with western hospitals (Whang, 1978). Forty new cases were seen annually at the Chinese Academy of Medical Sciences, Tienjin, China and 18 annually at Kyungpook National University Hospital, Korea. In contrast, the annual number of new patients seen in hospital in the West is much lower, being 2.3 at the University of Virginia Hospital, 4.2 at the University of Utah and Salt Lake City Veterans Administration Hospital, and 3.9 at St Vincent's Hospital, Melbourne (Whang, 1978). In the UK the average population served by a district hospital is 250 000, and such district hospitals may see one new patient every 2 years. On the other hand, St George's Hospital, London is a referral centre for aplastic anaemia patients and between 20 and 30 new patients are seen each year. In the French study (Mary et al, 1990), 83 hospitals saw 250 patients over a 3-year period, an average of one new patient per hospital per year. The average population served by these 83 hospitals would be theoretically 660 000. The number of patients seen at a major referral centre, such as the Hôpital St Louis in Paris, is higher: 15–20 per annum (Professor E. Gluckman, personal communication). Thus, the use of hospital admissions as an indicator of the incidence of disease has to be viewed with some caution.

Based on the autopsy rate of patients with aplastic anaemia, the disease might be at least three times higher in the Far East than in the West. It was reported that the autopsy rate for the disease in Japan was 0.7%, whereas that in Texas was 0.28% and in Vienna 0.21% (Corrigan, 1974). Comparison of age-adjusted mortality statistics revealed annual rates in Japan of 9.2 per million of the population, compared with 3 per million in western Europe and 5 per million in north America (Aoki et al, 1980), although the wide range reported from Europe and the USA should be considered. Young et al (1986) reported that aplastic anaemia appears to be almost as common as acute myeloid leukaemia in the Far East, whereas in most western hospitals acute leukaemia is five to ten times more common than aplastic anaemia.

In Thailand the prevalence of aplastic anaemia appears to be high. At Siriraj Hospital in Bangkok, between 49 and 82 new cases of aplastic anaemia are seen annually and more than 1000 cases have been documented in the haematological clinic. Siriraj Hospital is one of the two large teaching hospitals in Mahidol University and one of ten major Medical Schools in Thailand. The hospital has 2400 beds and serves half the population of Bangkok. In addition, nearly half the patients are self-referred or referred by physicians from other regions of the country. Table 2 shows the distribution of aplastic anaemia and related disorders compared with haematological malignancies seen during the period 1971–1989 at the Division of Haematology, Department of Medicine, Siriraj Hospital. The number of cases of aplastic anaemia in proportion to the number of cases of acute leukaemia is strikingly high. Of course this may reflect selective referral

Table 2. Number of patients with aplastic anaemia, related disorders and haematologic malignancies seen at the Division of Haematology, Siriraj Hospital, Bangkok.

	1971	1972	1973	1974	1975	1976	1977	1978	1979	1980	1981	1982	1983	1984	1985	1986	1987	1988	1989
Aplastic anaemia	60	64	64	71	49	65	57	54	61	61	82	62	59	68	67	54	60	74	62
PNH	4	4	4	3	7	7	3	2	1	1	7	5	5	8	7	12	9	9	14
Agranulocytosis	1	1	2	3	2	4	7	5	2	2	5	6	1	5	3	1	7	5	7
Acute leukaemia	54	65	75	65	73	77	65	93	106	106	130	113	106	114	162	138	151	134	135
CML/CLL	18/1	25/3	17/4	25/3	30/3	25/4	27/4	35/2	34/3	30/2	32/2	37/8	35/5	37/3	44/1	37/11	25/6	33/9	27/12
Malignant lymphoma	71	65	58	61	74	70	90	93	96	97	115	115	151	125	159	165	168	179	167
Multiple myeloma	4	5	3	7	3	6	16	10	17	17	19	19	17	24	22	26	22	14	19
Ratio AA:AL	1.11	0.99	0.85	1.09	0.67	0.84	0.88	0.58	0.58	0.58	0.63	0.55	0.56	0.60	0.41	0.39	0.40	0.55	0.46

AA, aplastic anaemia; AL, acute leukaemia; CLL, chronic lymphocytic leukaemia; CML, chronic myeloid leukaemia; PNH, paroxysmal nocturnal haemoglobinuria.

from other hospitals in Bangkok and the rural areas. However, if it can be assumed that the case population for aplastic anaemia and acute leukaemia is similar, then the data in Table 2 suggests that the incidence of aplastic anaemia is indeed higher in Thailand, although it will be noticed that the ratio of aplastic anaemia to acute leukaemia cases has been falling, mainly due to an increase in referred leukaemia cases.

Population-based studies

Accurate figures on the incidence of aplastic anaemia in the Far East have hitherto been lacking. In Japan, an industry-based National survey found an annual incidence of 14 per million (Aoki et al, 1980; Shima and Kato, 1986). Since September 1988 a population-based case control study of aplastic anaemia has been underway in Bangkok, Thailand. The methods employed are similar to those used in the IAAAS (1986) publication. In 1982, 32 cases from the study region that met the diagnostic criteria were identified. Based on the total population of 8.7 million, this revealed an overall incidence of 3.7 per million (Issaragrisil et al, 1991). The age and sex of specific rates are shown in Table 3. The annual incidence rates for age groups 0–24, 25–59 and

Table 3. Incidence of aplastic anaemia in Bangkok in 1989 according to age and sex.

	Males		Females		Total	
Age interval (years)	Rate/million	*n*	Rate/million	*n*	Rate/million	*n*
0–14	3.8	12	0.8	1	2.4	6
15–24	8.4	7	6.0	5	7.2	12
25–39	4.6	6	0.8	1	2.0	7
40–59	4.4	3	4.3	3	4.3	6
>60	0	0	3.8	1	2.1	1
Total	4.8	28	2.5	11	3.7	32

60 years or over were 4.3, 3.2 and 1.1 per million respectively, the rate being highest (7.2 per million) in those aged 15–24 years. There was only one patient whose age was more than 59 years. In most age groups, the incidence was higher in males than females; the overall sex specific rates were 4.8 and 2.5 per million respectively. It will be noticed that although the overall incidence falls within the reported range from Europe and the USA, there is an important and striking difference between the Bangkok study and those from the West. In Bangkok, aplastic anaemia is largely a disease of young adults and the incidence amongst those aged 15–24 was considerably higher than that seen in any of the European studies. This age distribution is similar to that observed in previous years in Siriraj Hospital. Among 1110 patients seen during the period 1968–1987, 62% were aged between 11 and 30 years. By contrast, in all western studies rates have been highest in the older age groups. The differences could reflect an extreme variation in hospital referral practice, but may also indicate a genuine difference in the age distribution in the two populations.

The explanation for the high incidence of aplastic anaemia in Thailand is unknown. The high incidence among young males favours an environmental aetiology, possibly occupational exposure. Other explanations may include genetic variation in susceptibility and different exposure to other aetiological factors, such as drugs and infections, particularly viral infections.

Drug exposure

In Thailand drugs can be purchased without a physician's prescription and there are many kinds, including herbal medicines. A history of drug or chemical exposure was elicited in 487 of 744 patients with aplastic anaemia (65%) from whom adequate history was available during the period 1968–1987 (Table 4). Most common drugs and chemicals were analgesics/antipyretics, Yachood (a combination of analgesics and antibiotics), chloramphenicol, insecticides and herbal medicines. However, if the sole criterion for the definition of a drug-induced aplastic anaemia is that the disease develops whilst the patient is receiving, or has received a drug, patients might well have been taking the drugs by chance alone. The proper and unbiased way to proceed is to identify all cases and carry out a case-controlled study. Preliminary results on a case-controlled study based on 41 cases and 162 controls have shown an inverse association with height and income with regard to factors other than drugs and chemicals. One possible explanation is that this is a reflection of poor nutritional status, which perhaps contributes to the risk by increasing susceptibility to the effects of environmental factors, such as drugs or viruses. Another finding is the possible association with work in the textile industry where there can be heavy exposure to dyes and cleaning agents.

Table 4. History of drug and chemical exposure in 744 Thai patients with aplastic anaemia.

Drug/chemical	*n*
Analgesics, antipyretics	230 (30.9)
Yachood (combination of drugs; antibiotics and analgesics)	92 (12.4)
Insecticide	61 (8.2)
Chloramphenicol	40 (5.4)
Herbal medicine	28 (3.8)
Benzene	8 (1.1)
Antituberculous drugs	8 (1.1)
Dye	8 (1.1)
Dichlorodiphenyltrichloroethane (DDT)	8 (1.1)
Sulphonamide	3 (0.4)
Hair dye	1 (0.1)
No history of drug or chemical exposure	257 (34.5)

Values in parentheses are percentages.

With regard to drugs, data were too limited to reach any firm conclusion. The results were consistent with an association with NSAIDs and some antibiotics; such an association has been reported previously (Kaufman et al, 1991). The greater use of antibiotics by aplastic anaemia cases, whilst not informative for specific drugs, may be consistent with a viral aetiology, inasmuch as viral infections manifesting as a sore throat, gastroenteritis and so on, are commonly if mistakenly treated with antibiotics. Chloramphenicol was used rarely, being taken by one case and three controls. This demonstrates that declining use of chloramphenicol has not been associated with changes in the incidence of aplastic anaemia in the Far East, observations in line with those in western Europe. With regard to insecticides, the results so far do not suggest a strong association, but the data are too sparse to rule out such an effect.

Viral infections

Viral infections may be a cause of aplastic anaemia (Young and Mortimer, 1984). In Taiwan, posthepatitic aplastic anaemia was found in 23.9% of all cases (Liang et al, 1990). Lin et al (1989) found that the carrier rate of the hepatitis B surface antigen (HBsAg) in patients with aplastic anaemia was similar to that in the general population in Taiwan, and chronic hepatitis B infection was not considered a major aetiological factor.

Viral hepatitis is an endemic disease in Thailand. Both hepatitis A and B as well as hepatitis C are common. A carrier rate of hepatitis B surface antigen (HBsAg) is 10%, which is about 100 times higher than that in Europe and the USA (Chainuvati, 1984). Previous studies in Thais show that 10% were HBsAg-positive, 30–46% had antibody to HBsAg (anti-HBs), and 75% had antibody to hepatitis B core antigen (anti-HBc). About 85% had antibody to hepatitis A (anti-HAV of IgG class) (Viranuvatti et al, 1982; Seidl and Chandanayingyong, 1984).

Serological assays for hepatitis A, B and C were performed on samples from 27 aplastic anaemia cases and 27 controls. Anti-HAV-IgG was positive in 26 of 27 cases and 18 of 27 controls, but no cases or controls were positive for anti-HAV-IgM. HBsAg was positive in only one case and two controls. Anti-HBsAg was present in 15 cases and 12 controls. Anti-HBcAg was evident in eight cases and five controls. Only one case was positive for antibody to hepatitis C, whereas all controls were negative. These findings suggest that viral hepatitis may not be a major cause of the higher incidence of aplastic anaemia in Thailand, but do not rule out the possibility that there is an interaction between viruses and other factors which produce the disease.

CONCLUSIONS

Studies on the epidemiology of aplastic anaemia have proved to be difficult and sometimes produce conflicting evidence. These difficulties arise because of the rarity of the disorder and the possibility of confusion in diagnosis. It seems probable that there is an excess incidence of aplastic anaemia in the Far East compared to western Europe and north America, but that this excess may not be marked, except perhaps in young males. Evidence for occupational hazards in the incidence of aplastic anaemia is suggestive for exposure to paint and benzene compounds. Epidemiological evidence also supports an association with NSAIDs and certain antibiotics in the aetiology of aplastic anaemia, but the restricted use of chloramphenicol seems to have removed this drug as a major cause of the disease in the population at large. Bearing in mind the difficulties of population studies, one approach for the future may be to ensure that serum and cellular material is stored from cases of aplastic anaemia, so that they may be examined as new possibilities for aetiological factors become available.

REFERENCES

Aggio MC, Alvarez RV, Bartomioli MA & Maguitman O (1988) Incidence and etiology of aplastic anemia in a defined population of Argentina (1966–1977). *Medicina (Buenos Aires)* **48:** 231–233.

Aladjem S (1969) Chloramphenicol in South America. *New England Journal of Medicine* **281:** 1369.

Aoki K, Ohtani M & Shimizu H (1978) Epidemiological approach to the etiology of aplastic anemia. In Hibino S, Takaku F & Shahidi NT (eds) *Aplastic Anemia*, pp 155–170. Baltimore: University Park Press.

Aoki K, Fujiki N, Shimizu H & Ohno Y (1980) Geographic and ethnic differences of aplastic anemia in humans. In Najean Y (ed.) *Medullary Aplasia*. New York: Masson.

Askoy M & Erdem S (1978) Follow up study on the mortality and development of leukemia in 44 pancytopenic patients with chronic exposure to benzene. *Blood* **52:** 285–292.

Askoy M, Erdem S & Dincol G (1974) Leukemia in shoe workers exposed chronically to benzene. *Blood* **44:** 837–841.

Baranski B & Young N (1987) Hematologic consequences of viral infections. *Hematology/Oncology Clinics of North America* **1:** 167–183.

Böttiger LE & Westerholm B (1972) Aplastic anaemia I. Incidence and aetiology. *Acta Medica Scandinavica* **192:** 315–318.

Cartwright RA, McKinney PA, Williams L et al (1988) Aplastic anaemia incidence in parts of the United Kingdom in 1985. *Leukaemia Research* **6:** 459–463.

Chainuvati T (1984) Epidemiology of hepatitis B in Thailand. *Proceedings of the 2nd International Symposium in Viral Hepatitis*. Japan, pp 111–119.

Clausen N (1986) A population study of severe aplastic anemia in children. *Acta Paediatrica Scandinavica* **75:** 58–63.

Cone TE & Abelson SM (1952) Aplastic anemia following two days of chloramphenicol therapy. *Journal of Pediatrics* **41:** 340–342.

Corrigan GE (1974) An autopsy survey of aplastic anemia. *American Journal of Clinical Pathology* **62:** 488–490.

Custer RP (1946) Aplastic anemia in soldiers treated with atabrine (quinacrine). *American Journal of Medical Sciences* **212:** 211–224.

Davies SM & Walker DJ (1986) Aplastic anaemia in the Northern Region 1971–1978 and follow up of long term survivors. *Clinical and Laboratory Haematology* **8:** 307–313.

de Planque MM, Kluin-Nelemans JC, Van Krieken JM et al (1988) Evolution of acquired severe aplastic anaemia to myelodysplasia and subsequent leukaemia in adults. *British Journal of Haematology* **70:** 55–62.

Forbes G, O'Grady HG & Williams R (1989) Aplastic anemia after liver transplantation for non-A, non-B hepatitis. *New England Journal of Medicine* **320:** 122.

Fraunfelder FT, Bagby GC & Kelly DJ (1982) Fatal aplastic anemia following topical administration of ophthalmic chloramphenicol. *American Journal of Ophthalmology* **93:** 356–360.

Ghitis J (1970) Chloramphenicol in South America. *New England Journal of Medicine* **282:** 813–814.

Hagler L, Pastore RA, Bergin JJ & Wrensch MR (1975) Aplastic anemia following viral hepatitis: report of two fatal cases and literature review. *Medicine (Baltimore)* **54:** 139–164.

IAAAS (International Agranulocytosis and Aplastic Anemia Study) (1986) Risks of agranulocytosis and aplastic anemia. A first report of their relation to drug use with special reference to analgesics. *Journal of the American Medical Association* **256:** 1749–1757.

IAAAS (International Agranulocytosis and Aplastic Anemia Study) (1987) Incidence of aplastic anaemia: the relevance of diagnostic criteria. *Blood* **70:** 1718–1721.

Issaragrisil S, Sriratanasatavorn C, Piankijagum A et al (1991) Incidence of aplastic anemia in Bangkok. *Blood* **77:** 2166–2168.

Josten K, Tooze JA, Borthwick-Clarke C et al (1991) Acquired aplastic anemia and paroxysmal nocturnal hemoglobinuria. *Blood* **78:** 3162–3167.

Kansu B & Erslev AJ (1976) Aplastic anaemia with 'hot pockets'. *Scandinavian Journal of Haematology* **17:** 326–334.

Kaufman DW, Kelly JP, Levy M & Shapiro S (1991) *The Drug Etiology of Agranulocytosis and Aplastic Anemia*. New York: Oxford University Press.

Lewis SM (1965) Course and prognosis in aplastic anaemia. *British Medical Journal* **i:** 1027–1030.

Liang DC, Lin KH, Lin DT et al (1990) Post-hepatitic anaemia in children in Taiwan, a hepatitis prevalent area. *British Journal of Haematology* **74:** 487–491.

Lin CK, Gau JP, Ho CH & Wang SY (1989) Aplastic anemia in Taiwan and its etiological factors. *Taiwan I Hsueh Hui Tsa Chih (Journal of the Formosan Medical Association)* **88:** 1123–1127.

Linet MS, Tielsch JM, Markowitz JA et al (1985) An apparent cluster of aplastic anemia in a small population of teenagers. *Archives of Internal Medicine* **145:** 635–640.

Linet MS, McCaffrey LD, Morgan WF et al (1986) Incidence of aplastic anemia in a three county area of South Carolina. *Cancer Research* **46:** 426–429.

Linet MS, Markowitz JA, Sensenbrenner LL et al (1989) A case-controlled study of aplastic anemia. *Leukemia Research* **13:** 3–11.

Mary JY, Baumelou E, Guiguet M & the French Cooperative Group for Epidemiological Study of Aplastic Anaemia (1990) Epidemiology of aplastic anemia in France: a prospective multicentre study. *Blood* **75:** 1646–1653.

Modan B, Segal S, Shani M & Sheva C (1975) Aplastic anemia in Israel: evaluation of the etiological role of chloramphenicol on a community-wide basis. *American Journal of Medical Sciences* **270:** 441–445.

Mukiibi JM, Paul B & Nkrumah FK (1987) Aplastic anaemia in Zimbabweans. *Central African Journal of Medicine* **33:** 1–8.

Paci E, Buiatti E, Costantini AS et al (1989) Aplastic anemia leukemia and other cancer mortality in a cohort of shoe workers exposed to benzene. *Scandinavian Journal of Work, Environment and Health* **15:** 313–318.

Rich ML, Ritterhoff RJ & Hoffmann RJ (1950) A fatal case of aplastic anemia following chloramphenicol (chloromycetin) therapy. *Annals of Internal Medicine* **33:** 1459–1467.

Rugman FP & Cosstick R (1990) Aplastic anaemia associated with organochlorine pesticide: case reports and review of evidence. *Journal of Clinical Pathology* **43:** 98–101.

Sarasti H (1970) Chloramphenicol in South America. *New England Journal of Medicine* **282:** 813.

Seidl S & Chandanayingyong D (1984) Viral hepatitis markers in Thai blood donors. *Vox Sanguinis* **47:** 54–59.

Shima S & Kato Y (1986) Incidence of aplastic anemia among workers in major industries in Japan and suspected causal factors. In Aoki K, Hosoda Y, Yanagowa H et al (eds) *Epidemiology of Intractable Diseases in Japan, Nagoya*, pp 53. Nagoya: Department of Preventive Medicine, Nagoya University School of Medicine.

Smadel JE (1949) Chloramphenicol (chloromycetin) in the treatment of infectious diseases. *American Journal of Medicine* **7:** 671–685.

Smick KM, Condit PK, Proctor RL & Sutcher V (1964) Fatal aplastic anaemia. An epidemiological study of its relationship to the drug chloramphenicol. *Journal of Chronic Diseases* **17:** 899–914.

Szklo M, Sensenbrenner L, Markowitz J et al (1985) Incidence of aplastic anemia in metropolitan Baltimore: a population-based study. *Blood* **66:** 115–119.

Tichelli A, Gratwohl A, Würsch A, Nissen C & Speck B (1988) Late haematological complications in severe aplastic anaemia. *British Journal of Haematology* **69:** 413–418.

Tzakis AG, Arditi M, Whitington PF et al (1988) Aplastic anemia complicating orthotopic liver transplantation for non-A, non-B hepatitis. *New England Journal of Medicine* **319:** 393–396.

Viranuvatti V, Hemindra P & Chainuvati T (1982) Anti-HAV in Thai population. *Journal of the Medical Association of Thailand* **65:** 379–382.

Wallerstein RO, Condit PK, Kasper CK, Brown JW & Morrison FR (1969) A statewide study of chloramphenicol therapy and fatal aplastic anemia. *Journal of the American Medical Association* **208:** 2045–2050.

Wang HH & Grufferman S (1981) Aplastic anemia and occupational pesticide exposure: a case control study. *Journal of Occupational Medicine* **23:** 364–366.

Welch H, Lewis CN & Kerlan I (1954) Blood dyscrasias: a nationwide survey. *Antibiotics and Chemotherapy* **4:** 607–623.

Whang KS (1978) Aplastic anemia in Korea: a clinical study of 309 cases. In Hibino S, Takaku F & Shahidi NT (eds) *Aplastic Anemia*, pp 225–242. Baltimore: University Park Press.

Wilkinson C (1988) Is the treatment of scabies hazardous? *Journal of the Royal College of General Practitioners* **38:** 460–469.

Williams DM, Lynch R & Cartwright GF (1973) Drug induced aplastic anemia. *Seminars in Hematology* **10:** 195–223.

Young N & Mortimer PP (1984) Viruses and bone marrow failure. *Blood* **63:** 729–737.

Young NS, Issaragrisil S, Chieh CW & Takaku F (1986) Aplastic anaemia in the Orient. *British Journal of Haematology* **62:** 1–6.

Index

Note: Page numbers of article titles are in **bold** type.